Hot Topics in Reproductive Medicine Research

Hot Topics in Reproductive Medicine Research

Editors

Aldo E. Calogero
Claudio Manna

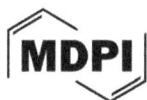

Basel • Beijing • Wuhan • Barcelona • Belgrade • Novi Sad • Cluj • Manchester

Editors
Aldo E. Calogero
University of Catania
Catania, Italy

Claudio Manna
Biofertility IVF and Infertility Center
Rome, Italy

Editorial Office
MDPI
St. Alban-Anlage 66
4052 Basel, Switzerland

This is a reprint of articles from the Special Issue published online in the open access journal *Journal of Clinical Medicine* (ISSN 2077-0383) (available at: https://www.mdpi.com/journal/jcm/special_issues/Hot_Topics_Reproductive_Medicine_Research).

For citation purposes, cite each article independently as indicated on the article page online and as indicated below:

Lastname, A.A.; Lastname, B.B. Article Title. *Journal Name* **Year**, *Volume Number*, Page Range.

ISBN 978-3-0365-9967-0 (Hbk)
ISBN 978-3-0365-9968-7 (PDF)
doi.org/10.3390/books978-3-0365-9968-7

© 2024 by the authors. Articles in this book are Open Access and distributed under the Creative Commons Attribution (CC BY) license. The book as a whole is distributed by MDPI under the terms and conditions of the Creative Commons Attribution-NonCommercial-NoDerivs (CC BY-NC-ND) license.

Contents

Marko Bašković, Dajana Krsnik, Marta Himelreich Perić, Ana Katušić Bojanac, Nino Sinčić,
Zdenko Sonicki and Davor Ježek
Astaxanthin Relieves Testicular Ischemia-Reperfusion Injury—Immunohistochemical and
Biochemical Analyses
Reprinted from: *J. Clin. Med.* **2022**, *11*, 1284, doi:10.3390/jcm11051284 1

Vincenzo De Leo, Claudia Tosti, Giuseppe Morgante, Rosetta Ponchia, Alice Luddi,
Laura Governini and Paola Piomboni
Positive Effect of a New Combination of Antioxidants and Natural Hormone Stimulants for the
Treatment of Oligoasthenoteratozoospermia
Reprinted from: *J. Clin. Med.* **2022**, *11*, 1991, doi:10.3390/jcm11071991 15

Romualdo Sciorio and Nady El Hajj
Epigenetic Risks of Medically Assisted Reproduction
Reprinted from: *J. Clin. Med.* **2022**, *11*, 2151, doi:10.3390/jcm11082151 25

Giuseppe Morgante, Ilenia Darino, Amelia Spanò, Stefano Luisi, Alice Luddi,
Paola Piomboni, et al.
PCOS Physiopathology and Vitamin D Deficiency: Biological Insights and Perspectives for
Treatment
Reprinted from: *J. Clin. Med.* **2022**, *11*, 4509, doi:10.3390/jcm11154509 43

Rossella Cannarella, Andrea Crafa, Laura M. Mongioì, Loredana Leggio, Nunzio Iraci,
Sandro La Vignera, et al.
DNA Methylation in Offspring Conceived after Assisted Reproductive Techniques: A
Systematic Review and Meta-Analysis
Reprinted from: *J. Clin. Med.* **2022**, *11*, 5056, doi:10.3390/jcm11175056 57

Serena Resta, Gaia Scandella, Ilenia Mappa, Maria Elena Pietrolucci, Pavjola Maqina and
Giuseppe Rizzo
Placental Volume and Uterine Artery Doppler in Pregnancy Following In Vitro Fertilization: A
Comprehensive Literature Review
Reprinted from: *J. Clin. Med.* **2022**, *11*, 5793, doi:10.3390/jcm11195793 81

Muzi Li, Yan Kang, Qianfei Wang and Lei Yan
Efficacy of Autologous Intrauterine Infusion of Platelet-Rich Plasma in Patients with
Unexplained Repeated Implantation Failures in Embryo Transfer: A Systematic
Review and Meta-Analysis
Reprinted from: *J. Clin. Med.* **2022**, *11*, 6753, doi:10.3390/jcm11226753 93

Maha H. Daghestani, Huda A. Alqahtani, AlBandary AlBakheet, Mashael Al Deery,
Khalid A. Awartani, Mazin H. Daghestani, et al.
Global Transcriptional Profiling of Granulosa Cells from Polycystic Ovary Syndrome Patients:
Comparative Analyses of Patients with or without History of Ovarian Hyperstimulation
Syndrome Reveals Distinct Biomarkers and Pathways
Reprinted from: *J. Clin. Med.* **2022**, *11*, 6941, doi:10.3390/jcm11236941 105

Federica Barbagallo, Rossella Cannarella, Andrea Crafa, Claudio Manna, Sandro La Vignera,
Rosita A. Condorelli and Aldo E. Calogero
The Impact of a Very Short Abstinence Period on Conventional Sperm Parameters and Sperm
DNA Fragmentation: A Systematic Review and Meta-Analysis
Reprinted from: *J. Clin. Med.* **2022**, *11*, 7303, doi:10.3390/jcm11247303 117

Qiumin Wang, Dan Qi, Lixia Zhang, Jingru Wang, Yanbo Du, Hong Lv and Lei Yan
Association of the Cumulative Live Birth Rate with the Factors in Assisted Reproductive
Technology: A Retrospective Study of 16,583 Women
Reprinted from: *J. Clin. Med.* **2023**, *12*, 493, doi:10.3390/jcm12020493 . . . . **137**

Claudio Manna, Federica Barbagallo, Francesca Sagnella, Ashraf Farrag and Aldo E. Calogero
Assisted Reproductive Technology without Embryo Discarding or Freezing in Women ≥40
Years: A 5-Year Retrospective Study at a Single Center in Italy
Reprinted from: *J. Clin. Med.* **2023**, *12*, 504, doi:10.3390/jcm12020504 . . . . **149**

Ana Navarro-Gomezlechon, María Gil Juliá, Irene Hervás, Laura Mossetti, Rocío Rivera-Egea and Nicolás Garrido
Advanced Paternal Age Does Not Affect Medically-Relevant Obstetrical and Perinatal
Outcomes following IVF or ICSI in Humans with Donated Oocytes
Reprinted from: *J. Clin. Med.* **2023**, *12*, 1014, doi:10.3390/jcm12031014 . . . . **163**

Houjin Dongye, Yizheng Tian, Dan Qi, Yanbo Du and Lei Yan
The Impact of Endometrioma on Embryo Quality in In Vitro Fertilization: A Retrospective
Cohort Study
Reprinted from: *J. Clin. Med.* **2023**, *12*, 2416, doi:10.3390/jcm12062416 . . . . **175**

Clara Serrano-Novillo, Laia Uroz and Carmen Márquez
Novel Time-Lapse Parameters Correlate with Embryo Ploidy and Suggest an Improvement in
Non-Invasive Embryo Selection
Reprinted from: *J. Clin. Med.* **2023**, *12*, 2983, doi:10.3390/jcm12082983 . . . . **185**

Vanessa Machado, Madalena Ferreira, Luísa Lopes, José João Mendes and João Botelho
Adverse Pregnancy Outcomes and Maternal Periodontal Disease: An Overview on
Meta-Analytic and Methodological Quality
Reprinted from: *J. Clin. Med.* **2023**, *12*, 3635, doi:10.3390/jcm12113635 . . . . **199**

Antonio Franco, Flavia Proietti, Veronica Palombi, Gabriele Savarese, Michele Guidotti, Costantino Leonardo, et al.
Varicocele: To Treat or Not to Treat?
Reprinted from: *J. Clin. Med.* **2023**, *12*, 4062, doi:10.3390/jcm12124062 . . . . **211**

Romualdo Sciorio, Claudio Manna, Patricia Fauque and Paolo Rinaudo
Can Cryopreservation in Assisted Reproductive Technology (ART) Induce Epigenetic Changes
to Gametes and Embryos?
Reprinted from: *J. Clin. Med.* **2023**, *12*, 4444, doi:10.3390/jcm12134444 . . . . **225**

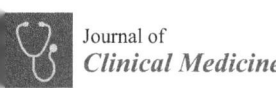

Article

Astaxanthin Relieves Testicular Ischemia-Reperfusion Injury—Immunohistochemical and Biochemical Analyses

Marko Bašković [1,2,*], Dajana Krsnik [1,3], Marta Himelreich Perić [1,3], Ana Katušić Bojanac [1,3], Nino Sinčić [1,3], Zdenko Sonicki [1,4] and Davor Ježek [1,5,6]

1. Scientific Centre of Excellence for Reproductive and Regenerative Medicine, School of Medicine, University of Zagreb, Šalata 3, 10000 Zagreb, Croatia; dajana.krsnik@mef.hr (D.K.); marta.himelreich@mef.hr (M.H.P.); ana.katusic@mef.hr (A.K.B.); nino.sincic@mef.hr (N.S.); zdenko.sonicki@snz.hr (Z.S.); davor.jezek@mef.hr (D.J.)
2. Department of Pediatric Urology, Children's Hospital Zagreb, Ulica Vjekoslava Klaića 16, 10000 Zagreb, Croatia
3. Department of Biology, School of Medicine, University of Zagreb, Šalata 3, 10000 Zagreb, Croatia
4. Department of Medical Statistics, Epidemiology and Medical Informatics, School of Public Health Andrija Štampar, School of Medicine, University of Zagreb, Johna Davidsona Rockfellera 4, 10000 Zagreb, Croatia
5. Department of Histology and Embryology, School of Medicine, University of Zagreb, Šalata 3, 10000 Zagreb, Croatia
6. Department of Transfusion Medicine and Transplantation Biology, University Hospital Centre Zagreb, Kišpatićeva 12, 10000 Zagreb, Croatia
* Correspondence: baskovic.marko@gmail.com; Tel.: +385-1-3636-379

Abstract: Testicular torsion potentially leads to acute scrotum and testicle loss, and requires prompt surgical intervention to restore testicular blood flow, despite the paradoxical negative effect of reperfusion. While no drug is yet approved for this condition, antioxidants are promising candidates. This study aimed to determine astaxanthin's (ASX), a potent antioxidant, effect on rat testicular torsion−detorsion injury. Thirty-two prepubertal male Fischer rats were divided into four groups. Group 1 underwent sham surgery. In group 2, the right testis was twisted at $720°$ for 90 min. After 90 min of reperfusion, the testis was removed. ASX was administered intraperitoneally at the time of detorsion (group 3) and 45 min after detorsion (group 4). Quantification of caspase-3 positive cells and oxidative stress markers detection were determined immunohistochemically, while the malondialdehyde (MDA) value, superoxide dismutase (SOD), and glutathione peroxidase (GPx) activities were determined by colorimetric assays. The number of apoptotic caspase-3 positive cells and the MDA value were lower in group 4 compared to group 2. A significant increase in the SOD and GPx activity was observed in group 4 compared to groups 2 and 3. We conclude that ASX has a favorable effect on testicular ischemia-reperfusion injury in rats.

Keywords: astaxanthin; testicular torsion; acute scrotum; ischemia-reperfusion injury; antioxidants; carotenoids; apoptosis; infertility; rats

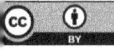

1. Introduction

Testicular torsion is a condition of acute scrotum, starting with the rotation of the testis around a longitudinal axis by at least 180 degrees, and followed by an interruption of circulation inside the organ. Despite the possibility of manual detorsion, surgery is usually required and should be performed as soon as possible after the onset of symptoms. If not recognized in time, it can result in ischemic injuries and testicular loss, but if the operation is performed within 6 h, most testicles can be saved [1–3]. The incidence of testicular torsion is 1 in 4000 males younger than 25 years, while the prevalence of testicular torsion out of a total of all acute scrotal conditions is 25–50% [4–6]. It can occur at any age, but most often shows a bimodal distribution, i.e., it most often occurs in infants and boys at puberty [7,8], usually occurring after some stimulus event (e.g., trauma or increased physical activity) or spontaneously [9]. Clinical features of testicular torsion include the acute onset of moderate to severe testicular pain with the possibility of the presence of redness and swelling with a negative cremaster reflex during physical examination. Nausea, vomiting, and diffuse pain in the lower abdomen may be associated with this condition. The classic clinical finding is an asymmetrically (transversely) highly laid testis [10,11].

Ischemia-reperfusion injury (IRI) exacerbates cell dysfunction observed after restoring blood flow in previously ischemic tissues. Hence, reperfusion paradoxically causes further damage, endangering the organ vitality and function despite the necessity for blood flow restoration. Reperfusion injury is a multifactorial process that results in tissue destruction [12]. During reperfusion, the influx of oxygen leads to the degradation of hypoxanthine to uric acid by enzyme xanthine oxidase. This reaction releases highly reactive anion superoxide (O^{2-}), which is then converted to hydrogen peroxide (H_2O_2) and hydroxyl radical (OH·). The main unwanted consequence of the production of hydroxyl radicals is membrane lipid peroxidation. Lipid peroxidation causes the systemic release of proinflammatory eicosanoids, disruption of cell permeability, and ultimately cell death [13–16]. The increase in the concentration of free oxygen radicals most often occurs if the mechanisms in charge of removing them become insufficient. This upsets the balance between prooxidants and antioxidants, favoring prooxidants (a state of oxidative stress). Cell damage is reversible up to one point, but with intense and prolonged stress, the cell is subject to irreversible damage [17]. While low concentrations of free oxygen radicals induce apoptosis, high ones result in necrosis. Cysteine proteases that form a large family of enzymes known as caspases cause most cell morphological changes [18,19].

Antioxidants are molecules that, by inhibiting the oxidation of other molecules, defend the body's system against potential damage by free oxygen radicals [20]. In recent decades, interest in natural sources of antioxidants has risen sharply. Algae constitute a significant source of molecules with an antioxidant activity, as they often grow in extreme environmental conditions, resulting in the production of large numbers of free oxygen radicals. To ameliorate their effect, algae create various secondary metabolites with antioxidant activities such as phycobilins, polyphenols, carotenoids, and vitamins [21].

The carotenoid pigment astaxanthin (ASX) ($C_{40}H_{52}O_4$), found in the microalgae *Haematococcus pluvialis*, has anti-inflammatory, immunomodulatory, and antioxidant effects [22]. ASX is also found in salmon, shrimp, and crabs, giving them a specific shade of red [23]. Compared to other carotenoids such as beta-carotene, zeaxanthin, and canthaxanthin, ASX shows higher levels of antioxidant activity [24]. The antioxidant activity of ASX is ten times higher than zeaxanthin, canthaxanthin, β-carotene, and lutein, and 100 times higher than α-tocopherol [25].

For these benefits, we decided to investigate the ASX's effect on testicular IRI. We previously published comprehensive histological results showing that ASX has a protective effect [26,27]. Still, only a multimodal approach can strengthen the hypothesis, we showed the results of immunohistochemical and biochemical analyses in this study. There is no drug in clinical practice that can be given to patients with torsion−detorsion testicular injury to date. We believe this study gives a new insight into the possible treatment of this urgent condition and its consequences (subfertility and infertility).

2. Materials and Methods

2.1. Animals

The study was performed on 32 male Fischer rats (weight 160–210 g, 35 days old) of prepubertal age. The animals were housed under the conditions following good laboratory practice (GLP), which included a temperature of 20–24 °C, relative humidity 55% +/− 10%, controlled lighting, and light dark cycle of 12 h/12 h. The noise level did not exceed 60 dB.

2.2. Ethics Approvals

The research was approved by the School of Medicine, University of Zagreb (classification; 641-01/19-02/01/registry number; 380-59-10106-19-111/162) and the Croatian

National Ethics Committee (EP 217/2019). The 3R principles were used—"reduction", "refinement", and "replacement"—and the concept of five freedoms was respected.

2.3. Experimental Groups and Surgical Procedure

Rats were randomly divided into four groups with eight individuals in each group, namely: sham-operated (S) group, torsion−detorsion (T/D) group, and torsion−detorsion + astaxanthin (T/D + ASX) groups.

Group 1 (S) underwent sham surgery. After the intraperitoneal injection of anesthetic, an incision was made in the right inguinal region, to pull out the ipsilateral testis, which was immediately returned to its natural position and the skin sutured. After suture removal, orchidectomy was performed after 3 h. In group 2 (T for 90 min/D for 90 min), the ipsilateral testis was twisted around its axis by 720° in a clockwise direction. It was fixed in that position for 90 min. After 90 min, detorsion was performed. The skin was sutured twice (0 min and 90 min). Orchidectomy was performed 90 min from the moment of detorsion. At the time of detorsion, group 3 (T for 90 min/D for 90 min + ASX at the time of detorsion) was administered pure ASX intraperitoneally (75 mg/kg, Sigma-Aldrich®, St. Louis, MO, USA, from *Blakeslea trispora*). In group 4 (T for 90 min/D for 90 min + ASX 45 min from the moment of detorsion) ASX was administered 45 min after detorsion.

All surgical procedures were performed under aseptic conditions. After shaving the right inguinoscrotal region, washing with chlorhexidine gluconate (PLIVA®sept, Pliva d.o.o., Zagreb, Croatia), and drying, the area was treated with a povidone-iodine solution (Betadine®10%, Alkaloid, Skopje, North Macedonia). In the midline of the scrotum, an incision was made. Upon opening the tunica vaginalis, the testis was twisted manually around its axis by 720° in a clockwise direction. The testis was fixed to the inner wall of the scrotum with a monofilament polyglactin suture 6/0 (Vicryl; Ethicon Inc., Johnson and Johnson Co., Somerville, NJ, USA). By removing the suture, the right testicle was manually returned to its natural position. The skin of the scrotum was also sutured with a monofilament polyglactin suture 6/0. All surgical procedures were performed under general anesthesia induced by intraperitoneal injection of ketamine (90 mg/kg) and xylazine (10 mg/kg). The animals were constantly monitored. In case of movement, twitching, or other signs of awakening, intraperitoneal anesthesia was supplemented in a smaller dose. No animals died during the experiment. After orchidectomy, the rats were euthanized using the T-61 solution (1 mL/kg) iv. (Intervet International GmbH®, Unterschleißheim, Germany).

2.4. Immunohistochemical Method and Analysis

The immunohistochemical method was used to evaluate the cell damage exhibited by apoptosis and oxidative stress in the testicular tubules after treatment. Anti-cleaved caspase-3 antibody (1:100, #9664, Cell Signaling Technology®, Danvers, MA, USA) was used as an apoptotic marker, while anti-8-oxo-2′-deoxyguanosine (anti 8-OHdG), anti-nitrotyrosine (anti-NT) (1:300, sc-66036 and 1:100, sc-32757, respectively, Santa Cruz Biotechnology, Inc., Dallas, TX, USA) and anti-4-hydroxy-2-nonenal (anti-HNE) antibodies (MAB3249 R&D Systems, Inc., Minneapolis, MN, USA) were used as oxidative stress markers. After overnight incubation with primary antibody at 4 °C, the sections were treated with appropriate secondary antibodies. The signal was visualized using 3,3′-diaminobenzidine-tetrahydrochloride (DAB) and hematoxylin for counterstaining. Positive control tissues were used, as recommended by the manufacturer of the antibodies, while the negative controls were gained by omitting the primary antibody in the buffer. To detect caspase-3 positive cells as clearly as possible, the "invert" option was used in the ImageJ® software (software package developed by the National Institutes of Health). The number of caspase-3-positive cells was determined by counting 100 random seminiferous tubules (apoptotic index) (x400). Caspase-3 positive cells were counted by visual observation from two independent researchers. If the numbers differed, the opinion of a third researcher was sought. Data are expressed as the mean of caspase-3-positive cells per 100 seminiferous tubules. Descriptive analysis of antibodies against oxidative stress markers was performed to evaluate the histological localization on six samples per group.

2.5. Biochemical Analysis

The values of malondialdehyde (MDA) and enzymatic antioxidants (superoxide dismutase (SOD) and glutathione peroxidase (GPx)) were determined by colorimetric assays using the testicular tissue homogenates as the samples. The MDA Assay Kit (MAK085, Sigma-Aldrich®, St. Louis, MO, USA) was used to measure lipid peroxidation. According to the manufacturer's protocol, the MDA in the homogenized sample makes a complex with thiobarbituric acid (TBA), which could be quantified colorimetrically (532 nm) on a spectrophotometer (Tecan Spark, Tecan, Life Sciences). The SOD activity was analyzed with the colorimetric SOD determination kit (19160, Sigma-Aldrich®, St. Louis, MO, USA). Tetrazolium salt was used as a substrate (WST), which produces a water-soluble formazan dye after reduction with a superoxide anion. The rate of WST reduction was linearly related to the xanthine oxidase (XO) activity, but concomitantly inhibited by SOD. IC50 (50% SOD inhibition activity) was determined by the colorimetric method. As the absorption at 440 nm is proportional to the amount of superoxide anion, the activity of SOD as an inhibitory activity was quantified by measuring the decrease in color development at 440 nm. The GPx Assay Kit (353919; Sigma-Aldrich®, St. Louis, MO, USA) measured GPx activity. The main reaction catalyzed by GPx is $2GSH + H_2O_2 \rightarrow GS-SG + 2H_2O$, where GSH is the reduced monomeric glutathione and GS–SG glutathione disulfide. The mechanism involves the oxidation of selenol in the selenocysteine residue via hydrogen peroxide. Glutathione reductase then reduces oxidized glutathione and completes the following cycle: $GS-SG + NADPH + H+ \rightarrow 2GSH + NADP+$. Oxidation of NADPH to NADP+ was accompanied by a decrease in absorption to 340 nm. Under conditions where GPx activity is limited, the rate of decrease in A_{340} is directly proportional to the GPx activity in the sample. The amount of NADPH in the reaction mixture was determined kinetically by reading the ΔA_{340} absorbance value at 340 nm at 1 min intervals over the 7 min time frame.

2.6. Statistical Analysis

Microsoft Excel® software program (XLSTAT®) for Windows, version 2020.5.1 (Microsoft Corporation, Redmond, DC, USA), was used to analyze the experimental data. Before the study, power analysis was performed where a sample of four groups of eight animals was shown to be required (for $\alpha = 0.05$, power = 95% and effect ≥ 0.9) in order to obtain high-quality data. The Shapiro–Wilk test was used for the normal distribution assessment of collected measurements mainly presented by the interquartile range (median). Differences between groups were analyzed by the nonparametric Kruskal–Wallis test. The data were presented as follows; chi-square (χ^2) = observed value (critical value), degrees of freedom (DF), and p-value. The Mann–Whitney U test with Bonferroni correction was used for the pairwise comparisons. A significance level of 0.05 was used.

3. Results

3.1. Caspase-3 Positive Cells Quantification

The number of caspase-3-positive cells was statistically significantly lower ($p = 0.016$) in group 4, in which ASX was administered 45 min from the time of detorsion (mean = 11.84) compared to the untreated torsion–detorsion group 2 (mean = 22,700). Compared to group 2, group 3, in which ASX was administered at the time of detorsion, recorded a far lower mean (mean = 12.50), but there was no statistically significant difference ($p = 0.077$; Table S1 and Figure 1).

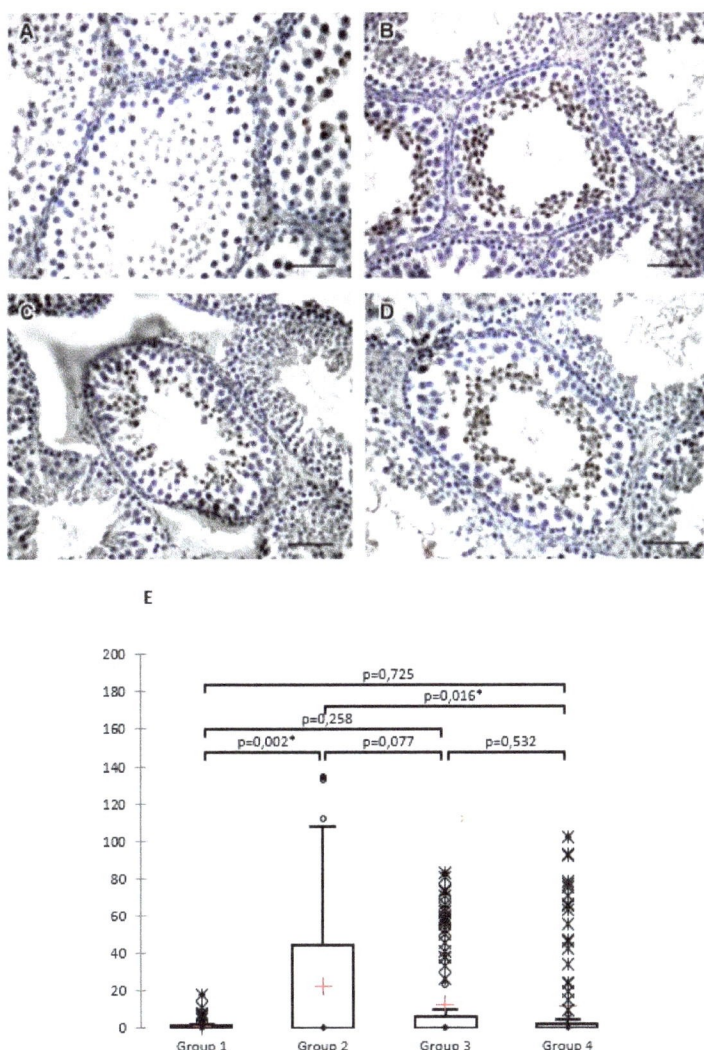

Figure 1. Caspase-3 positive cells on representative, randomly selected cross-sections on which the measurements were performed: (**A**) group 1, (**B**) group 2, (**C**) group 3, and (**D**) group 4. DAB, hematoxylin counterstain, scale bar 50 μm. (**E**) Box plots for caspase-3 positive cells (data are presented as mean ± SD). A Kruskal–Wallis test revealed a statistically significant difference in the number of caspase-3 positive cells between the different groups (at a significance level of 5%); (χ^2 = 10.441 (7.815), DF = 3, p = 0.015), * $p < 0.05$.

3.2. Histological Assessment of Oxidative Stress

8-hydroxy-2′deoxyguanosine (8-OHdG), the marker of oxidative DNA damage, was found in most tubules of all groups, although it was more intensely stained in group 3, and was without visible tubules with no affection in the same group. The signal was cytoplasmic, limited to the basal layer of the Sertoli cells and spermatogonia, near the tubular wall. In all groups except group 3, there were completely unaffected tubules next to those with a damaged histological appearance (Figure 2G).

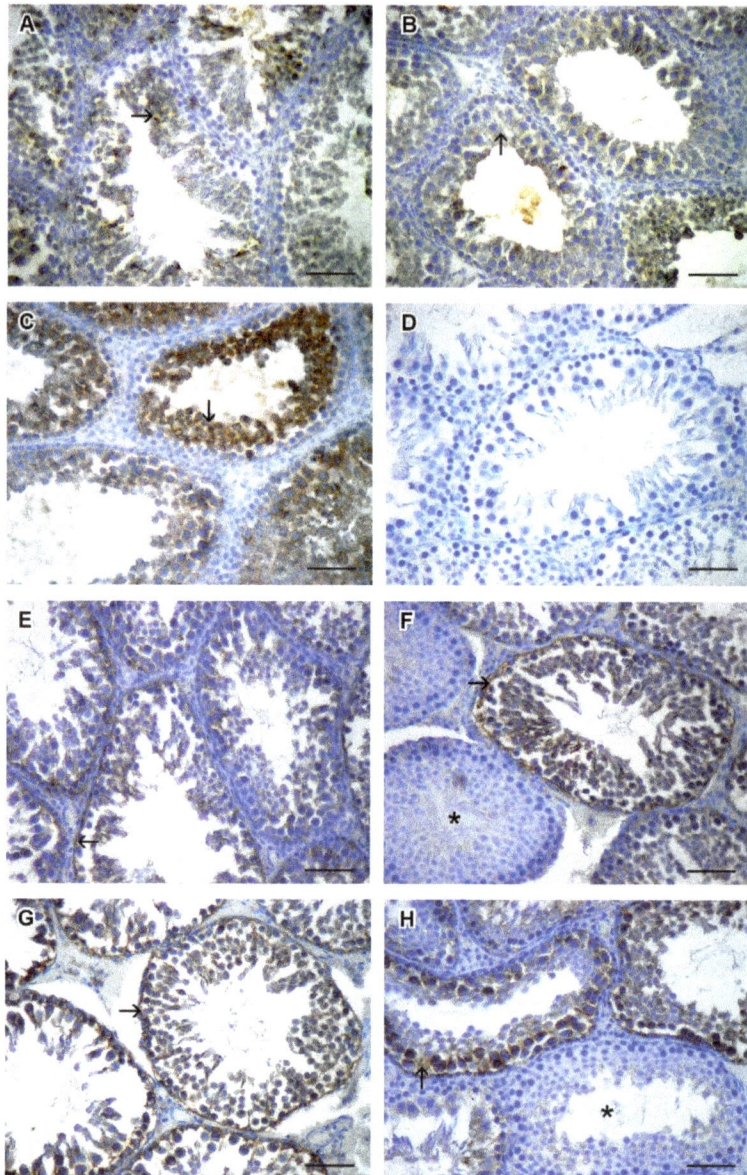

Figure 2. Representative images of HNE (**A–D**) and 8-OHdG (**E–H**) expression (→) in the rat testes of groups 1 (**A,E**), 2 (**B,F**), 3 (**C,G**), and 4 (**D,H**). Note the difference in the expression on neighboring tubules in images F and H (*- nonaffected tubule). DAB, hematoxylin counterstain, scale bar 50 μm.

4-hydroxy-2-nonenal (HNE), the marker of lipid peroxidation, showed the strongest staining intensity in group 3, affecting the entire height of the seminiferous epithelium (Figure 2C). Group 4 had a staining signal similar to the negative control (Figure 2D).

Nitrotyrosine staining showed no positive signal in the specimens, while the positive control was stained as expected.

3.3. Values of Malondialdehyde (MDA)

Malondialdehyde values decreased in the group in which ASX was administered 45 min from the moment of detorsion (Mdn = 0.187) compared to the untreated torsion−detorsion group (Mdn = 0.222), but the difference was not statistically significant ($p = 0.574$). The median values between group 2 (Mdn = 0.222) and group 3 (Mdn = 0.227) were almost identical ($p = 0.798$). The MDA values in group 2 in relation to the negative control group increased significantly ($p = 0.001$) (Table S2 and Figure 3).

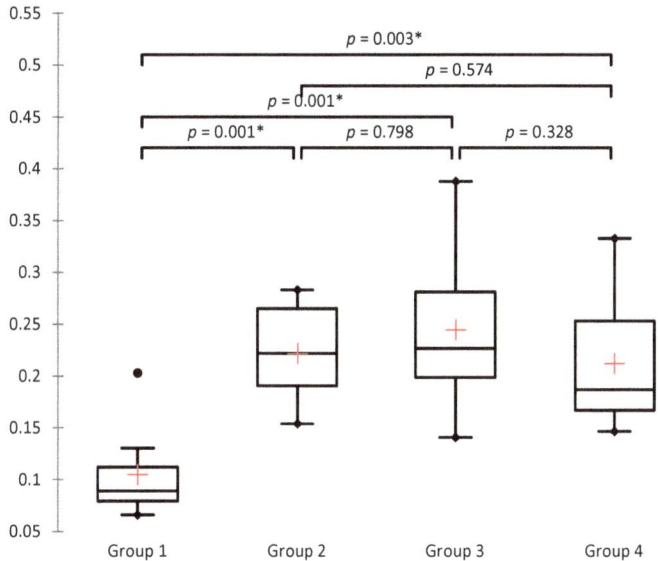

Figure 3. Box plots for malondialdehyde (nmol/µg). The Kruskal−Wallis test shows a statistically significant difference in the observed parameters between different groups (at a significance level of 5%); ($\chi^2 = 14.395$ (7.815), DF = 3, $p = 0.002$), * $p < 0.05$.

3.4. Values of Superoxide Dismutase (SOD)

Following the results, a statistically significant increase in the enzyme activity of superoxide dismutase (SOD) was observed in group 4, in which ASX was administered 45 min from the moment of detorsion (Mdn = 89.61) compared to untreated torsion−detorsion group 2 (Mdn = 88.39) ($p = 0.01$) and group 3, in which ASX was administered at the time of detorsion (Mdn = 85.30) ($p = 0.000$). It is interesting to note a statistically significant decrease in the enzyme activity of SOD in group 3 compared to group 2 ($p = 0.001$; Table S3 and Figure 4).

3.5. Values of Glutathione Peroxidase (GPx)

The Kruskal−Wallis test showed a statistically significant difference in the observed parameters between different groups (at a significance level of 5%); first minute ($\chi^2 = 17.020$ (7.815), DF = 3, $p = 0.001$), second minute ($\chi^2 = 13.497$ (7.815), DF = 3, $p = 0.004$), third minute ($\chi^2 = 14.838$ (7.815), DF = 3, $p = 0.002$), fourth minute ($\chi^2 = 17.701$ (7.815), DF = 3, $p = 0.001$), fifth minute ($\chi2 = 18.637$ (7.815), DF = 3, $p = 0.000$), sixth minute ($\chi^2 = 19.431$ (7.815), DF = 3, $p = 0.000$) (Table S4, Figures S1–S6, and Figure 5).

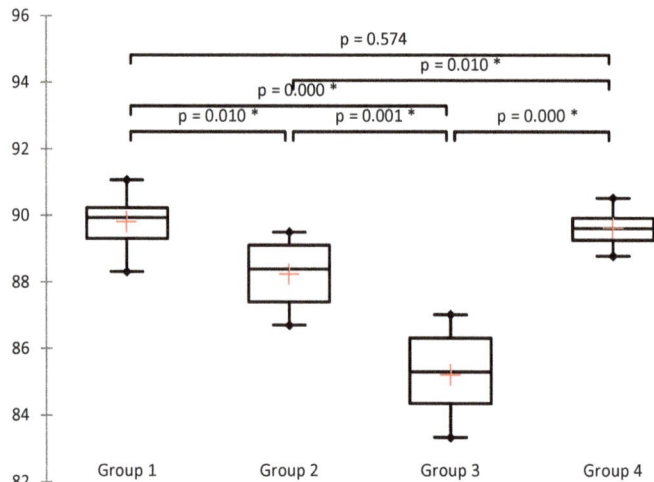

Figure 4. Box plots for SOD activity (inhibition rate %). The Kruskal–Wallis test shows a statistically significant difference in the observed parameter between different groups (at a significance level of 5%); (χ^2 = 22.023 (7.815), DF = 3, $p < 0.0001$), * $p < 0.05$.

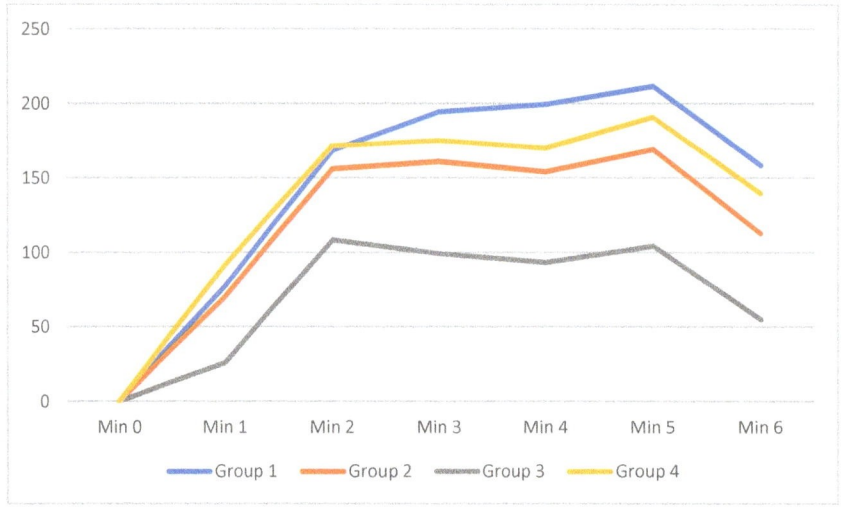

Figure 5. Linear graph of GPx activity (nmol/min/mL) over time from the first to the sixth minute.

4. Discussion

The results of this study showed that ASX has a favorable effect on ischemia-reperfusion testicular injury (IRI) in rats. In the immunohistochemical part of the study, we found that there was a decrease in the number of apoptotic caspase-3 positive cells in the ASX groups compared to the torsion–detorsion group in which ASX was not applied (group 2) and statistically significant when ASX was applied 45 min from the moment of detorsion (group 4). Furthermore, biochemical studies showed a decrease in malondialdehyde values and an increase in the enzyme activity of superoxide dismutase and glutathione peroxidase in group 4. Although the malondialdehyde values did not decrease significantly, the observed median decreased. The superoxide dismutase enzyme activity increased significantly in group 4 compared to groups 2 and 3. The same pattern of results was observed for the glutathione peroxidase enzyme activity in the first six minutes. It is also interesting to note statistically significant decreases in group 3 compared to group 2 in the superoxide dismutase and glutathione peroxidase enzyme activity. We expected the ameliorating effect of ASX on the torsion to be stronger in group 3 compared to group 4 because, in group 3, ASX was applied concomitantly with detorsion. Still, the results of all measured variables were closer to the negative control in group 4. This may be due to the sluggish return of the blood flow, which can limit vascular capacity to deliver appropriate doses of antioxidants to the testes during the immediate post-torsion period. By prolonging the duration of torsion, the return of blood after detorsion is slower. It is important to note that the first 60–90 min after the initial reperfusion is a critical time, for a toxic outbreak of free oxygen radicals [28].

Several studies have reported a cytoplasmic 8-OHdG expression [29–31], in concordance with our study and reports of 8-OHdG accumulating in mitochondrial DNA, although it is known to be found in the nuclei [32]. The finding of unaffected tubules shows that some tubules avoid ischemia and necrosis if the torsion persists, and these findings are in concordance with the expression pattern of oxidative stress markers 8-OHdG and NT. The strongest signal, being in group 3, treated with ASX at the time of the torsion, may be due to the induction of oxidative stress markers expression as signaling molecules in different cascades of tissue repair [33] or the edema, which prevents the transport of ASX to the testicular tissues.

This study focused on the acute effect and acute changes after IRI, but in everyday clinical practice, the average time from torsion to surgery often exceeds 90 min. To mimic real-life settings, the study would benefit from extending the time from torsion to surgery. Prolonging the time from torsion to reperfusion can be considered in future studies. ASX was administered intraperitoneally, as this route of administration was most appropriate for this model. We are aware that oral and intravenous routes of administration are more applicable for human administration, but as more detailed pharmacokinetic and pharmacodynamic studies are ongoing, we believe that intraperitoneal administration is more than satisfactory for testing ASX as a potentially potent antioxidant in preventing IRI. We opted for a dose of 75 mg/kg, but believe that in future studies, the dose may be reduced to keep the dose within the range currently recommended for use in humans, even though no adverse effects have been found in recent toxicological studies and at much higher doses. Next, we show that the slow return of blood could influence the effectiveness of the applied antioxidant, but we also point to the more beneficial effect of ASX when applied 45 min after detorsion than at the time of detorsion. Additional experimental groups should be included in the study to determine the optimal time for the ASX administration. Each group would be given ASX at a successively different time from the moment of detorsion. For example, regarding the already known harmful effect of IRI of the ipsilateral on the contralateral testis, one would also have to explore the ASX potential in ameliorating this effect.

The effects of ASX on testicular torsion have not been investigated prior to our study, although the effects regarding its precursor lycopene have been. Hekimoglu et al. [34] investigated changes after one-hour vascular clamp ischemia, and after three-hour and twenty-four-hour reperfusions. Analogous to our results in the previous study [26,27], the group receiving lycopene statistically significantly improved the Johnsen score in the testis, compared to the group in which only torsion–detorsion was performed. Analogous to the results presented here, Hekimoglu et al. showed that the values of GPx activity in the lycopene group approached the values of the sham group, demonstrating a protective effect. Malondialdehyde values, analogous to our results, were similar in all groups, with no statistically significant difference, but the mean values were lower in the groups in which lycopene was administered, supporting its protective effect. We must point out that in preclinical studies, ischemia should be performed by manual torsion rather than by vascular ligation with a vascular clamp. The torsion initially clogs veins but not arteries, and thus causes partial ischemia in the early torsion period. Güzel et al. [35] investigated the effect of intraperitoneal lycopene administration. In their model, torsion of 720° lasted for two hours, after which lycopene was given for three and ten days at a dose of 20 mg/kg/day. The mean seminiferous tubule diameter and Johnsen score were higher in the group receiving lycopene for three days intraperitoneally compared with the group without lycopene. In addition, in the groups in which lycopene was administered, a smaller number of apoptotic cells were observed by the TUNEL method, while the MDA values decreased in both groups that received lycopene for three and ten days. The SOD values did not show this tendency, while in our study, in group 4, the SOD values showed a statistically significant increase compared to group 2. From this, it undoubtedly follows that ASX has a far more potent effect than its precursor, but we must keep in mind that lycopene was administered at a dose of 20 mg/kg/day, while we administered ASX at a dose of 75 mg/kg. Compared to the studies mentioned earlier [34,35], we must note that we used prepubertal rats in our study due to the well-known fact that testicular torsion in humans occurs primarily in adolescence and preadolescence [36]. It is also important to note that Hekimoglu et al., compared to Güzel et al., gave lycopene by gavage. The route of administration of the potential drugs is of great importance, as some studies have shown limitations after oral administration, such as low stability, bioavailability, and bio-efficiency with ASX, revealing the need for new biomaterials acting as carriers in vivo [37]. Given the results of previous research as well as our research, it would certainly be interesting to investigate the possible beneficial effects of other compounds from the biosynthetic pathway of ASX, such as β-carotene, zeaxanthin, canthaxanthin, and violaxanthin [38].

Although it has been known for centuries that certain natural derivatives (exogenous factors) have beneficial effects on human health and the male reproductive system, it is only in recent decades that they have become increasingly important. Many are already registered as dietary supplement and are presented on the pharmaceutical market as supplements [21,39,40]. Currently, the main carotenoids of market interest are β-carotene, ASX, lutein, zeaxanthin, lycopene, and canthaxanthin. ASX and β-carotene are the two most well-known carotenoids in the global market and make up almost half of the carotenoid market (according to *Business Communications Company*, 2015). The total carotenoid market in 2019 was $1.8 billion, and β-carotene, lutein, and ASX accounted for more than 60% of the market share [22,41–43]. The beneficial effects of ASX are reflected in several studies. Otsuka et al. [44] concluded that the use of ASX could effectively protect against neurodegeneration during ischemic retinopathy. ASX has shown optimistic results in IRI of the liver and muscles [45,46], while the myocardium had a beneficial effect regarding IRI from disodium disuccinate ASX [47]. The preservation of renal function has been observed in a mouse kidney model [48]. While Tripathi and Jena [49] observed a protective effect on the germ cells protector in cyclophosphamide-treated mice, the positive effect of ASX on steroidogenesis in Leydig cells was described by Wang et al. [50].

Within the European Union, ASX from natural sources is currently sold in daily doses of up to 12 mg and is approved by national authorities worldwide in daily doses of up to 24 mg. Critical determinants of ASX's ability to properly integrate into its molecular environment to increase its activity are structural features such as size, shape, and polarity [51]. To date, studies in more than 2000 participants have found no significant toxicity at any dose for natural ASX, which has shown an excellent clinical safety profile at short-term (up to 100 mg) and long-term daily doses (8 to 12 mg) [52]. In rats, safety was assessed by the daily oral administration of ASX-rich biomass at concentrations up to 500 mg/kg/day for 90 days, or synthetic ASX ranging between 880 and 1240 mg/kg/day for 13 weeks [53,54]. Katsumata et al. investigated a subchronic toxicity of daily administration of natural ASX by oral gavage at doses up to 1000 mg/kg/day for 13 weeks. The only observed result was the excretion of dark red color feces [55]. Given these results and the current knowledge, it is unlikely that there will be an obstacle to recommending higher than current doses for human use in the future.

Given the potential ethical issues and research length, to date, no clinical studies have been conducted on the effect of ASX on testicular IRI in humans. The effects of ASX on humans are being explored, showing its beneficial effect on the human body (e.g., ASX inhibits LDL oxidation and increases HDL levels, modulates the immune response, protects against UV radiation, is used in anti-aging treatments, inhibits proliferation of human gastric cancer cell lines, has genoprotective properties) [56–62]. As for male infertility, Comhaire et al. [63] observed positive effects on sperm parameters and fertility. Research on the pharmacokinetics and pharmacodynamics of ASX has not been completed, so we will have to wait for the optimal administration route determination [64,65]. The existence of the blood–testis barrier, as well as its changes due to ischemia during torsion, should not be overlooked [66].

5. Conclusions

Our study promotes ASX treatment on testicular ischemia-reperfusion injury. Given the rapid growth of research in the field of antioxidants and testicular ischemia-reperfusion injury, we believe that one day the powerful antioxidants, especially ASX, will be applicable in clinical settings, given that, to date, there is no cure given to patients.

Supplementary Materials: The following are available online at https://www.mdpi.com/article/10.3390/jcm11051284/s1, Figure S1: Box plots for for GPx activity in the 1st minute, Figure S2: Box plots for for GPx activity in the 2nd minute, Figure S3: Box plots for for GPx activity in the 3rd minute, Figure S4: Box plots for for GPx activity in the 4th minute, Figure S5: Box plots for for GPx activity in the 5th minute, Figure S6: Box plots for for GPx activity in the 6th minute, Table S1: Means, standard deviations, medians, Q1, Q3, and interquartile ranges by groups for caspase-3 positive cells, Table S2: Median, Q1, Q3, and interquartile range values by groups for MDA, Table S3: Median, Q1, Q3, and interquartile range values by groups for SOD, Table S4: Median, Q1, Q3, and interquartile ranges by groups for GPx activity in the 1st, 2nd, 3rd, 4th, 5th, and 6th minutes.

Author Contributions: Conceptualization, M.B. and D.J.; methodology, M.B., A.K.B., N.S. and D.J.; validation, A.K.B., N.S., Z.S. and D.J.; formal analysis, M.B., A.K.B., N.S., M.H.P., D.K., Z.S. and D.J.; investigation, M.B., A.K.B., N.S., M.H.P., D.K. and D.J.; resources, A.K.B., N.S., and D.J.; data curation, M.B., M.H.P., D.K. and Z.S.; writing—original draft preparation, M.B., M.H.P., D.K. and D.J.; writing—review and editing, M.B., A.K.B., N.S., and D.J.; visualization, M.B., M.H.P., D.K. and Z.S.; supervision, D.J.; project administration, D.J.; funding acquisition, D.J. All authors have read and agreed to the published version of the manuscript.

Funding: The research was supported by the Scientific Center of Excellence for Reproductive and Regenerative Medicine, Republic of Croatia, and the European Union through the European Regional Development Fund, under the contract KK.01.1.1.01.0008, project "Regenerative and Reproductive Medicine—Exploring New Platforms and Potentials".

Institutional Review Board Statement: The research was approved by the School of Medicine, University of Zagreb (classification; 641-01/19-02/01/registry number; 380-59-10106-19-111/162) and the Croatian National Ethics Committee (EP 217/2019).

Informed Consent Statement: Not applicable.

Data Availability Statement: The data that support the findings of this study are available upon request from the corresponding author.

Acknowledgments: We thank Milan Kopač for taking care of the animals. We thank Mariana Dragojević for preparing the histological sections.

Conflicts of Interest: The authors declare no conflict of interest. The funders had no role in the design of the study; in the collection, analyses, or interpretation of data; in the writing of the manuscript; or in the decision to publish the results.

References

1. Mäkelä, E.; Lahdes-Vasama, T.; Rajakorpi, H.; Wikström, S. A 19-year review of paediatric patients with acute scrotum. *Scand. J. Surg.* **2007**, *96*, 62–66. [CrossRef] [PubMed]
2. Bowlin, P.R.; Gatti, J.M.; Murphy, J.P. Pediatric Testicular Torsion. *Surg. Clin. N. Am.* **2017**, *97*, 161–172. [CrossRef] [PubMed]

3. Ta, A.; D'Arcy, F.T.; Hoag, N.; D'Arcy, J.P.; Lawrentschuk, N. Testicular torsion and the acute scrotum: Current emergency management. *Eur. J. Emerg. Med.* **2016**, *23*, 160–165. [CrossRef]
4. Watkin, N.A.; Reiger, N.A.; Moisey, C.U. Is the conservative management of the acute scrotum justified on clinical grounds? *Br. J. Urol.* **1996**, *78*, 623–627. [CrossRef] [PubMed]
5. Tajchner, L.; Larkin, J.O.; Bourke, M.G.; Waldron, R.; Barry, K.; Eustace, P.W. Management of the acute scrotum in a district general hospital: 10-year experience. *Sci. World J.* **2009**, *9*, 281–286. [CrossRef]
6. Hegarty, P.K.; Walsh, E.; Corcoran, M.O. Exploration of the acute scrotum: A retrospective analysis of 100 consecutive cases. *Ir. J. Med. Sci.* **2001**, *170*, 181–182. [CrossRef] [PubMed]
7. Molokwu, C.N.; Somani, B.K.; Goodman, C.M. Outcomes of scrotal exploration for acute scrotal pain suspicious of testicular torsion: A consecutive case series of 173 patients. *BJU Int.* **2011**, *107*, 990–993. [CrossRef]
8. Zhao, L.C.; Lautz, T.B.; Meeks, J.J.; Maizels, M. Pediatric testicular torsion epidemiology using a national database: Incidence, risk of orchiectomy and possible measures toward improving the quality of care. *J. Urol.* **2011**, *186*, 2009–2013. [CrossRef]
9. Ben-Chaim, J.; Leibovitch, I.; Ramon, J.; Winberg, D.; Goldwasser, B. Etiology of acute scrotum at surgical exploration in children, adolescents and adults. *Eur. Urol.* **1992**, *21*, 45–47.
10. Schick, M.A.; Sternard, B.T. Testicular Torsion. In *StatPearls*; StatPearls Publishing: Treasure Island, FL, USA, 2021.
11. Bašković, M.; Župančić, B.; Vukasović, I.; Štimac-Rojtinić, I.; Ježek, D. Validation of a TWIST Score in Diagnosis of Testicular Torsion—Single-Center Experience. *Klin. Padiatr.* **2019**, *231*, 217–219. [CrossRef]
12. Kalogeris, T.; Baines, C.P.; Krenz, M.; Korthuis, R.J. Cell biology of ischemia/reperfusion injury. *Int. Rev. Cell. Mol. Biol.* **2012**, *298*, 229–317. [PubMed]
13. Carden, D.L.; Granger, D.N. Pathophysiology of ischaemia-reperfusion injury. *J. Pathol.* **2000**, *190*, 255–266. [CrossRef]
14. Grace, P.A.; Mathie, R.T. *Ischemia-Reperfusion Injury*; Blackwell Science: London, UK, 1999.
15. Bellanti, F. Ischemia-reperfusion injury: Evidences for translational research. *Ann. Transl. Med.* **2016**, *4*, S55. [CrossRef] [PubMed]
16. Slegtenhorst, B.R.; Dor, F.J.; Rodriguez, H.; Voskuil, F.J.; Tullius, S.G. Ischemia/reperfusion Injury and its Consequences on Immunity and Inflammation. *Curr. Transplant. Rep.* **2014**, *1*, 147–154. [CrossRef]
17. Rahal, A.; Kumar, A.; Singh, V.; Yadav, B.; Tiwari, R.; Chakraborty, S.; Dhama, K. Oxidative stress, prooxidants, and antioxidants: The interplay. *Biomed. Res. Int.* **2014**, *2014*, 761264. [CrossRef]
18. Chandra, J.; Samali, A.; Orrenius, S. Triggering and modulation of apoptosis by oxidative stress. *Free. Radic. Biol. Med.* **2000**, *29*, 323–333. [CrossRef]
19. Hengartner, M.O. The biochemistry of apoptosis. *Nature* **2000**, *407*, 770–776. [CrossRef]
20. Miguel, M.G. Antioxidant and anti-inflammatory activities of essential oils: A short review. *Molecules* **2010**, *15*, 9252–9287. [CrossRef]
21. Manivannan, K.; Karthikai Devi, G.; Anantharaman, P.; Balasubramanian, T. Antimicrobial potential of selected brown seaweeds from Vedalai coastal waters, Gulf of Mannar. *Asian Pac. J. Trop. Biomed.* **2011**, *1*, 114–120. [CrossRef]
22. Guerin, M.; Huntley, M.E.; Olaizola, M. Haematococcus astaxanthin: Applications for human health and nutrition. *Trends Biotechnol.* **2003**, *21*, 210–216. [CrossRef]
23. Kidd, P. Astaxanthin, cell membrane nutrient with diverse clinical benefits and anti-aging potential. *Altern. Med. Rev.* **2011**, *16*, 355–364.
24. Pashkow, F.J.; Watumull, D.G.; Campbell, C.L. Astaxanthin: A novel potential treatment for oxidative stress and inflammation in cardiovascular disease. *Am. J. Cardiol.* **2008**, *101*, 58–68. [CrossRef]
25. Miki, W. Biological functions and activities of animal carotenoids. *Pure. Appl. Chem.* **1991**, *63*, 141–146. [CrossRef]
26. Bašković, M.; Bojanac, A.K.; Sinčić, N.; Perić, M.H.; Krsnik, D.; Ježek, D. The effect of astaxanthin on testicular torsion-detorsion injury in rats-detailed morphometric evaluation of histological sections. *J. Pediatr. Urol.* **2021**, *17*, 439.e1–439.e12. [CrossRef] [PubMed]
27. Bašković, M.; Ježek, D. Response to Letter to the Editor re 'The effect of astaxanthin on testicular torsion-detorsion injury in rats-detailed morphometric evaluation of histological sections'. *J. Pediatr. Urol.* **2021**. Epub ahead of print. [CrossRef] [PubMed]
28. Prillaman, H.M.; Turner, T.T. Rescue of testicular function after acute experimental torsion. *J. Urol.* **1997**, *157*, 340–345. [CrossRef]
29. Conlon, K.A.; Zharkov, D.O.; Berrios, M. Immunofluorescent localization of the murine 8-oxoguanine DNA glycosylase (mOGG1) in cells growing under normal and nutrient deprivation conditions. *DNA Repair.* **2003**, *2*, 1337–1352. [CrossRef] [PubMed]
30. Nakayama, S.; Kajiya, H.; Okabe, K.; Ikebe, T. Effects of oxidative stress on the expression of 8-oxoguanine and its eliminating enzymes in human keratinocytes and squamous carcinoma cells. *Oral Sci. Int.* **2011**, *8*, 11–16. [CrossRef]
31. Sheng, Z.; Oka, S.; Tsuchimoto, D.; Abolhassani, N.; Nomaru, H.; Sakumi, K.; Yamada, H.; Nakabeppu, Y. 8-Oxoguanine causes neurodegeneration during MUTYH-mediated DNA base excision repair. *J. Clin. Investig.* **2012**, *122*, 4344–4361. [CrossRef]
32. Sobočan, N.; Katušić Bojanac, A.; Sinčić, N.; Himelreich-Perić, M.; Krasić, J.; Majić, Ž.; Jurić-Lekić, G.; Šerman, L.; Vlahović, M.; Ježek, D.; et al. A Free Radical Scavenger Ameliorates Teratogenic Activity of a DNA Hypomethylating Hematological Therapeutic. *Stem Cells Dev.* **2019**, *28*, 717–733. [CrossRef]
33. Sharma, P.; Jha, A.B.; Dubey, R.S.; Pessarakli, M. Reactive oxygen species, oxidative damage, and antioxidative defense mechanism in plants under stressful conditions. *J. Bot.* **2012**, *2012*, 217037. [CrossRef]
34. Hekimoglu, A.; Kurcer, Z.; Aral, F.; Baba, F.; Sahna, E.; Atessahin, A. Lycopene, an antioxidant carotenoid, attenuates testicular injury caused by ischemia/reperfusion in rats. *Tohoku J. Exp. Med.* **2009**, *218*, 141–147. [CrossRef] [PubMed]

55. Güzel, M.; Sönmez, M.F.; Baştuğ, O.; Aras, N.F.; Öztürk, A.B.; Küçükaydın, M.; Turan, C. Effectiveness of lycopene on experimental testicular torsion. *J. Pediatr. Surg.* **2016**, *51*, 1187–1191. [CrossRef] [PubMed]
56. Becker, E.J., Jr.; Turner, T.T. Endocrine and exocrine effects of testicular torsion in the prepubertal and adult rat. *J. Androl.* **1995**, *16*, 342–351.
57. Zuluaga, M.; Gueguen, V.; Letourneur, D.; Pavon-Djavid, G. Astaxanthin-antioxidant impact on excessive Reactive Oxygen Species generation induced by ischemia and reperfusion injury. *Chem. Biol. Interact.* **2018**, *279*, 145–158. [CrossRef]
58. Sathasivam, R.; Ki, J.S. A Review of the Biological Activities of Microalgal Carotenoids and Their Potential Use in Healthcare and Cosmetic Industries. *Mar. Drugs* **2018**, *16*, 26. [CrossRef]
59. Mishra, R.K.; Singh, S.; Singh, S.K. Natural products in regulation of male fertility. *Indian J. Med. Res.* **2018**, *148*, S107–S114.
60. Dias, T.R.; Alves, M.G.; Oliveira, P.F.; Silva, B.M. Natural products as modulators of spermatogenesis: The search for a male contraceptive. *Curr. Mol. Pharmacol.* **2014**, *7*, 154–166. [CrossRef]
61. Li, J.; Zhu, D.; Niu, J.; Shen, S.; Wang, G. An economic assessment of astaxanthin production by large scale cultivation of Haematococcus pluvialis. *Biotechnol. Adv.* **2011**, *29*, 568–574. [CrossRef]
62. Sung, Y.J.; Sim, S.J. Multifaceted strategies for economic production of microalgae Haematococcus pluvialis-derived astaxanthin via direct conversion of CO_2. *Bioresour. Technol.* **2021**, *344*, 126255. [CrossRef]
63. Bauer, A.; Minceva, M. Techno-economic analysis of a new downstream process for the production of astaxanthin from the microalgae Haematococcus pluvialis. *Bioresour. Bioprocess.* **2021**, *8*, 111. [CrossRef]
64. Otsuka, T.; Shimazawa, M.; Inoue, Y.; Nakano, Y.; Ojino, K.; Izawa, H.; Tsuruma, K.; Ishibashi, T.; Hara, H. Astaxanthin Protects Against Retinal Damage: Evidence from In Vivo and In Vitro Retinal Ischemia and Reperfusion Models. *Curr. Eye Res.* **2016**, *41*, 1465–1472. [CrossRef]
65. Curek, G.D.; Cort, A.; Yucel, G.; Demir, N.; Ozturk, S.; Elpek, G.O.; Savas, B.; Aslan, M. Effect of astaxanthin on hepatocellular injury following ischemia/reperfusion. *Toxicology* **2010**, *267*, 147–153. [CrossRef] [PubMed]
66. Zuluaga Tamayo, M.; Choudat, L.; Aid-Launais, R.; Thibaudeau, O.; Louedec, L.; Letourneur, D.; Gueguen, V.; Meddahi-Pellé, A.; Couvelard, A.; Pavon-Djavid, G. Astaxanthin Complexes to Attenuate Muscle Damage after In Vivo Femoral Ischemia-Reperfusion. *Mar. Drugs* **2019**, *17*, 354. [CrossRef] [PubMed]
67. Lauver, D.A.; Lockwood, S.F.; Lucchesi, B.R. Disodium Disuccinate Astaxanthin (Cardax) attenuates complement activation and reduces myocardial injury following ischemia/reperfusion. *J. Pharmacol. Exp. Ther.* **2005**, *314*, 686–692. [CrossRef]
68. Qiu, X.; Fu, K.; Zhao, X.; Zhang, Y.; Yuan, Y.; Zhang, S.; Gu, X.; Guo, H. Protective effects of astaxanthin against ischemia/reperfusion induced renal injury in mice. *J. Transl. Med.* **2015**, *13*, 28. [CrossRef] [PubMed]
69. Tripathi, D.N.; Jena, G.B. Astaxanthin inhibits cytotoxic and genotoxic effects of cyclophosphamide in mice germ cells. *Toxicology* **2008**, *248*, 96–103. [CrossRef]
70. Wang, J.Y.; Lee, Y.J.; Chou, M.C.; Chang, R.; Chiu, C.H.; Liang, Y.J.; Wu, L.S. Astaxanthin protects steroidogenesis from hydrogen peroxide-induced oxidative stress in mouse Leydig cells. *Mar. Drugs* **2015**, *13*, 1375–1388. [CrossRef] [PubMed]
71. Britton, G. Structure and properties of carotenoids in relation to function. *FASEB J.* **1995**, *9*, 1551–1558. [CrossRef] [PubMed]
72. Brendler, T.; Williamson, E.M. Astaxanthin: How much is too much? A safety review. *Phytother. Res.* **2019**, *33*, 3090–3111. [CrossRef]
73. Stewart, J.S.; Lignell, A.; Pettersson, A.; Elfving, E.; Soni, M.G. Safety assessment of astaxanthin-rich microalgae biomass: Acute and subchronic toxicity studies in rats. *Food. Chem. Toxicol.* **2008**, *46*, 3030–3036. [CrossRef] [PubMed]
74. Vega, K.; Edwards, J.; Beilstein, P. Subchronic (13-week) toxicity and prenatal developmental toxicity studies of dietary astaxanthin in rats. *Regul. Toxicol. Pharmacol.* **2015**, *73*, 819–828. [CrossRef]
75. Katsumata, T.; Ishibashi, T.; Kyle, D. A sub-chronic toxicity evaluation of a natural astaxanthin-rich carotenoid extract of Paracoccus carotinifaciens in rats. *Toxicol. Rep.* **2014**, *1*, 582–588. [CrossRef]
76. Kishimoto, Y.; Yoshida, H.; Kondo, K. Potential Anti-Atherosclerotic Properties of Astaxanthin. *Mar. Drugs* **2016**, *14*, 35. [CrossRef]
77. Park, J.S.; Chyun, J.H.; Kim, Y.K.; Line, L.L.; Chew, B.P. Astaxanthin decreased oxidative stress and inflammation and enhanced immune response in humans. *Nutr. Metab.* **2010**, *7*, 18. [CrossRef]
78. Ito, N.; Seki, S.; Ueda, F. The Protective Role of Astaxanthin for UV-Induced Skin Deterioration in Healthy People-A Randomized, Double-Blind, Placebo-Controlled Trial. *Nutrients* **2018**, *10*, 817. [CrossRef]
79. Davinelli, S.; Scapagnini, G.; Marzatico, F.; Nobile, V.; Ferrara, N.; Corbi, G. Influence of equol and resveratrol supplementation on health-related quality of life in menopausal women: A randomized, placebo-controlled study. *Maturitas* **2017**, *96*, 77–83. [CrossRef]
80. Eren, B.; Tuncay Tanrıverdi, S.; Aydın Köse, F.; Özer, Ö. Antioxidant properties evaluation of topical astaxanthin formulations as anti-aging products. *J. Cosmet. Dermatol.* **2019**, *18*, 242–250. [CrossRef]
81. Kim, J.H.; Park, J.J.; Lee, B.J.; Joo, M.K.; Chun, H.J.; Lee, S.W.; Bak, Y.T. Astaxanthin Inhibits Proliferation of Human Gastric Cancer Cell Lines by Interrupting Cell Cycle Progression. *Gut Liver* **2016**, *10*, 369–374. [CrossRef] [PubMed]
82. Pilinska, M.A.; Kurinnyi, D.A.; Rushkovsky, S.R.; Dybska, O.B. Genoprotective properties of astaxanthin revealed by ionizing radiation exposure in vitro on human peripheral blood lymphocytes. *Probl. Radiac. Med. Radiobiol.* **2016**, *21*, 141–148. [CrossRef] [PubMed]
83. Comhaire, F.H.; El Garem, Y.; Mahmoud, A.; Eertmans, F.; Schoonjans, F. Combined conventional/antioxidant "Astaxanthin" treatment for male infertility: A double blind, randomized trial. *Asian J. Androl.* **2005**, *7*, 257–262. [CrossRef] [PubMed]

64. Reboul, E. Mechanisms of Carotenoid Intestinal Absorption: Where Do We Stand? *Nutrients* **2019**, *11*, 838. [CrossRef] [PubMed]
65. Parker, R.S. Absorption, metabolism, and transport of carotenoids. *FASEB J.* **1996**, *10*, 542–551. [CrossRef] [PubMed]
66. Mel'man, E.P.; Gritsulyak, B.V.; Shutka, B.V. Changes in the ultrastructure of components of the blood-testis barrier in circulatory hypoxia. *Bull. Exp. Biol. Med.* **1979**, *88*, 928–931. [CrossRef]

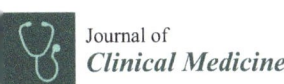

Communication

Positive Effect of a New Combination of Antioxidants and Natural Hormone Stimulants for the Treatment of Oligoasthenoteratozoospermia

Vincenzo De Leo [1,2], Claudia Tosti [2], Giuseppe Morgante [1,2], Rosetta Ponchia [1,2], Alice Luddi [1,*], Laura Governini [1,*] and Paola Piomboni [1,2]

1. Department of Molecular and Developmental Medicine, Siena University, 53100 Siena, Italy; vincenzo.deleo@unisi.it (V.D.L.); giuseppe.morgante@unisi.it (G.M.); ponchia2@student.unisi.it (R.P.); paola.piomboni@unisi.it (P.P.)
2. Assisted Reproduction Unit, Siena University Hospital, 53100 Siena, Italy; claudia.tosti@ao-siena.toscana.it
* Correspondence: luddi@unisi.it (A.L.); laura.governini@unisi.it (L.G.); Tel.: +39-0577-233521 (A.L.); +39-0577-586810 (L.G.)

Abstract: Oligoasthenoteratozoospermia (OAT) accounts for about 90% of male infertility; in many cases this disorder may be associated with oxidative stress, a condition that decreases the success of fertilization. Therefore, the empirical treatment of male infertility is often based on the use of antioxidants. The aim of the present study was to assess the effectiveness of three months' administration of a new nutraceutical preparation on hormone profile, sperm parameters and fertilization capability in men undergoing in vitro fertilization (IVF). A total of 36 OAT patients were daily treated for 3 months with a dose of a formulation containing: Inositol, L-Carnitine, Vitamins C, D, E, Coenzyme Q10 and Selenium. Selected parameters were analysed before (T0) and after (T1) treatment, and IVF outcomes were evaluated. We observed an improvement of sperm concentration, motility, morphology and vitality; blood level of testosterone also showed an increase. A significant increase of fertilization rate was detected in 14 couples, whose male partner were treated with the nutraceutical preparation. The present results indicate that a formulation containing antioxidant and energy supply substances was effective in the treatment of sperm alterations and led to significant recovery of fertilizing capacity.

Keywords: male infertility; oligoasthenoteratozoospermia; clinical-therapeutic strategies; antioxidant treatment

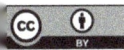

1. Introduction

The World Health Organization (WHO) estimates that in advanced industrial countries, couples with fertility problems constitute about 15–20% of the population of reproductive age, with the male factor contributing to almost half of the cases [1,2]. The problem seems to be increasing for reasons such as postponing parenthood, negative environmental factors, unhealthy life-styles and various social conditions.

Excluding anatomical defects, a low sperm count combined with poor sperm motility and morphology (oligoasthenoteratozoospermia, OAT) is considered one of the most common causes of male infertility. Of these, about 30% are unexplained; the others are linked to causes that range from hormonal alterations, genetic anomalies, iatrogenic factors and unhealthy life-style (diet, smoking, alcohol) [3–5] and oxidative stress by reactive oxygen species (ROS) [6]. In semen there is a homeostasis between free radicals, produced by leukocytes and spermatozoa [7], and protective enzymatic and non-enzymatic antioxidants. Some pathophysiology conditions, environmental factors or unhealthy lifestyles may alter this equilibrium and lead to an accumulation of ROS in seminal fluid, causing a harmful oxidative damage [8–10].

Regarding the hormonal component, infertile men are characterized by low plasma concentrations of testosterone and LH, almost invariably combined with a lack of energizing factors and antioxidants, all of which contribute to the onset of OAT.

With increasing recognition of the role of oxidative stress energy release in the pathophysiology of male infertility, the use of antioxidants/energizing compounds is one of the therapeutic options adopted for the treatment of idiopathic infertility. An ideal supplement should provide substances that affect plasma concentrations of testosterone, as well as energizing ingredients and antioxidants to improve sperm vitality and protect them against oxidative injury [11,12].

Many substances found in nature have such effects [5,13]. In particular, inositol seems to have specific effects on certain hormonal markers, favouring an increase in plasma concentrations of LH, followed by those of testosterone, through stimulation of Leydig cells in the testicles interstitium [14]. In vitro supplementation of myo-inositol is able to significantly improve sperm motility in a dose-dependent manner [15], demonstrating a protective role during sperm cryopreservation [16].

Another interesting substance is L-carnitine, which promotes energy and makes sperm more vital by improving their post-gonadic maturation. Arginine is also indicated as an amino acid useful for spermatogenesis and formation of nitric oxide, an energy source for sperm cells [17]. A major role among the antioxidants is played by the vitamin C and E, normally present in seminal fluid, which ensures the stability of cell structures and contributes to sperm motility [18]. Vitamin E (α-tocopherol) is an important lipid-soluble antioxidant molecule in the cell membrane. It is thought to interrupt lipid peroxidation and enhance the activity of various antioxidants that scavenge free radicals generated during the univalent reduction of molecular oxygen and during normal activity of oxidative enzymes [19]. The results of in vitro experiments suggest that vitamin E may protect spermatozoa from oxidative damage and loss of motility as well as enhance the sperm performance in the hamster egg penetration assay [20]. The ability of Vitamin C in suppressing the endogenous oxidative damage is also well documented [21]. Vitamin C concentration in the seminal plasma, is 10-fold higher than that in the serum [22]. And its levels in seminal plasma negatively correlated with the sperm DNA fragmentation index. Indeed, vitamin C supplementation has been reported improve sperm parameters in infertile men [23,24]. Vitamin D3 supplementation is increasingly accepted, since deficiencies have been correlated with the onset of certain male and female reproductive disorders. The enzyme responsible for vitamin D metabolism in the human sperm flagellum is correlated with the quality, vitality and function of mature sperm [25]. The antioxidant effects of coenzyme Q10 are well known, and although seminal fluid seems to protect sperm against oxidative stress, treatment with this coenzyme improves sperm motility [26,27]. Zinc is a fundamental trace element for reproductive processes, since it is involved in cell reproduction and protection against oxidative stress.

The present study aimed to investigate the impact of an oral antioxidant supplementation, composed of natural substances, on seminal and hormonal parameters of infertile men with OAT.

2. Materials and Methods
2.1. Study Design and Patients Recruitment

This prospective study was performed on a total of 36 Caucasian males undergoing semen evaluation at the Unit of Medically Assisted Reproduction, Siena University Hospital, after 12–18 months of unprotected sexual intercourse without conception.

A comprehensive clinical history of patients was obtained; we excluded patients with possible causes of male infertility such as varicocele, cryptorchidism, endocrine disorders or systemic diseases and patients with intake of spermiotoxic drugs, smoking, alcohol or drugs abuse. All patients underwent microbiological analysis of seminal fluid and urine for common bacteria such as *Mycoplasma*, *Trichomonas vaginalis* and *Chlamydia trachomatis*. The median age of the patients was 34 years (range: 25–47 years); the BMI ranged between

18 and 25. All participants signed a written informed consent, and the study protocol was approved by the Ethic Committee of the Siena University Hospital (approval ID: CEASVE 191113).

In the selected patients, the diagnosis of oligoasthenoteratozoospermia (OAT) was confirmed by performing two spermiogram at one month (T0) from the first investigation (T-1). Recruited patients were asked to take orally, once a day, for three consecutive months, a preparation (Gomotil®, Gofarma, Italy) containing a cocktail of nutraceutical substances: Inositol, L-Carnitine, Acetyl L-Carnitine Hydrochloride, Vitamin E, Vitamin C, Coenzyme Q10, Selenium, and Vitamin D3 (Table 1).

Table 1. Composition, Dosage and Nutrient Reference Values (NRVs) of the administered nutraceutical preparation.

Nutraceutical Composition	Per 1 Packet	NRV
Inositol	1000 mg	-
L-Carnitine	250 mg	-
Acetyl L-Carnitine Hydrochloride	250 mg	-
Vitamin E	60 mg	500%
Vitamin C	100 mg	125%
Vitamin D3	5 mcg	100%
Coenzyme Q10	20 mg	-
Selenium	50 mcg	90.90%

At T0, the hormone profile of enrolled patients has been performed, including Testosterone, Follicle Stimulating Hormone (FSH), Luteinizing Hormone (LH), Sex hormone binding globulin (SHBG), Prolactin and Estradiol. The main blood-metabolic parameters were also measured: Glucose, Insulin, Creatinine, Total Cholesterol, Triglycerides, Oxaloacetic Transaminase, Pyruvic Transaminase and C-Reactive Protein. Sperm evaluation, hormone and metabolic profiles were tested after 3 months of treatment (T1; Table 2).

Table 2. Study Timeline.

Required Examination	T-1	T0 Basal	T1 Post Treatment
Spermiogram	X	X	X
Hormonal panel		X	X
Hemato-Metabolic panel		X	X

2.2. Semen Analysis

At T-1, T0 and T1 the ejaculate samples were collected, by masturbation, in sterile containers after a period of abstinence between 2 and 5 days. Semen samples were assessed according to WHO (2010) parameters [28].

Seminal analysis was carried out, within 30 min after fluidification. The volume, viscosity, pH, and appearance of the semen were evaluated together with sperm concentration, progressive and total motility, and morphology. Sperm concentration was evaluated using a Makler counting chamber (Irvine Scientific, Santa Ana, CA, USA), under an optical microscope (Nikon, Nikon Europe B.V., Amsterdam, The Netherlands) at 200× magnification. Sperm morphology was evaluated by using pre-coloured glasses (Testsimplets) and the eosin Y test was applied to evaluate sperm vitality.

2.3. Assisted Reproduction Techniques

The main reproductive outcomes were retrospectively evaluated in 14 couples (Group A) undergoing IVF at the Unit of Medically Assisted Reproduction, Siena University Hospital, whose male partners received the nutraceutical supplementation for three months, before an IVF cycle. The control group (Group B) was composed by 14 couples where male, with a diagnosis of OAT, didn't receive any supplementation before IVF.

Inclusion criteria were male infertility (OAT); exclusion criteria were female fertility factor and/or couple or idiopathic infertility.

We included homolog cycles (no egg or sperm donors) using fresh oocytes and ejaculated sperm. Standard controlled ovarian stimulation protocols were used. Stimulation with gonadotrophins was monitored by measuring serum estradiol levels and follicle growth. Human chorionic gonadotropin was administered when patients reached the individual clinic's trigger point for follicular growth. Cumulus–oocyte complexes were collected 36 h later, by ultrasound-guided transvaginal follicular aspiration. To perform ICSI, after 2 h of incubation the oocytes were denuded. Sperm injection was performed immediately after denudation according to conventional procedure. Fertilization was assessed 16–18 h after injection.

2.4. Statistical Analysis

A statistical analysis was performed by means of the GraphPad Prism 5.0 (GraphPad Software, San Diego, CA, USA) using nonparametric tests. The differences among groups of data, before (T0) and after (T1) the treatment with the nutraceutical preparation, were tested by the Kruskal–Wallis test. The data are reported as mean ± standard deviation (SD). The differences observed have been considered statistically significant at $p < 0.05$.

3. Results

3.1. Effect on Hormone and Metabolic Profile

The patients enrolled in the study did not have a history of endocrine, metabolic or anatomical alterations. Microbiological tests were all negative for Chlamydia trachomatis, Mycoplasma and Trichomonas vaginalis.

The comparison of values before the beginning of the treatment (T0) and after three months (T1) shows an increase, although not statistically significant, of the blood levels of testosterone and in general an improvement of the hormonal profile (Table 3).

Table 3. Evaluation of the hormone levels before treatment with the nutraceutical preparation (T0) and after three months of administration (T1).

Test Parameters	T0 Basal	T1 Post Treatment	*Reference Values*
Testosterone (ng/mL)	4.5 ± 1.6	5.2 ± 1.8	2.8–8.0
FSH (mUI/mL)	5.2 ± 1.3	4.8 ± 0.9	0.7–11.0
LH (mUI/mL)	6.1 ± 1.7	5.5 ± 0.6	0.8–8.0
SHBG (nmol/mL)	48.0 ± 12.0	55 ± 16	10.0–57.0
Prolactin (ng/mL)	11.2 ± 3.0	10.6 ± 2.0	2.0–13.0
Estradiol (pg/mL)	32.0 ± 6.0	25.0 ± 4.0	<32.0

The effects of the nutraceutical preparation were evaluated at the T1 and compared with the T0 (Table 4). The analysis shows an improvement, even if not statistically significant, of the main metabolic parameters. This result, together with the absence of side effects, evidences the safety of the product making it suitable also for a large-scale use and for prolonged periods.

Table 4. Main blood values of patients before the beginning of the treatment with nutraceutical preparation (T0) and after three months of treatment (T1).

Test Parameters	T0 Basal	T1 Post Treatment	*Reference Values*
Glucose (mg/dL)	98 ± 7	91 ± 3	60–110
Insulin (microU/mL)	12.7 ± 4.2	9.3 ± 2.6	2.6–24.9
Creatinine (mg/dL)	0.88 ± 0.2	0.80 ± 0.3	0.55–1.40

Table 4. Cont.

Test Parameters	T0 Basal	T1 Post Treatment	Reference Values
Total Cholesterol (mg/dL)	218 ± 9	202 ± 5	140–220
Triglycerides (mg/dL)	160 ± 8	154 ± 7	<200
Oxaloacetic Transaminase *(AST)(GOT)* (U/L)	24 ± 5	22 ± 6	<30
Pyruvic Transaminase *(ALT)(GPT)* (U/L)	19 ± 3	18 ± 4	<41
C Reactive Protein (CRP) (mg/L)	0.8 ± 0.3	0.7 ± 0.4	0.0–5.0

3.2. Effect on Sperm Parameters

The data analysis shows that the treatment with nutraceutical preparation significantly improve the main sperm parameters: a statistically significant rise of sperm concentration was evident, with an increase of 71.7% (* $p < 0.05$) (Figure 1A).

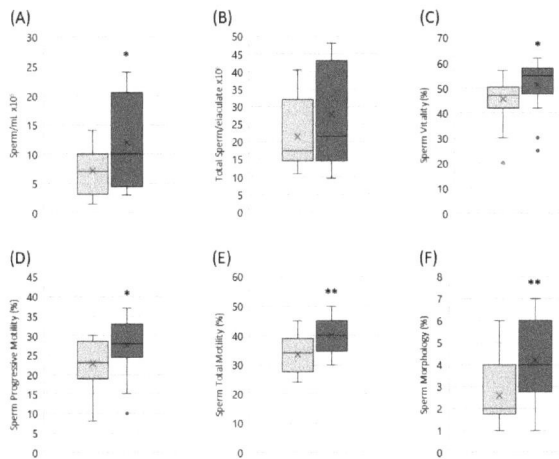

Figure 1. Sperm concentration (**A**); total sperm number (**B**); sperm vitality (**C**); progressive (**D**) and total (**E**) sperm motility; sperm morphology (**F**) before (T0; light grey) and after 3 months (T1; dark grey) treatment with nutraceutical preparation. Graphical diagrams are plotted as box–whisker plots, where boxes show the interquartile range with median and mean values, and whiskers represent min and max confidence intervals, outliers are represented as single dots (* $p < 0.05$; ** $p < 0.01$).

The total sperm number was increased of 28.6%, in a non-statistically significant manner (Figure 1B). Indeed, this parameter is closely related to contingent conditions such as ejaculate volume at the time of sample collection, which may be influenced by psychological stress or hydration of the patient. The effect of treatment on both progressive (Figure 1D) and total sperm motility (Figure 1E) showed an increase of 20.6% (* $p < 0.05$) and 19.6% (** $p < 0.01$) respectively. Sperm morphology evaluation demonstrated that the integrity and shape of the acrosome, the head morphology and the flagellum profile significantly changed after treatment with an increase of 61.5% (** $p < 0.01$; Figure 1F). Spermiogram data are summarised in Table 5.

Table 5. Seminal parameters investigated at basal conditions (T0) and after three months of nutraceutical administration (T1) (* $p < 0.05$; ** $p < 0.01$).

Semen Parameters	T0 Basal	T1 Post Treatment	*p* Value
Concentration ($\times 10^6$/mL)	7.13 ± 4.24	12.24 ± 7.83	*
Total sperm count ($\times 10^6$/ejaculate)	21.54 ± 10.15	27.70 ± 14.87	ns

Table 5. Cont.

Semen Parameters	T0 Basal	T1 Post Treatment	p Value
Vitality (%)	45.4 ± 8.2	51.2 ± 9.5	*
Progressive Motility (%)	22.8 ± 5.9	27.5 ± 6.4	*
Total motility (%)	33.6 ± 5.5	40.2 ± 5.8	**
Morphology (%)	2.6 ± 1.4	4.2 ± 1.9	**

ns: not significant.

3.3. Reproductive Outcomes

At the end of 3 months of treatment with the nutraceutical preparation 14 patients (Group A) out of 36 underwent an IVF cycle at the UOSA PMA–University Hospital of Siena. The number of retrieved oocytes, MII injected oocytes, fertilization and pregnancy rate were registered and are reported in Table 6, in comparison with Group B.

Table 6. Reproductive Outcomes of IVF cycle between Group A and Group B (* p < 0.05).

Reproductive Outcomes	Group A	Group B	p Value
Male patient's age (years)	34.4 ± 6.8	35.2 ± 6.3	ns
Female patient'age at pick-up (years)	33.7 ± 2.5	34.1 ± 3.2	ns
Number retrieved oocytes	9.8 ± 3.5	9.2 ± 3.3	ns
Number MII oocytes	7.9 ± 2.7	7.5 ± 2.4	ns
Fertilization rate (%)	87.3 ± 15.7	74.3 ± 22.6	*
Pregnancy rate (%)	19.6 ± 3.7	17.2 ± 2.9	ns

4. Discussion

Male infertility is a significant social problem with a strong impact on well-being as well as an unbroken medical challenge. A large number of recent studies have focused on the ability of many substances, generally termed as *nutraceuticals*, to improve the hormonal status and sperm parameters by different mechanisms [29,30]. The supplementation with natural compound for the treatment of male infertility is greatly debated on literature. The evaluation of the effectiveness and safety of supplementary oral antioxidants in subfertile men put in evidence some important bias of the published studies, first of all the selection of patients and control groups. Results from observational studies might have been confounded by lifestyle factors such as age, weight, physical health and/or medication use. The administration of individual antioxidants or combinations of them, the dosage and formulation of the nutraceutical and the duration of treatment, can create discordant and non-significant results [11,31,32]. Apart from cases with a specific aetiology (genetic, hormonal, infectious etc.), which are readily diagnosed and treated medically and/or surgically, idiopathic alterations of the main sperm characteristics, as in the case of OAT, can benefit from the use of oral supplements based on amino acids (L-carnitine), antioxidants, such as vitamins A, C and E, folic acid and elements such as selenium [33,34]. This is not surprising, since oxidative stress resulting from an imbalance between ROS and antioxidants systems usually present in seminal fluid is fundamental in male fertility. Indeed, ROS abundance has been implicated in sperm abnormalities [35,36], while the exact impact on fertilization and pregnancy has long been the subject of considerable discussion. On the other end, reactive oxygen species mediate certain physiological processes such as sperm maturation, capacitation and acrosome reaction, two key events for the acquisition of fertilizing ability; therefore their fine balancing is fundamental to assure a proper redox microenvironment [37]. This is also supported by growing evidence demonstrating that the abuse of antioxidant treatments may induce sperm damage as a result of a reductive-stress-induced state. Therefore the phenomenon known as "antioxidant paradox" should be kept in mind and absolutely not underestimated in order to avoid that the uncontrolled supplementation may indirectly cause fertility health risks [38].

The results of this study show that the administration of a nutraceutical cocktail, containing amino acids able to provide energy, Vitamins C, D3 and E, Selenium and Coenzyme Q10 with a strong antioxidant action and other natural substances, can be considered an effective treatment for OAT men, showing a significant increase in all sperm parameters and thus suggesting a recovery of the fertilizing capability.

The effects of the antioxidant therapy on seminal fluid have been studied in many clinical trials that have demonstrated individual and synergic action of compounds used in the nutraceutical formulation administered in this study.

Indeed, vitamin E and coenzyme Q10 have been reported to be effectives in protecting sperm against oxidative stress in cases of idiopathic infertility [34]. Several studies demonstrated that vitamin D3 plays key roles in the acquisition of hyperactivated motility, capacitation, and acrosome reaction. Despite these reports, there is no unanimous agreement on the effectiveness of vitamin D administration in recovering poor semen parameters. Indeed, some authors reported a beneficial effect of supplementation with vitamin D on sperm progressive motility and morphology in men with OAT, while others did not [39,40].

Carnitine is a key antioxidant involved in cell energy production, thus directly involved in recruiting ATP for sperm motility. To this regard, men with OAT have significantly lower levels of carnitine in their semen [34]. The combination of carnitine and acetyl-L-carnitine is effective in improving total motility in idiopathic asthenozoospermia [41].

Last but not the least, the most abundant component of the mix we used in this study is Inositol, whose effectiveness in improving sperm motility and morphology, along with a significant protective role against oxidative damage to DNA has been already demonstrated [15,16]. Data form literature show the beneficial effects of inositol on sperm motility and mitochondrial function, due to insulin-sensitizing properties, antioxidant activity and hormonal regulatory effects [42].

The effectiveness of this supplementation is definitively demonstrated by the positive effects on the fertilization rate, one of the most important parameter to evaluate the impact of male partner in the outcome of assisted reproduction cycles. Indeed, male partner received the aforesaid antioxidant supplementation for three months before the cycle obtained a higher fertilization rates obtained in ICSI cycles. The absence of side effects proves the safety of the product and provides specialists working in the field of assisted reproduction with alternative tools to classic hormonal therapies for the treatment of male infertility.

5. Conclusions

In conclusion, the present results demonstrate that a formulation containing amino acids as energy source, vitamin E and coenzyme Q10 with strong antioxidant effects, and natural substances that influence androgen production is an ideal therapy for OAT.

Anyway, further studies in a larger cohort of patients are needed to confirm the effectiveness of this nutraceutical formulation in ameliorating sperm parameters.

Author Contributions: Conceptualization, V.D.L. and P.P.; methodology, L.G., A.L., R.P. and G.M.; formal analysis, L.G. and A.L.; writing—original draft preparation, L.G. and C.T.; writing—review and editing, A.L., V.D.L. and P.P.; supervision, V.D.L. and P.P. All authors have read and agreed to the published version of the manuscript.

Funding: This research received no external funding.

Institutional Review Board Statement: The study was conducted according to the guidelines of the Declaration of Helsinki, and approved by the Institutional Ethics Committee of University of Siena (approval ID: CEAVSE 191113).

Informed Consent Statement: Informed consent was obtained from all subjects involved in the study.

Data Availability Statement: Not applicable.

Conflicts of Interest: The authors declare no conflict of interest.

References

1. Hamada, A.; Esteves, S.C.; Agarwal, A. Unexplained Male Infertility: Potential Causes and Management. *Hum. Androl.* **2011**, *1*, 2–16. [CrossRef]
2. Rouchou, B. Consequences of Infertility in Developing Countries. *Perspect. Public Health* **2013**, *133*, 174–179. [CrossRef]
3. Vine, M.F. Smoking and Male Reproduction: A Review. *Int. J. Androl.* **1996**, *19*, 323–337. [CrossRef]
4. Auger, J.; Eustache, F.; Andersen, A.G.; Irvine, D.S.; Jørgensen, N.; Skakkebaek, N.E.; Suominen, J.; Toppari, J.; Vierula, M.; Jouannet, P. Sperm Morphological Defects Related to Environment, Lifestyle and Medical History of 1001 Male Partners of Pregnant Women from Four European Cities. *Hum. Reprod.* **2001**, *16*, 2710–2717. [CrossRef]
5. Silva, T.; Jesus, M.; Cagigal, C.; Silva, C. Food with Influence in the Sexual and Reproductive Health. *Curr. Pharm. Biotechnol.* **2019**, *20*, 114–122. [CrossRef] [PubMed]
6. Agarwal, A.; Majzoub, A. Role of Antioxidants in Assisted Reproductive Techniques. *World J. Men's Health* **2017**, *35*, 77–93. [CrossRef]
7. Baker, H.W.; Brindle, J.; Irvine, D.S.; Aitken, R.J. Protective Effect of Antioxidants on the Impairment of Sperm Motility by Activated Polymorphonuclear Leukocytes. *Fertil. Steril.* **1996**, *65*, 411–419. [CrossRef]
8. Sabeti, P.; Pourmasumi, S.; Rahiminia, T.; Akyash, F.; Talebi, A.R. Etiologies of Sperm Oxidative Stress. *Int. J. Reprod. Biomed.* **2016**, *14*, 231–240. [CrossRef]
9. Henkel, R.R. Leukocytes and Oxidative Stress: Dilemma for Sperm Function and Male Fertility. *Asian J. Androl.* **2011**, *13*, 43–52. [CrossRef] [PubMed]
10. Eskenazi, B.; Kidd, S.A.; Marks, A.R.; Sloter, E.; Block, G.; Wyrobek, A.J. Antioxidant Intake Is Associated with Semen Quality in Healthy Men. *Hum. Reprod.* **2005**, *20*, 1006–1012. [CrossRef]
11. Garolla, A.; Petre, G.C.; Francini-Pesenti, F.; De Toni, L.; Vitagliano, A.; Di Nisio, A.; Foresta, C. Dietary Supplements for Male Infertility: A Critical Evaluation of Their Composition. *Nutrients* **2020**, *12*, 1472. [CrossRef]
12. Buhling, K.J.; Laakmann, E. The Effect of Micronutrient Supplements on Male Fertility. *Curr. Opin. Obstet. Gynecol.* **2014**, *26*, 199–209. [CrossRef] [PubMed]
13. Sinclair, S. Male Infertility: Nutritional and Environmental Considerations. *Altern. Med. Rev.* **2000**, *5*, 28–38.
14. Dinicola, S.; Unfer, V.; Facchinetti, F.; Soulage, C.O.; Greene, N.D.; Bizzarri, M.; Laganà, A.S.; Chan, S.-Y.; Bevilacqua, A.; Pkhaladze, L.; et al. Inositols: From Established Knowledge to Novel Approaches. *Int. J. Mol. Sci.* **2021**, *22*, 10575. [CrossRef]
15. Governini, L.; Ponchia, R.; Artini, P.G.; Casarosa, E.; Marzi, I.; Capaldo, A.; Luddi, A.; Piomboni, P. Respiratory Mitochondrial Efficiency and DNA Oxidation in Human Sperm after In Vitro Myo-Inositol Treatment. *J. Clin. Med.* **2020**, *9*, 1638. [CrossRef]
16. Ponchia, R.; Bruno, A.; Renzi, A.; Landi, C.; Shaba, E.; Luongo, F.P.; Haxhiu, A.; Artini, P.G.; Luddi, A.; Governini, L.; et al. Oxidative Stress Measurement in Frozen/Thawed Human Sperm: The Protective Role of an In Vitro Treatment with Myo-Inositol. *Antioxidants* **2021**, *11*, 10. [CrossRef]
17. Appleton, J. Arginine: Clinical Potential of a Semi-Essential Amino Acid. *Altern. Med. Rev.* **2002**, *7*, 512–522.
18. Rolf, C.; Cooper, T.G.; Yeung, C.H.; Nieschlag, E. Antioxidant Treatment of Patients with Asthenozoospermia or Moderate Oligoasthenozoospermia with High-Dose Vitamin C and Vitamin E: A Randomized, Placebo-Controlled, Double-Blind Study. *Hum. Reprod.* **1999**, *14*, 1028–1033. [CrossRef]
19. Sabetian, S.; Jahromi, B.N.; Vakili, S.; Forouhari, S.; Alipour, S. The Effect of Oral Vitamin E on Semen Parameters and IVF Outcome: A Double-Blinded Randomized Placebo-Controlled Clinical Trial. *BioMed Res. Int.* **2021**, *2021*, 5588275. [CrossRef]
20. Mortazavi, M.; Salehi, I.; Alizadeh, Z.; Vahabian, M.; Roushandeh, A.M. Protective Effects of Antioxidants on Sperm Parameters and Seminiferous Tubules Epithelium in High Fat-Fed Rats. *J. Reprod. Infertil.* **2014**, *15*, 22–28.
21. Fraga, C.G.; Motchnik, P.A.; Shigenaga, M.K.; Helbock, H.J.; Jacob, R.A.; Ames, B.N. Ascorbic Acid Protects against Endogenous Oxidative DNA Damage in Human Sperm. *Proc. Natl. Acad. Sci. USA* **1991**, *88*, 11003–11006. [CrossRef]
22. Jacob, R.A.; Pianalto, F.S.; Agee, R.E. Cellular Ascorbate Depletion in Healthy Men. *J. Nutr.* **1992**, *122*, 1111–1118. [CrossRef]
23. Ahmadi, S.; Bashiri, R.; Ghadiri-Anari, A.; Nadjarzadeh, A. Antioxidant Supplements and Semen Parameters: An Evidence Based Review. *Int. J. Reprod. Biomed.* **2016**, *14*, 729–736. [CrossRef]
24. Akmal, M.; Qadri, J.Q.; Al-Waili, N.S.; Thangal, S.; Haq, A.; Saloom, K.Y. Improvement in Human Semen Quality after Oral Supplementation of Vitamin C. *J. Med. Food* **2006**, *9*, 440–442. [CrossRef] [PubMed]
25. Blomberg Jensen, M. Vitamin D and Male Reproduction. *Nat. Rev. Endocrinol.* **2014**, *10*, 175–186. [CrossRef]
26. Alahmar, A.T.; Singh, R. Comparison of the Effects of Coenzyme Q10 and Centrum Multivitamins on Semen Parameters, Oxidative Stress Markers, and Sperm DNA Fragmentation in Infertile Men with Idiopathic Oligoasthenospermia. *Clin. Exp. Reprod. Med.* **2022**, *49*, 49–56. [CrossRef]
27. Sharma, A.P.; Sharma, G.; Kumar, R. Systematic Review and Meta-Analysis on Effect of Carnitine, Coenzyme Q10 and Selenium on Pregnancy and Semen Parameters in Couples with Idiopathic Male Infertility. *Urology* **2021**, *161*, 4–11. [CrossRef] [PubMed]
28. World Health Organization (Ed.) *WHO Laboratory Manual for the Examination and Processing of Human Semen*, 5th ed.; World Health Organization: Geneva, Switzerland, 2010; ISBN 978-92-4-154778-9.
29. Calogero, A.E.; Aversa, A.; La Vignera, S.; Corona, G.; Ferlin, A. The Use of Nutraceuticals in Male Sexual and Reproductive Disturbances: Position Statement from the Italian Society of Andrology and Sexual Medicine (SIAMS). *J. Endocrinol. Investig.* **2017**, *40*, 1389–1397. [CrossRef]

30. Duca, Y.; Calogero, A.E.; Cannarella, R.; Condorelli, R.A.; La Vignera, S. Current and Emerging Medical Therapeutic Agents for Idiopathic Male Infertility. *Expert Opin. Pharmacother.* **2019**, *20*, 55–67. [CrossRef]
31. Smits, R.M.; Mackenzie-Proctor, R.; Yazdani, A.; Stankiewicz, M.T.; Jordan, V.; Showell, M.G. Antioxidants for Male Subfertility. *Cochrane Database Syst. Rev.* **2019**, CD007411. [CrossRef] [PubMed]
32. Amorini, A.M.; Listorti, I.; Bilotta, G.; Pallisco, R.; Saab, M.W.; Mangione, R.; Manca, B.; Lazzarino, G.; Tavazzi, B.; Lazzarino, G.; et al. Antioxidant-Based Therapies in Male Infertility: Do We Have Sufficient Evidence Supporting Their Effectiveness? *Antioxidants* **2021**, *10*, 220. [CrossRef]
33. Agarwal, A.; Sekhon, L.H. The Role of Antioxidant Therapy in the Treatment of Male Infertility. *Hum. Fertil.* **2010**, *13*, 217–225. [CrossRef]
34. Majzoub, A.; Agarwal, A. Antioxidant Therapy in Idiopathic Oligoasthenoteratozoospermia. *Indian J. Urol.* **2017**, *33*, 207–214. [CrossRef] [PubMed]
35. Helli, B.; Kavianpour, M.; Ghaedi, E.; Dadfar, M.; Haghighian, H.K. Probiotic Effects on Sperm Parameters, Oxidative Stress Index, Inflammatory Factors and Sex Hormones in Infertile Men. *Hum. Fertil.* **2020**, 1–9. [CrossRef]
36. Lanzafame, F.M.; La Vignera, S.; Vicari, E.; Calogero, A.E. Oxidative Stress and Medical Antioxidant Treatment in Male Infertility. *Reprod. Biomed. Online* **2009**, *19*, 638–659. [CrossRef]
37. Aitken, R.J.; Drevet, J.R.; Moazamian, A.; Gharagozloo, P. Male Infertility and Oxidative Stress: A Focus on the Underlying Mechanisms. *Antioxidants* **2022**, *11*, 306. [CrossRef] [PubMed]
38. Symeonidis, E.N.; Evgeni, E.; Palapelas, V.; Koumasi, D.; Pyrgidis, N.; Sokolakis, I.; Hatzichristodoulou, G.; Tsiampali, C.; Mykoniatis, I.; Zachariou, A.; et al. Redox Balance in Male Infertility: Excellence through Moderation-"Μέτρον ἄριστον". *Antioxidants* **2021**, *10*, 1534. [CrossRef]
39. Blomberg Jensen, M.; Lawaetz, J.G.; Petersen, J.H.; Juul, A.; Jørgensen, N. Effects of Vitamin D Supplementation on Semen Quality, Reproductive Hormones, and Live Birth Rate: A Randomized Clinical Trial. *J. Clin. Endocrinol. Metab.* **2018**, *103*, 870–881. [CrossRef] [PubMed]
40. Maghsoumi-Norouzabad, L.; Zare Javid, A.; Mansoori, A.; Dadfar, M.; Serajian, A. The Effects of Vitamin D3 Supplementation on Spermatogram and Endocrine Factors in Asthenozoospermia Infertile Men: A Randomized, Triple Blind, Placebo-Controlled Clinical Trial. *Reprod. Biol. Endocrinol.* **2021**, *19*, 102. [CrossRef]
41. Mongioì, L.; Calogero, A.E.; Vicari, E.; Condorelli, R.A.; Russo, G.I.; Privitera, S.; Morgia, G.; La Vignera, S. The Role of Carnitine in Male Infertility. *Andrology* **2016**, *4*, 800–807. [CrossRef]
42. Condorelli, R.A.; Barbagallo, F.; Calogero, A.E.; Cannarella, R.; Crafa, A.; La Vignera, S. D-Chiro-Inositol Improves Sperm Mitochondrial Membrane Potential: In Vitro Evidence. *J. Clin. Med.* **2020**, *9*, 1373. [CrossRef]

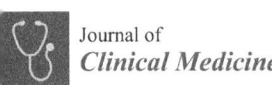

Review

Epigenetic Risks of Medically Assisted Reproduction

Romualdo Sciorio [1,*] and Nady El Hajj [2]

[1] Edinburgh Assisted Conception Programme, Royal Infirmary of Edinburgh, Edinburgh EH16 4SA, UK
[2] College of Health and Life Sciences, Hamad Bin Khalifa University, Doha P.O. Box 34110, Qatar; nelhajj@hbku.edu.qa
* Correspondence: sciorioromualdo@hotmail.com

Abstract: Since the birth of Louise Joy Brown, the first baby conceived via in vitro fertilization, more than 9 million children have been born worldwide using assisted reproductive technologies (ART). In vivo fertilization takes place in the maternal oviduct, where the unique physiological conditions guarantee the healthy development of the embryo. During early embryogenesis, a major wave of epigenetic reprogramming takes place that is crucial for the correct development of the embryo. Epigenetic reprogramming is susceptible to environmental changes and non-physiological conditions such as those applied during in vitro culture, including shift in pH and temperature, oxygen tension, controlled ovarian stimulation, intracytoplasmic sperm injection, as well as preimplantation embryo manipulations for genetic testing. In the last decade, concerns were raised of a possible link between ART and increased incidence of imprinting disorders, as well as epigenetic alterations in the germ cells of infertile parents that are transmitted to the offspring following ART. The aim of this review was to present evidence from the literature regarding epigenetic errors linked to assisted reproduction treatments and their consequences on the conceived children. Furthermore, we provide an overview of disease risk associated with epigenetic or imprinting alterations in children born via ART.

Keywords: human in vitro fertilization; assisted reproductive technology; epigenetics; imprinting disorders

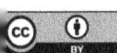

1. Introduction

Over the past 40 years, the use of ART for infertility treatment has been continuously on the rise and has resulted in the birth of more than 9 million children globally [1,2]. The number of couples facing infertility problems has steadily increased over the last decades, particularly since a growing number of individuals are postponing the desire to have children further into older age. Many of those couples ultimately need in vitro fertilization (IVF) to be able to conceive a baby [3]. Nowadays, nearly 3.3 million ART cycles are performed annually, resulting in over 500,000 deliveries worldwide [1]. ART procedures are considered relatively safe; however, in the last decade, novel concerns have been raised due to increased prevalence of epigenetic errors and imprinting defects in ART-born children [4]. This was first observed in cattle and sheep, where incidence of large offspring syndrome (LOS) increased following transfer of in vitro fertilized embryos [5]. In 2001, Young et al. reported that epigenetic alterations in *IGF2R* was responsible for LOS following embryo culture in sheep [6]. Epigenetic alterations in various imprinted genes were also observed in preimplantation mouse embryos cultured in M16 or Whitten's medium [7]. In vivo fertilization takes place in the oviduct, which is a natural environment with optimal physiological conditions including all the metabolic requirements for early embryo development. Even though embryology laboratories try to mimic those natural conditions to the best extent possible, during in vitro fertilization, the embryo is exposed to five or six days of diverse environmental conditions (Figure 1) [8]. Since about 3–5% of children are conceived following ART cycles [1], it is important to determine the potential negative effects of the procedure on the conceived baby. Epidemiological data revealed increased incidence of low and very low birth weight in ART born babies following fresh embryo replacement [9]. Similar results were recently published by Sunkara et al., who analyzed UK registry data (Human Fertilization and Embryology Authority, HFEA) from 1991 to 2016 including about 117,000 singleton live births following ART. The authors showed that the causes of infertility had a negative impact on preterm birth and low birth weight following fresh embryo transfer [10]. However, the opposite scenario was reported following frozen-thawed embryo transfer (FET) in ART. A large study performed by Terho et al. suggested that FET is linked with higher birth weights and higher risk of large-for-gestational-age [11]. In 2002, a case report [12] was published describing two unrelated patients with Angelman syndrome with sporadic imprinting defects following intracytoplasmic sperm injection (ICSI). A year later, DeBaun et al. reported increased incidence of Beckwith–Wiedemann syndrome with imprinting alterations in *H19* and *LIT1* in children born after ART [13]. Subsequently, several studies tried to determine possible culprits behind the observed epigenetic errors including controlled ovarian stimulation (COS), in vitro oocyte maturation, intracytoplasmic sperm injection (ICSI), in vitro embryo culture, couple infertility, and more recently, preimplantation embryo manipulation for genetic assessment.

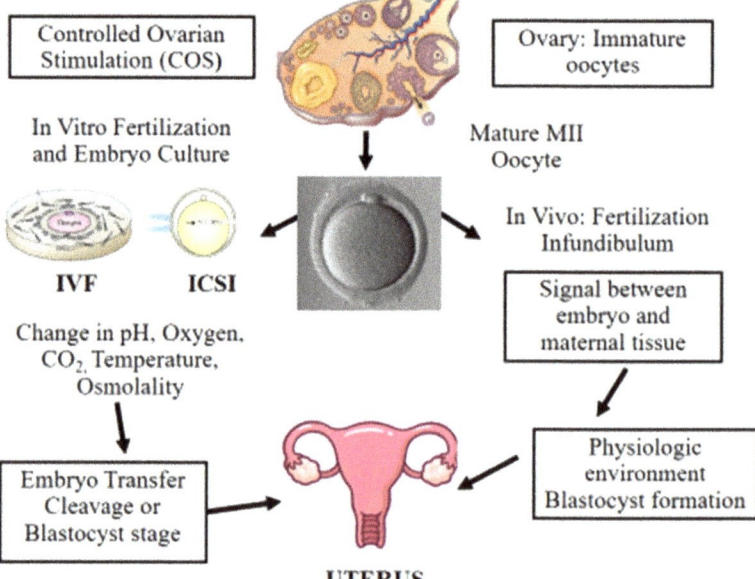

Figure 1. Scheme illustrating in vitro and in vivo fertilization. Controlled ovarian stimulation (COS) is used to promote follicle growth, maturation, and ovulation. ART adopts either IVF or ICSI for fertilization. Following fertilization, the preimplantation embryo is cultured in incubators, where suboptimal culture conditions such as pH, oxygen, temperature, and osmolality may affect its further development. Finally, the in vitro-produced embryo is transferred to the uterus at the cleavage or blastocyst stage. On the other hand, in vivo the female and male gametes interact together and the sperm fertilizes the oocyte in the infundibulum. Next, the developing embryo moves towards the uterus interacting with the female reproductive system in a physiologic and optimal environment.

2. Epigenetics in Development and Imprinted Genes

In 1942, Conrad Waddington highlighted the importance of environmental interactions with genes during early stages of embryo development. Although at that time, only limited information was available about the mechanisms of early embryogenesis, Waddington emphasized the importance of studying features that control embryo development that can mediate the correlations between genotype and phenotype. Waddington introduced the term "*Epigenetics*", which he described as the "the branch of biology that studies the causal interactions between genes and their products which bring the phenotype into being" [14]. Epigenetic regulation is essential for normal mammalian development and is described as the study of heritable changes in gene function that are not associated with changes to the DNA sequence itself [15]. In mammals, two waves of epigenetic reprogramming occur during development that reset epigenetic marks in germ cells and preimplantation embryos. During early embryogenesis, epigenetic marks are reprogrammed to prepare the embryo for development; however, parental-specific DNA methylation patterns at imprinted genes are maintained. The second phase occurs during germ cell development when primordial germ cells (PGCs) enter the fetal gonadal ridge. Here, DNA methylation patterns are globally erased including marks at imprinted genes. Parental imprinting marks are later established during germ cell differentiation with distinct imprints in male and female germ cells. During reprogramming, the epigenome is highly susceptible to external and internal cues that can alter the reprogramming process and induce long-term disease risk in the future generation [16,17]. One of the most studied epigenetic modifications is DNA methylation [18], where a methyl group is added at the 5′ carbon position of the cytosine pyrimidine ring in the context of CG dinucleotide (CpG sites) [19]. Those epigenetic modifications are maintained by daughter cells throughout cell divisions by DNA methyltransferase 1 (DNMT1) [20]. Epigenetic modifications are crucial in regulating gene expression during embryo development, whereby any disruption to epigenetic states during this sensitive time window can lead to future consequences for development and disease [21,22]. Genomic imprinting is an epigenetic process resulting in monoallelic expression of either the maternally or the paternally inherited allele. This mechanism of parent-of-origin-specific expression is restricted to a limited number of ~200 imprinted genes described in humans [23,24]. Genomic imprinting has been mainly reported in eutherian mammals; however, similar phenomena were identified in flowering plants and in some insects indicating independent evolutionary origins [25]. Imprinted genes are regulated by cis-acting elements known as imprinting control regions (ICRs). For example, in the *H19-Igf2* locus, the ICR located upstream of *H19* along with enhancers controls the expression of *H19* from the maternal allele and of the insulin-like growth factor (*IGF2*) gene from the paternal allele [26,27]. This exclusive monoallelic expression is controlled by specific epigenetic marks and regulatory elements such as DNA methylation, histone modifications, long non-coding RNA (lncRNA), and CCCTC binding factor (CTCF)-mediated boundaries [28]. The parental-specific imprints established in the germ line escape epigenetic reprogramming in preimplantation embryos, where imprinted genes play an important role in early development [29] and are essential for the regulation of energy balance between the mother and the developing fetus [30]. In humans, genetic mutations, copy number aberrations, and epigenetic alterations affecting imprinted genes have been linked to a number of disorders, e.g., Beckwith–Wiedemann syndrome (BWS), Angelman syndrome (AS), Silver–Russell syndrome (SRS), and Prader-Willi syndrome (PWS), Ref [31] characterized by clinical features affecting development, metabolism, and growth.

3. Epigenetic Alterations and Imprinting Disorders in ART

Following fertilization, the zygote develops into a structure called the "blastocyst" (Figure 2). At this stage, the embryo encloses about 150 or 200 cells differentiated into two types: the trophectoderm (TE), an epithelial sheet surrounding the fluid filled cavity (i.e., the blastocoele) and the inner cell mass (ICM), a group of cells attached to the inside of the trophectoderm that eventually give rise to the fetus. TE cells facilitate implantation into the uterine lining and form extraembryonic tissues including the placenta. During early development, embryonic cells are guided toward their future lineages through epigenetic reprogramming and subsequent re-establishment of cell-type-specific epigenetic signatures. This corresponds to the period when gametes and embryos are being in vitro manipulated and cultured inside the embryology laboratory. Therefore, such artificial intrusions during this critical time window might lead to epigenetic aberrations in the resultant offspring (Figures 1 and 3). Several studies reported imprinted loci to be vulnerable to external envi ronmental cues during in vitro embryo culture. For example, *KvDMR1* has been observed to be abnormally methylated in ART-related BWS in humans [32,33] and hypomethylated in ART-produced bovine conceptuses with LOS [34]. Several studies have also shown that ART-related procedures including COS, ICSI, and embryo manipulation might induce epigenetic abnormalities [29,31,35]. A systematic review published by Lazaraviciute et al. compared the incidence of imprinting disorders and DNA methylation alterations at key imprinted genes in children conceived via ART versus those conceived naturally. A total of 18 papers were included in this review, and the combined odds ratio (95% confidence intervals) for the incidence of imprinting disorders in children conceived through ART was 3.67 in comparison to spontaneously conceived children. The authors concluded that an increased risk of imprinting disorders occurs in babies born via IVF and ICSI; nevertheless, there was limited evidence for a link between epigenetic alterations at imprinted genes and ART [36]. Another review summarizing data from eight studies on BWS and ART reported a significant positive association between IVF and ICSI procedures and BWS with increased relative risk of about 5.2 times (95% CI 1.6–7.4) [37]. However, the authors did not observe an association for either AS or PWS with IVF and ICSI, but rather a positive association with fertility problems. Regarding SRS, the number of children born following ART was small ($n = 13$); therefore, probable significance for SRS incidences could not be inferred. A more recent epidemiological study investigated the risk of imprinting disorders in IVF children born in Denmark and Finland, where the authors compared the incidence rate of PWS, SRS, BWS, and AS in ART-conceived babies in Denmark ($n = 45,393$ born 1994–2014) and Finland ($n = 29,244$ born 1990–2014). They observed an increased odds rate for BWS (OR 3.07, 95% CI: 1.49–6.31) in ART-conceived children; however, no significant difference was evident for PWS, SRS, and AS [38]. Similarly, a nation-wide study in Japan found a 4.46-fold increase in BWS and an 8.91-fold increase in SRS following ART including several with aberrant DNA methylation at imprinted genes [39]. The effect of altered epigenetics marks and epimutations on human health is just beginning to be understood. Further research in this area is needed help clarify whether ART-induced epigenetic changes affect growth, development, and health of future offspring. In the next sections, we discuss specific procedures applied during ART treatments to provide examples on how certain treatments may lead to epigenetic alterations.

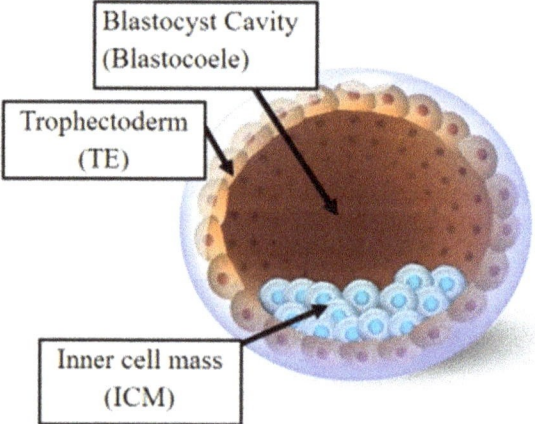

Figure 2. The human blastocyst. The structure comprises two differentiated cell types and a central cavity filled with fluid (blastocoel cavity). The inner cell mass (ICM) becomes the fetus and the trophectoderm (TE) cells later develop into the placenta.

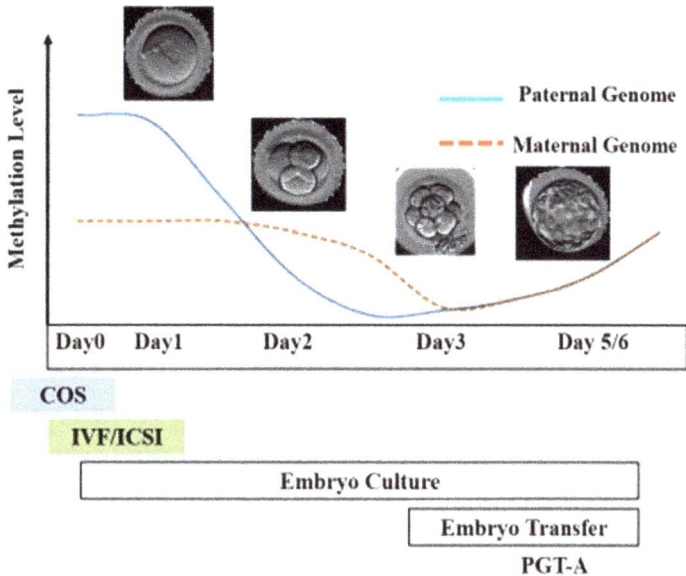

Figure 3. Epigenetic reprogramming during the early stage of embryo development. Post-fertilization, the paternal genome undergoes active demethylation, whereas the maternal genome is passively demethylated. The scheme illustrates the stage of development at which different ART techniques are employed.

4. Controlled Ovarian Stimulation in ART

Ovarian stimulation is one procedure likely responsible for epigenetic aberrations in the oocyte and embryo [40]. COS may lead to the selection of poor quality oocytes that are usually excluded in a natural cycle, and those oocytes might induce perturbed genomic imprinting during the early stage of embryo development and later in the placenta [41,42]. Medical records of women who gave birth to children with BWS following ART revealed ovarian stimulation medication as the only common factor among those patients [43]. Each month, the human ovaries typically produce a single dominant follicle which ovulates and releases a single oocyte. To increase the number of fertilized oocytes and improve IVF outcome, COS is applied using exogenous gonadotropins to stimulate the ovary and promote multifollicular development yielding multiple oocytes. Typically, a pharmacological dose of FSH is used to induce the growth of multiple follicles. As follicles grow and reach a specific width, LH is administered to produce the mid-cycle LH surge, which promotes oocyte maturation and later ovulation. Oocyte retrieval is precisely timed following LH administration to retrieve mature oocytes prior to ovulation. LH exposure initiates meiosis and leads to oocyte maturation from the immature "metaphase I" (MI) stage to the mature "metaphase II" (MII) stage of development. During this time, the first polar body is extruded and the oocyte reaches the metaphase II stage, which indicates its competence to be fertilized [44]. Following ovulation, the rest of the follicle forms the corpus luteum, which produces high levels of progesterone to prepare the endometrium for the process of embryo implantation. Since the expected number of oocytes is low in patients with reduced ovarian reserve, several strategies mainly based on increased gonadotropin dose have been applied to collect more oocytes. In certain cases, it is only possible to retrieve immature oocytes after COS where in vitro maturation might be adopted to obtain matured MII oocytes. Culture systems for in vitro maturation of human oocytes holds great potential but is still considered experimental for clinical use in ART [45]. In the last decade, there has been a growing concern over an association between COS and epigenetic aberrations in oocytes and embryos, which further increases the risk of imprinting disorders in the offspring [46]. Indeed, DNA methylation analysis of imprinted genes revealed aberrations in *PEG1, KCNQ1OT1,* and *ZAC* in oocytes collected following COS when compared to oocytes obtained after natural ovulation [47,48]. Furthermore, reports described DNA methylation alterations and expression changes in the *H19* imprinted control region in embryos obtained from superovulated oocytes [49]. Mature oocytes obtained following superovulation were shown to have conserved DNA methylation patterns at ICRs; however, methylation aberrations were detected in genes involved in glucose metabolism, nervous system development, mRNA processing, cell cycle, and cell proliferation [50]. This is in contrary to a genome-wide DNA methylation study in superovulated mouse oocytes, which showed minor methylation differences between superovulated versus naturally ovulated oocytes [51]. DNA methylation was also studied in embryos generated from superovulated oocytes, where superovulation was shown to interfere with the genome-wide DNA methylation reprogramming process that occurs during early embryogenesis [52]. Multiple superovulation cycles were also shown to have adverse effects on the structure and function of the ovaries, causing lower fertilization rate and decreased rate of early embryo development. In addition, repeated superovulation affected expression of pluripotency genes and led to aberrant histone modifications in early embryos and in the future offspring [53,54]. However, the effect of the ovarian superovulation on various epigenetic mechanisms are still to be fully elucidated. In animal models, reports have largely described that COS might alter the correct activities of DNA methyltransferases [53,54]. One of the first studies to determine that superovulation modifies expression levels of the DNMT proteins was published by Uysal et al. [55]. In this study, the authors compared DNMT protein levels in three groups (control, high dose, and normal dose of gonadotropins) and found that DNMT1, DNMT3A, and DNMT3B protein expression in the oocytes and developed embryos differed significantly when compared with controls. Similar data have been published by other groups confirming those results [53,54,56,57].

5. Fertilization Procedures: In Vitro Fertilization (IVF) and Intracytoplasmic Sperm Injection (ICSI)

There are two techniques used for oocyte fertilization in vitro: (1) the standard insemination where sperm and oocyte are placed together overnight in a culture dish for the sperm to fertilize the oocyte and (2) the intra-cytoplasmic sperm injection (ICSI) where an embryologist adopting an inverted microscope and a micromanipulator with a slim injection pipette collects and immobilizes a single sperm before slowly releasing it into the oocyte's cytoplasm. ICSI was first performed by Palermo et al. in 1992 [58] and it was introduced in clinical practice without prior experimental testing or clinical validation in animal models. Since then, it has been one of the major advances in ART for infertile couples diagnosed with severe male factor infertility. Natural fertilization usually follows specific physiological events including natural sperm selection and capacitation as well as acrosome reaction and membrane fusion before the sperm nucleus is released into the oocyte cytoplasm. Nevertheless, all these processes that occur during fertilization are basically omitted when ICSI is applied [59]. The usage of ICSI is increasing recently, where the technique is even applied in couples with men having semen analysis within reference ranges. Currently, ICSI is the main insemination technique in several infertility centers and in the Middle East, it is adopted in ~96% of all ART cycles [60]. Several researchers have put forward the idea that imprinting errors may originate due to abnormal spermatogenesis, which are later transmitted to the embryo following ICSI. For example, DNA hypomethylation at the *H19* gene locus in sperm has been associated with oligozoospermia and azoospermia [61]. Similarly, Kobayashi et al. studied imprinting in sperm of 97 infertile men where they identified errors at paternally imprinted genes in 14.4% of patients and errors at maternally imprinted genes in 20.6% of patients. The majority of imprinting defects were in oligospermic men, which led the authors to conclude that infertile men with abnormal sperm parameters have an increased risk of transmitting incorrect imprints to their offspring [62]. Similarly, Marques et al. observed increased risk for *H19* hypomethylation in testicular spermatozoa from men with abnormal spermatogenesis, indicating a possible link between disruptive spermatogenesis and imprinting errors [63]. During ICSI, natural sperm selection is omitted where sperm from men with severe male factor infertility might lead to the transmission of imprinting errors to the offspring. Furthermore, sperm following testicular sperm extraction (TESE) from men with non-obstructive azoospermia have been also used in ICSI procedures. In contrast to the previously mentioned studies, several reports showed no increased risk of epigenetic alterations in children born following ART. For example, a retrospective cohort study measuring DNA methylation in the *PEG3*, *IGF2*, *SNRPN*, and *INS* genes as well as the long interspersed nuclear element I (LINE-1) observed no significant DNA methylation differences in ART-conceived children [64]. Another study by Rancourt et al. investigated methylation levels of *GRB10*, *MEST*, *H19*, *SNRPN*, *KCNQ1*, and *IGF2DMR0* where they found no association between epigenetic aberrations and ART [65]. Additional studies have similarly reported no significant global or imprint-specific differences when comparing children born following IVF, ICSI, and natural conception [66–68]. More recently, a genome-wide DNA methylation analysis could only identify DNA methylation changes of small effect size in cord blood of ICSI-born children including eight sites at imprinted control regions [69]. Following a targeted and genome-wide DNA methylation analysis, Barberet et al. found lower methylation levels in buccal smear DNA at the *H19/IGF2* DMR in ART children as well as higher *PEG3* DMR methylation. However, the authors could only observe lower DNA methylation levels at the *LINE-1* transposable elements when comparing ICSI children to their IVF counterparts [8]. Another study by Choux et al. investigated the relation between ART and DNA methylation alterations in imprinted genes. The authors analyzed DNA methylation and expression levels of three imprinted loci (*H19/IGF2*, *KCNQ1OT1*, and *SNURF DMRs*) in cord blood and placenta obtained at birth from 15 standard IVF and 36 ICSI singleton pregnancies versus their 48 spontaneously conceived counterparts. Results showed that DNA methylation levels of *H19/IGF2*, *KCNQ1OT1*, *LINE-1Hs*, and *ERVFRD-1* were significantly lower in IVF and ICSI placentas than in control placentas, while there was no difference for cord blood [70]. Recent studies have shown that the placenta is more susceptible to epigenetic alterations when compared to the embryo and can therefore be used as a proxy to measure early epigenetic alterations affecting the embryo [71–74]. For example, placentas from ICSI- but not IVF-born children were reported to have global *H3K4me3* differences when compared to natural conceptuses [75]. A comprehensive study by Choufani et al. examined placentas from singleton pregnancies in an ART group and matched controls enrolled in the Quebec-based Canadian 3D longitudinal cohort, where they observed outliers in placentas of ART conceptuses to be enriched for DNA hypomethylation at imprinted genes. Furthermore, they observed that paternal age and infertility further perturbed the placental epigenome of ART-born children [67]. They found hypomethylation at imprinted genes to be associated with lower *H3K9me3* (repressive) and higher *H3K4me2* (permissive) marks [76]. This is in line with other reports that identified age-related changes in the sperm epigenome that might be later transmitted to the offspring [77,78]. In addition, male obesity and paternal diet was associated with malleable changes in the sperm epigenome [79–82]. Recent evidence has shown that disruption to the paternal epigenome can induce male infertility and subsequently transfer epigenetic aberrations to the embryo and potentially to the offspring, especially when fertilization is achieved using ART or ICSI. An analysis published by Schon et al. observed an overall reduction in *H4* acetylation as well as alterations in *H4K20* and *H3K9* methylation in asthenoteratozoospermic men compared to normozoospermic samples [82]. Furthermore, a study by Vieweg et al. found that abnormal histone acetylation in gene promoters of infertile men is associated with insufficient sperm chromatin compaction, and this alteration could potentially be transmitted to the future offspring [83]. Similarly, other studies reported alterations in methylation imprints in sperm of men with abnormal sperm parameters as well as methylation differences at *ALu* repeats that could be even associated with ART outcome [84]. ICSI might increase the incidence of imprinting disorders, adversely affect embryo development, and eventually lead to adverse health consequences in the resulting children [83,85]. Several reports have challenged the extensive usage of ICSI as well as its advantages compared to traditional IVF [86]. As a result, the Practice Committee of the American Society for Reproductive Medicine (ASRM) has recently produced a committee opinion paper recommending against the extensive use of ICSI in couples undergoing MAR cycles without male factor infertility [87].

6. Epigenetic Alterations Following In Vitro Culture

Despite in vitro fertilization being routinely practiced in couples with infertility issues, the cause for the increased risk for perinatal problems in ART-conceived children is still poorly understood. Animal models have provided evidence suggesting that imprinting establishment in oocytes and embryos is sensitive to environmental changes. Several studies have described the effects of in vitro culture on gene expression in preimplantation embryos in different mammals [72–74,88–90]. Epigenetic marks necessary for optimal embryo development are acquired during gametogenesis (imprinting) and preimplantation embryo development. Correct establishment of epigenetic patterns is crucial for development; however, morphological assessment of gametes and/or embryo quality cannot identify epigenetic errors during ART treatment [91]. Several trials have shown disrupted methylation at a number of imprinted genes due to in vitro culture in certain media [7,49,92–95]. A comprehensive study by Schwarzer et al. analyzed IVF procedures and in vitro culture media versus in vivo controls. In total 5735 fertilized mouse oocytes were cultured in vitro or in the female oviduct and scored for developmental parameters at the blastocyst stage (around 96 h). The authors reported that culture media might induce a wide range of changes in cellular, developmental, and metabolic pathways [96]. Similar results were observed by Gad et al. while investigating the effect of different culture media on the transcriptome profile of bovine preimplantation embryo development [97]. In humans, a handful of studies have explored the effects of culture media in preimplantation embryos. Kleijkers et al. cultured human embryos in two different culture media, where they observed differential expression of 951 genes involved in apoptosis, metabolism, protein processing, and cell cycle regulation diverged significantly when comparing blastocysts cultured in either G5 or human tubal fluid (HTF) [98]. Similarly, a more recent study reported differential expression of several genes between human cryopreserved embryos cultured using the same two media; however, expression differences were higher due to maternal age and developmental stage. The authors were not able to confirm whether the observed differences might be caused by confounding factors and concluded further research is needed to validate those results [99]. A randomized controlled trial compared DNA methylation at imprinted genes in IVF placentas from embryos cultured in HTF versus G5 medium, where no significant differences in DNA methylation were detected. Furthermore, no DNA methylation differences were observed when comparing IVF versus naturally conceived placentas, despite IVF placentas exhibiting a higher number of outliers [100]. A striking example of the negative effects of in vitro culture on embryo development was observed in cattle with LOS [5]. A study published by Chen et al. highlighted the concern that in vitro culture and ART induces misregulation of several imprinted genes in the kidney, brain, and liver of LOS fetuses. The magnitude of overgrowth in LOS fetuses is associated with the number of epigenetically altered imprinted genes [40].

7. Oxygen Tension

In vitro culture is thought to be one of the most important factors affecting epigenetic reprogramming as well as the developmental potential of embryos produced by ART. Since the 1950s, research has been conducted to determine the concentration of oxygen in the female reproductive tract. Historically, embryo culture has been performed at atmospheric oxygen levels of around 20%. Later, it was established that oxygen concentration in the female reproductive tract of mammalian species is between 2–8% [101], which indicates that embryos develop in vivo under low oxygen concentrations [101,102]. Several studies on mammals, including humans, suggested adverse effects of atmospheric oxygen levels on embryo development [103,104] as well as changes in the proteome [105], the transcriptome [106], and the epigenome of the embryo [29]. In the cytoplasm, oxidative stress resulting from the accumulation of reactive oxygen species (ROS) is likely a mechanism via which high oxygen concentration weakens the embryo, reducing its implantation potential and its capacity to generate a viable pregnancy. It has been proposed that in vitro culture of human embryos at reduced oxygen tension is an important feature to retain physiological evolution and increase reproductive competence. Indeed, there is plenty of evidence advocating in vitro culture of human embryos at 5% levels, rather than ambient oxygen, to improve pregnancy outcomes [105–107]. A recent prospective randomized multicenter study performed on 1563 oocytes confirmed that inclusion of antioxidants to the culture media significantly increases embryo viability, implantation, and pregnancy rates, possibly via oxidative stress reduction [108]. Similarly, the Cochrane Database review confirmed the results of several trials showing that in vitro culture of human embryos under conditions of low oxygen concentration improves ART outcomes [109].

8. In Vitro Culture and Human Birthweight

Birthweight is a useful and essential metric related to fetal growth and is suggested by some as a possible prognostic factor of long-term risk of metabolic disease. Low birthweight is known to be associated with increased rates of coronary heart disease as well as related disorders such as stroke, hypertension, and non-insulin dependent diabetes [110]. A study by Dumoulin et al. compared pregnancy rates and perinatal outcomes from singleton pregnancies born following 826 first IVF cycles, in which embryos were randomly cultured in two different sequential media. In total, 110 live-born singletons were analyzed where a significant difference in birthweight (3453 +/− 53 versus 3208 +/− 61 g, $p = 0.003$) adjusted for gestational age and sex was observed. This led the authors to conclude that in vitro culture of human embryos can affect the birth weight of live-born singletons [111]. This finding was confirmed by the same group in a separate report, where they studied a larger cohort of 294 live-born singletons [112]. Similarly, other groups reported comparable results to the previously mentioned studies [98,113–115]. IVF culture medium were also shown to be associated with postnatal weight changes during the first two years of life, suggesting that the early stage of human embryo development is susceptible to the external environment and that the culture medium might have long-term consequences [98,116]. On the other hand, a retrospective study published by Lin et al. comparing the effect of three commercially available culture media on the birthweight and length of newborns revealed no significant differences in mean birthweight [117]. Further studies using a different range of culture media also reported no significant differences in birthweight [118,119]. Despite conflicting results, the debate is still ongoing and no definite conclusion can be drawn. Therefore, it is essential to longitudinally follow-up IVF-born children and monitor their long-term growth, development, and health. Several other factors during in vitro culture might have an effect on birthweight such as the age of the culture media, storage time in the fridge or in the incubator [120], as well as the protein source and the used concentration [121]. Furthermore, one of the most debatable questions is related to culture period length, as well as to whether the embryo is transferred to the uterine cavity at the cleavage stage (day 2–3) or the blastocyst stage (day 5). This aspect has been investigated by Zhu et al. in a retrospective analysis of 2929 singletons, where the authors found that birthweight of singletons after blastocyst transfer was significantly higher than singletons from embryos at day three transfer (3465.31 ± 51.36 versus 3319.82 ± 10.04 g, respectively, $p = 0.009$) [122]. These questions were also addressed in a systematic review [123] that looked at several published human studies investigating the association between culture media and birthweight. The authors concluded that out of the 11 published studies, only six reported differences in birthweight while five observed no changes. As discussed earlier, epidemiological studies reported an increased incidence of low and very low birth weight in ART-born babies following fresh embryo transfer [9–11]. On the other hand, a different picture emerges following FET in ART. A recently published large scale study have analyzed live-born singletons born in Denmark, Norway, and Sweden between the years 2000 and 2015. The authors correlated singletons born after FET (n = 17,500) to singletons born after fresh embryo transfer (n = 69,510) and natural conception (n = 3311.588). Results showed that birth weights were significantly higher after FET compared to fresh ET for both boys and girls [11]. Comparable results have been also published by Litzky et al. using data from registries in the United States and analyzing the impact of FET (n = 55,898) versus fresh embryo transfer (n = 180,184) on birth weight of singletons conceived via ART between 2007–2014. Results found that FET was correlated with, on average, a 142 g increase in birthweight compared with infants born after fresh embryo transfer (p < 0.001) [124].

9. Cardiometabolic Complications in ART-Conceived Children

In addition to fetal growth restriction, prematurity, and low birth weight, certain studies have reported a possible association between ART cycles and a slightly increased risk of cardiovascular diseases [125]. A study conducted in Sweden compared the presence of congenital malformations in 15,570 infants born following ART versus all infants born in Sweden between 2001–2007. This analysis revealed a slightly increased risk of congenital malformations, cardiovascular disease, neural tube defects, and esophageal atresia after IVF [126]. Similarly, a trial was performed in Australia to determine disease risk in children (at least 1 year of age) born following IVF treatment. Results from this study suggested an increase in the incidence of raised blood pressure, elevated fasting glucose, and higher total body fat composition in IVF offspring. Nevertheless, it is still debatable whether these potential associations are related to the ART procedure itself or prior genetic susceptibility in the children [127]. A separate study assessed systemic and pulmonary vascular function in 65 healthy children born after ART, where they reported a 30% higher (p < 0.001) systolic pulmonary artery pressure in ART versus naturally conceived children (n = 57) [128]. Similarly, von Arx et al. compared the cardiac function and pulmonary artery pressure in 54 healthy children conceived via ART versus 54 age- and sex-matched control children. In this study, they observed increased right ventricular dysfunction in children and adolescents conceived by ART under stressful conditions of high-altitude pressure and hypoxia [129]. This concern has been also investigated in twin pregnancies following ART. Multiple pregnancies are common following ART and are normally linked with increased adverse perinatal outcomes such as hypertensive disorders, gestational diabetes, and preterm birth. In a recent study, Valenzuela-Alcaraz et al. investigated the presence of fetal cardiac remodeling and disruption in ART twin pregnancies [130]. The authors found that in comparison to non-ART conceptuses, twin pregnancies following ART showed significant cardiac changes, predominantly affecting the right heart, such as dilated atria, more globular ventricles, and thicker myocardial walls, as well as reduced longitudinal motion (p < 0.001). This study confirmed aberrations that are similar to those observed in ART singletons. Additional studies have reported similar results, thus reinforcing the evidence of an increased risk for metabolic and cardiovascular diseases following ART [131–133]. However, Bi et al. recently reported that changes associated with cardiac morphology and function seems to be limited to ART fetuses and do not persist towards early infanthood [134]. A more recent study on the Growing Up in Singapore Towards healthy Outcomes (GUSTO) prospective cohort observed no changes in metabolic biomarkers in ART conceived singletons; however, those children were shorter, weighed less, and had lower blood pressure and reduced skinfold thickness compared to their naturally conceived counterparts at ~6–6.5 years of age [135]. A recently published prospective study compared socioeconomic, psychosocial, and clinical measures in ART-conceived singletons who were 22–35 years of age during the time of the study. It was reassuring that the authors did not observe increased risk of cardiometabolic, growth, or respiratory problems in young adults conceived via ART when compared to the non-ART group [136]. An elegant follow-up study by Novakovic et al. performed genome-wide DNA methylation analysis in Guthrie spots and whole blood DNA in the same cohort, where ART procedures were shown to be associated with DNA methylation alterations at birth that did not persist into adulthood [137].

10. Epigenetic Alterations and Preimplantation Genetic Testing Following ART

Embryo biopsy for preimplantation genetic testing for aneuploidies (PGT-A) or further aspects related to preimplantation diagnostics might also have effects on the epigenome of the offspring [138,139]. PGT-A is used to avoid the transfer of chromosomally abnormal embryos to reduce implantation failures and miscarriages and is normally advised for advanced maternal age (AMA), repeated implantation failure (RIF), and recurrent pregnancy loss (RPL) [140]. The genetic assessment is linked to the biopsy procedure, which in the early days was based on blastomere aspiration collected from a cleavage stage embryo (day three). The method uses the acid Tyrode solution to make a hole in the zona pellucida (ZP) for subsequent aspiration of the cell. Later, laser-assisted zona drilling and calcium magnesium free media was introduced, which allows for easier blastomere removal. Trophectoderm biopsy (TEB) was suggested in 1990 [141], which allows the collection of more genetic material (~5–10 cells) for improved diagnostic accuracy [140,141]. However, considerations on the safety of PGT-A have been until now not well considered, particularly issues related to sampling strategy (i.e., blastomere biopsy at the cleavage stage or trophectoderm biopsy), as well as the manipulation and change in culture media during the procedure [101–104]. Specific settings such as temperature, culture media pH, and a reduced physiologic 5% oxygen tension have an effect on embryo quality and can mediate epigenetic dysregulation [103,105,106]. Similarly, the approach used to dissect the zona pellucida might harm the embryo and impair its development [29,142]. Recently, PGT-A is moving to TEB, normally performed on days five and six or even on day seven in certain cases. Although there is still limited evidence favoring blastocyst transfer in ART [143], extended in vitro culture beyond the embryonic genome activation (EGA) stage might have negative effects on the embryo. Several review studies raised the alarm over an increased incidence of negative obstetric and perinatal outcomes from extended embryo culture, pointing to possible epigenetic alterations in the embryo [8,69,88,89,91,94]. However, due to the limited number of studies on human embryos, it is difficult to delineate whether epigenetic alterations arise due to infertility (Figure 4), follicular stimulation, or embryo culture per se [96–99]. An elegant study in the bovine model allowed embryos to develop in vivo up to the 2, 8, and 16 cell stage followed by in vitro culture until the blastocyst stage to separate the epigenetic alterations sourced in the different phases of embryo development. This study demonstrated that every step of in vitro culture before and during embryonic genome activation (EGA) was contributing to epigenetic alterations. However, the majority of changes were occurring around the EGA phase with far less alterations after genome activation [144]. Furthermore, the sensitivity of embryo culture to oxygen drives the attention to preimplantation embryo metabolism and to a possible role of the culture media in improving outcomes following PGT-A. Cytogenetic composition and health of human embryos in vitro have been shown to be associated with metabolism, where aneuploid human embryos were reported to carry significant changes in amino acid turnover as measured in their spent culture medium [145,146]. This opens the possibility to measure embryo metabolism as a biomarker to assess embryo quality and for monitoring the effect of culture conditions to reduce mitotic error rate. Nevertheless, as long as our understanding of human preimplantation embryo metabolism is limited, one has to carefully consider that any additional day of in vitro culture has the potential to negatively affect the embryo and induce epigenetic alterations.

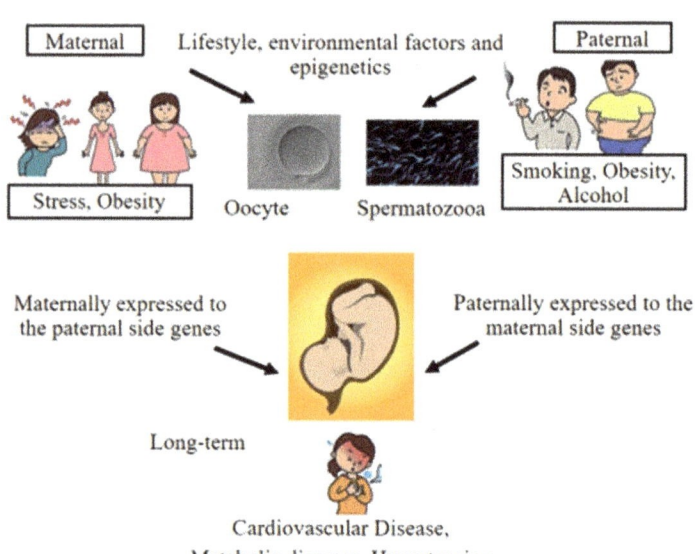

Figure 4. Paternal and maternal lifestyle prior to conception may affect sperm and oocyte epigenetic changes, offspring epigenetics, and phenotypic abnormalities, including increased risk of cardiovascular and metabolic disease in later life.

11. Conclusions and Future Perspectives

ART procedures have helped millions of infertile couples in having children; however, several concerns remain regarding the safety of these techniques on the health and well-being of the offspring at birth and in later adult life. The main aim of this review was to provide an overview of epigenetic alterations associated with in vitro fertilization and culture of human embryos. Several studies in animal models as well as retrospective follow-up studies of ART-born babies have reported an increased risk of epigenetic errors particularly affecting imprinted loci. Nevertheless, there is still no conclusive evidence of a strong link between ART and epigenetic modifications as well as increased disease risk in later adult life. It is important to mention that manipulation of oocytes and embryos should be restricted to a minimum, or in other words, the advantage of a specific technique such as extended culture to the blastocyst stage or preimplantation genetic assessment must outweigh the potential negative effects. Unfortunately, many decisions in human-assisted reproduction are not based on conclusive evidence, since longitudinal studies with a follow-up over several decades are still very limited. Therefore, large-scale epidemiological studies to evaluate the implications of various ART techniques on the health and well-being of the offspring not only at the time of delivery but also during later adult life are urgently needed.

Author Contributions: R.S. contributed to the conception and designed the manuscript. R.S. and N.E.H. wrote sections of the manuscript and revised it for content. Both the authors contributed to manuscript revision. All authors have read and agreed to the published version of the manuscript.

Funding: This research received no external funding.

Institutional Review Board Statement: All procedures performed in studies involving human participants were in accordance with the ethical standards of the institutional and with the 1964 Helsinki declaration and its later amendments. For this type of study, formal consent is not required.

Informed Consent Statement: Not applicable.

Data Availability Statement: No data are available.

Conflicts of Interest: The authors declare no conflict of interest.

References

1. De Geyter, C.; Wyns, C.; Calhaz-Jorge, C.; De Mouzon, J.; Ferraretti, A.P.; Kupka, M.; Andersen, A.N.; Nygren, K.G.; Goossens, V. 20 years of the European IVF-monitoring Consortium registry: What have we learned? A comparison with registries from two other regions. *Hum. Reprod.* **2020**, *35*, 2832–2849. [CrossRef]
2. Steptoe, P.; Edwards, R. Birth after the reimplantation of a human embryo. *Lancet* **1978**, *312*, 366. [CrossRef]
3. Thoma, M.E.; McLain, A.; Louis, J.F.; King, R.B.; Trumble, A.C.; Sundaram, R.; Louis, G.B. Prevalence of infertility in the United States as estimated by the current duration approach and a traditional constructed approach. *Fertil. Steril.* **2013**, *99*, 1324–1331. [CrossRef] [PubMed]
4. Ventura-Juncá, P.; Irarrázaval, I.; Rolle, A.J.; Gutiérrez, J.I.; Moreno, R.D.; Santos, M.J. In vitro fertilization (IVF) in mammals: Epigenetic and developmental alterations. Scientific and bioethical implications for IVF in humans. *Biol. Res.* **2015**, *48*, 68. [CrossRef]
5. Young, L.E.; Sinclair, K.D.; Wilmut, I. Large offspring syndrome in cattle and sheep. *Rev. Reprod.* **1998**, *3*, 155–163. [CrossRef] [PubMed]
6. Young, L.E.; Fernandes, K.; McEvoy, T.G.; Butterwith, S.C.; Gutierrez, C.G.; Carolan, C.; Broadbent, P.J.; Robinson, J.J.; Wilmut, I.; Sinclair, K. Epigenetic change in IGF2R is associated with fetal overgrowth after sheep embryo culture. *Nat. Genet.* **2001**, *27*, 153–154. [CrossRef] [PubMed]
7. Doherty, A.S.; Mann, M.R.; Tremblay, K.D.; Bartolomei, M.S.; Schultz, R.M. Differential Effects of Culture on Imprinted H19 Expression in the Preimplantation Mouse Embryo1. *Biol. Reprod.* **2000**, *62*, 1526–1535. [CrossRef]
8. Barberet, J.; Binquet, C.; Guilleman, M.; Doukani, A.; Choux, C.; Bruno, C.; Bourredjem, A.; Chapusot, C.; Bourc'his, D.; Duffourd, Y.; et al. Do assisted reproductive technologies and in vitro embryo culture influence the epigenetic control of imprinted genes and transposable elements in children? *Hum. Reprod.* **2021**, *36*, 479–492. [CrossRef]
9. Schieve, L.A.; Meikle, S.F.; Ferre, C.; Peterson, H.B.; Jeng, G.; Wilcox, L.S. Low and Very Low Birth Weight in Infants Conceived with Use of Assisted Reproductive Technology. *N. Engl. J. Med.* **2002**, *346*, 731–737. [CrossRef]
10. Sunkara, S.K.; Antonisamy, B.; Redla, A.C.; Kamath, M.S. Female causes of infertility are associated with higher risk of preterm birth and low birth weight: Analysis of 117 401 singleton live births following IVF. *Hum. Reprod.* **2020**, *36*, 676–682. [CrossRef]
11. Terho, A.M.; Pelkonen, S.; Opdahl, S.; Romundstad, L.B.; Bergh, C.; Wennerholm, U.B.; Henningsen, A.A.; Pinborg, A.; Gissler, M.; Tiitinen, A. High birth weight and large-for-gestational-age in singletons born after frozen compared to fresh embryo transfer, by gestational week: A Nordic register study from the CoNARTaS group. *Hum. Reprod.* **2021**, *36*, 1083–1092. [CrossRef] [PubMed]
12. Cox, G.F.; Bürger, J.; Lip, V.; Mau, U.A.; Sperling, K.; Wu, B.-L.; Horsthemke, B. Intracytoplasmic Sperm Injection May Increase the Risk of Imprinting Defects. *Am. J. Hum. Genet.* **2002**, *71*, 162–164. [CrossRef] [PubMed]
13. DeBaun, M.R.; Niemitz, E.L.; Feinberg, A.P. Association of In Vitro Fertilization with Beckwith-Wiedemann Syndrome and Epigenetic Alterations of LIT1 and H19. *Am. J. Hum. Genet.* **2003**, *72*, 156–160. [CrossRef] [PubMed]
14. Waddington, C.H. The epigenotype. *Int. J. Epidemiol.* **2012**, *411*, 10–13. [CrossRef] [PubMed]
15. Russo, V.E.A.; Martienssen, R.A.; Riggs, A.D. *Epigenetic Mechanisms of Gene Regulation*; Cold Spring Harbor Laboratory Press: Plainview, NY, USA, 1996.
16. Skinner, M.K. Environmental epigenomics and disease susceptibility. *EMBO Rep.* **2011**, *12*, 620–622. [CrossRef]
17. Santos, F.; Hyslop, L.; Stojkovic, P.; Leary, C.; Murdoch, A.; Reik, W.; Stojkovic, M.; Herbert, M.; Dean, W. Evaluation of epigenetic marks in human embryos derived from IVF and ICSI. *Hum. Reprod.* **2010**, *25*, 2387–2395. [CrossRef]
18. Klose, R.J.; Bird, A.P. Genomic DNA methylation: The mark and its mediators. *Trends Biochem. Sci.* **2006**, *31*, 89–97. [CrossRef]
19. Bannister, A.J.; Kouzarides, T. Regulation of chromatin by histone modifications. *Cell Res.* **2011**, *21*, 381–395. [CrossRef]
20. Rivera, C.M.; Ren, B. Mapping Human Epigenomes. *Cell* **2013**, *155*, 39–55. [CrossRef]
21. Hirst, M.; Marra, M.A. Epigenetics and human disease. *Int. J. Biochem. Cell Biol.* **2009**, *41*, 136–146. [CrossRef]
22. Weber, W. Cancer epigenetics. *Prog. Mol. Biol. Transl. Sci.* **2010**, *95*, 299–349.
23. Skaar, D.A.; Li, Y.; Bernal, A.J.; Hoyo, C.; Murphy, S.; Jirtle, R.L. The Human Imprintome: Regulatory Mechanisms, Methods of Ascertainment, and Roles in Disease Susceptibility. *ILAR J.* **2012**, *53*, 341–358. [CrossRef]
24. Allegrucci, C.; Thurston, A.; Lucas, E.; Young, L. Epigenetics and the germline. *Reproduction* **2005**, *129*, 137–149. [CrossRef]
25. Glaser, R.L.; Ramsay, J.P.; Morison, I.M. The imprinted gene and parent-of-origin effect database now includes parental origin of de novo mutations. *Nucleic Acids Res.* **2006**, *34*, D29–D31. [CrossRef] [PubMed]
26. Tremblay, K.D.; Duran, K.L.; Bartolomei, M.S. A 5′ 2-kilobase-pair region of the imprinted mouse H19 gene exhibits exclusive paternal methylation throughout development. *Mol. Cell. Biol.* **1997**, *17*, 4322–4329. [CrossRef] [PubMed]
27. Thorvaldsen, J.L.; Duran, K.L.; Bartolomei, M.S. Deletion of the H19 differentially methylated domain results in loss of im-printed expression of H19 and Igf2. *Genes Dev.* **1998**, *12*, 3693–3702. [CrossRef] [PubMed]
28. Koerner, M.V.; Pauler, F.M.; Huang, R.; Barlow, D.P. The function of non-coding RNAs in genomic imprinting. *Development* **2009**, *136*, 1771–1783. [CrossRef] [PubMed]
29. Marcho, C.; Cui, W.; Mager, J. Epigenetic dynamics during preimplantation development. *Reproduction* **2015**, *150*, R109–R120. [CrossRef]
30. Tunster, S.J.; Jensen, A.B.; John, R.M. Imprinted genes in mouse placental development and the regulation of fetal energy stores. *Reproduction* **2013**, *145*, R117–R137. [CrossRef]

31. Eggermann, T.; de Nanclares, G.P.; Maher, E.R.; Temple, I.K.; Tümer, Z.; Monk, D.; Mackay, D.J.; Grønskov, K.; Riccio, A.; Linglart, A.; et al. Imprinting disorders: A group of congenital disorders with overlapping patterns of molecular changes affecting imprinted loci. *Clin. Epigenet.* **2015**, *7*, 123. [CrossRef]
32. White, C.R.; Denomme, M.M.; Tekpetey, F.R.; Feyles, V.; Power, S.G.A.; Mann, M.R.W. High Frequency of Imprinted Methylation Errors in Human Preimplantation Embryos. *Sci. Rep.* **2015**, *5*, 17311. [CrossRef] [PubMed]
33. Huntriss, J.D.; Hemmings, K.E.; Hinkins, M.; Rutherford, A.J.; Sturmey, R.G.; Elder, K.; Picton, H.M. Variable imprinting of the MEST gene in human preimplantation embryos. *Eur. J. Hum. Genet.* **2012**, *21*, 40–47. [CrossRef] [PubMed]
34. Chen, Z.; Robbins, K.M.; Wells, K.D.; Rivera, R.M. Large offspring syndrome: A bovine model for the human loss-of-imprinting overgrowth syndrome Beckwith-Wiedemann. *Epigenetics* **2013**, *8*, 591–601. [CrossRef] [PubMed]
35. Hiura, H.; Okae, H.; Chiba, H.; Miyauchi, N.; Sato, F.; Sato, A.; Arima, T. Imprinting methylation errors in ART. *Reprod. Med. Biol.* **2014**, *13*, 193–202. [CrossRef]
36. Lazaraviciute, G.; Kauser, M.; Bhattacharya, S.; Haggarty, P.; Bhattacharya, S. A systematic review and meta-analysis of DNA methylation levels and imprinting disorders in children conceived by IVF/ICSI compared with children conceived spontane-ously. *Hum. Reprod. Update* **2014**, *20*, 840–852. [CrossRef]
37. Vermeiden, J.P.; Bernardus, R.E. Are imprinting disorders more prevalent after human in vitro fertilization or intracytoplasmic sperm injection? *Fertil. Steril.* **2013**, *99*, 642–651. [CrossRef]
38. Henningsen, A.A.; Gissler, M.; Rasmussen, S.; Opdahl, S.; Wennerholm, U.B.; Spangmose, A.L.; Tiitinen, A.; Bergh, C.; Romund-stad, L.B.; Laivuori, H.; et al. Imprinting disorders in children born after ART: A Nordic study from the CoNARTaS group. *Hum. Reprod.* **2020**, *35*, 1178–1184. [CrossRef]
39. Hattori, H.; Hiura, H.; Kitamura, A.; Miyauchi, N.; Kobayashi, N.; Takahashi, S.; Okae, H.; Kyono, K.; Kagami, M.; Ogata, T.; et al. Association of four imprinting disorders and ART. *Clin. Epigenet.* **2019**, *11*, 21. [CrossRef]
40. Chen, Z.; Hagen, D.E.; Elsik, C.G.; Ji, T.; Morris, C.J.; Moon, L.E.; Rivera, R.M. Characterization of global loss of imprinting in fetal overgrowth syndrome induced by assisted reproduction. *Proc. Natl. Acad. Sci. USA* **2015**, *112*, 4618–4623. [CrossRef]
41. Van der Auwera, I.; D'Hooghe, T. Superovulation of female mice delays embryonic and fetal development. *Hum. Reprod.* **2001**, *16*, 1237–1243. [CrossRef]
42. Market-Velker, B.A.; Zhang, L.; Magri, L.S.; Bonvissuto, A.C.; Mann, M.R. Dual effects of superovulation: Loss of maternal and paternal imprinted methylation in a dose-dependent manner. *Hum. Mol. Genet.* **2009**, *19*, 36–51. [CrossRef] [PubMed]
43. Chang, A.S.; Moley, K.H.; Wangler, M.; Feinberg, A.; DeBaun, M.R. Association between Beckwith-Wiedemann syndrome and assisted reproductive technology: A case series of 19 patients. *Fertil. Steril.* **2005**, *83*, 349–354. [CrossRef] [PubMed]
44. Voronina, E.; Wessel, G.M. The Regulation of Oocyte Maturation. *Curr. Top. Dev. Biol.* **2003**, *58*, 53–110. [PubMed]
45. Telfer, E. Progress and prospects for developing human immature oocytes in vitro. *Reproduction* **2019**, *158*, F45–F54. [CrossRef]
46. Mak, W.; Weaver, J.R.; Bartolomei, M.S. Is ART changing the epigenetic landscape of imprinting? *Anim. Reprod.* **2010**, *7*, 168–176.
47. Sato, A.; Otsu, E.; Negishi, H.; Utsunomiya, T.; Arima, T. Aberrant DNA methylation of imprinted loci in superovulated oo-cytes. *Hum. Reprod.* **2007**, *22*, 26–35. [CrossRef]
48. Laprise, S.L. Implications of epigenetics and genomic imprinting in assisted reproductive technologies. *Mol. Reprod. Dev.* **2009**, *76*, 1006–1018. [CrossRef]
49. Fauque, P.; Jouannet, P.; Lesaffre, C.; Ripoche, M.-A.; Dandolo, L.; Vaiman, D.; Jammes, H. Assisted Reproductive Technology affects developmental kinetics, H19 Imprinting Control Region methylation and H19 gene expression in individual mouse embryos. *BMC Dev. Biol.* **2007**, *7*, 116. [CrossRef]
50. Huo, Y.; Yan, Z.Q.; Yuan, P.; Qin, M.; Kuo, Y.; Li, R.; Yan, L.Y.; Feng, H.L.; Qiao, J. Single-cell DNA methylation sequencing reveals epigenetic alterations in mouse oocytes superovulated with different dosages of gonadotropins. *Clin. Epigenetics* **2020**, *12*, 75. [CrossRef]
51. Saenz-De-Juano, M.D.; Ivanova, E.; Billooye, K.; Herța, A.-C.; Smitz, J.; Kelsey, G.; Anckaert, E. Correction to: Genome-wide assessment of DNA methylation in mouse oocytes reveals effects associated with in vitro growth, superovulation, and sexual maturity. *Clin. Epigenet.* **2020**, *12*, 18. [CrossRef]
52. Yu, B.; Smith, T.H.; Battle, S.L.; Ferrell, S.; Hawkins, R.D. Superovulation alters global DNA methylation in early mouse embryo development. *Epigenetics* **2019**, *14*, 780–790. [CrossRef] [PubMed]
53. Kalthur, G.; Salian, S.R.; Nair, R.; Mathew, J.; Adiga, S.K.; Kalthur, S.G.; Zeegers, D.; Hande, M.P. Distribution pattern of cytoplasmic organelles, spindle integrity, oxidative stress, octamer-binding transcription factor 4 (Oct4) expression and de-velopmental potential of oocytes following multiple superovulation. *Reprod. Fertil. Dev.* **2016**, *28*, 2027–2038. [CrossRef] [PubMed]
54. Tang, S.-B.; Yang, L.-L.; Zhang, T.-T.; Wang, Q.; Yin, S.; Luo, S.-M.; Shen, W.; Ge, Z.-J.; Sun, Q.-Y. Multiple superovulations alter histone modifications in mouse early embryos. *Reproduction* **2019**, *157*, 511–523. [CrossRef] [PubMed]
55. Uysal, F.; Ozturk, S.; Akkoyunlu, G. Superovulation alters DNA methyltransferase protein expression in mouse oocytes and early em-bryos. *J. Assist. Reprod. Genet.* **2018**, *35*, 503–513. [CrossRef]
56. Kindsfather, A.J.; Czekalski, M.A.; Pressimone, C.A.; Erisman, M.P.; Mann, M.R. Perturbations in imprinted methylation from assisted reproductive technologies but not advanced maternal age in mouse preimplantation embryos. *Clin. Epigenet.* **2019**, *11*, 162. [CrossRef]

57. Chen, X.; Huang, Y.; Huang, H.; Guan, Y.; Li, M.; Jiang, X.; Yu, M.; Yang, X. Effects of superovulation, in vitro fertilization, and oocyte in vitro maturation on imprinted gene Grb10 in mouse blastocysts. *Arch. Gynecol. Obstet.* **2018**, *298*, 1219–1227. [CrossRef]
58. Palermo, G.; Joris, H.; Devroey, P.; Van Steirteghem, A.C. Pregnancies after intracytoplasmic injection of single spermatozoon into an oocyte. *Lancet* **1992**, *340*, 17–18. [CrossRef]
59. Hewitson, L.; Simerly, C.; Dominko, T.; Schatten, G. Cellular and molecular events after in vitro fertilization and intracyto-plasmic sperm injection. *Theriogenology* **2000**, *53*, 95–104. [CrossRef]
60. Sullivan, E.A.; Zegers-Hochschild, F.; Mansour, R.; Ishihara, O.; De Mouzon, J.; Nygren, K.G.; Adamson, G.D. International Committee for Monitoring Assisted Reproductive Technologies (ICMART) world report: Assisted reproductive technology 2004. *Hum. Reprod.* **2013**, *28*, 1375–1390. [CrossRef]
61. Minor, A.; Chow, V.; Ma, S. Aberrant DNA methylation at imprinted genes in testicular sperm retrieved from men with ob-structive azoospermia and undergoing vasectomy reversal. *Reproduction* **2011**, *141*, 749–757. [CrossRef]
62. Kobayashi, H.; Sato, A.; Otsu, E.; Hiura, H.; Tomatsu, C.; Utsunomiya, T.; Sasaki, H.; Yaegashi, N.; Arima, T. Aberrant DNA methylation of imprinted loci in sperm from oligospermic patients. *Hum. Mol. Genet.* **2007**, *16*, 2542–2551. [CrossRef] [PubMed]
63. Marques, C.J.; Francisco, T.; Sousa, S.; Carvalho, F.; Barros, A.; Sousa, M. Methylation defects of imprinted genes in human testicular spermatozoa. *Fertil. Steril.* **2010**, *94*, 585–594. [CrossRef] [PubMed]
64. Whitelaw, N.; Bhattacharya, S.; Hoad, G.; Horgan, G.W.; Hamilton, M.; Haggarty, P. Epigenetic status in the offspring of spontaneous and assisted conception. *Hum. Reprod.* **2014**, *29*, 1452–1458. [CrossRef] [PubMed]
65. Rancourt, R.; Harris, H.; Michels, K. Methylation levels at imprinting control regions are not altered with ovulation induction or in vitro fertilization in a birth cohort. *Hum. Reprod.* **2012**, *27*, 2208–2216. [CrossRef]
66. Xu, N.; Barlow, G.M.; Cui, J.; Wang, E.T.; Lee, B.; Akhlaghpour, M.; Kroener, L.; Williams, J.; Rotter, J.I.; Chen, Y.-D.I.; et al. Comparison of Genome-Wide and Gene-Specific DNA Methylation Profiling in First-Trimester Chorionic Villi From Pregnancies Conceived With Infertility Treatments. *Reprod. Sci.* **2016**, *24*, 996–1004. [CrossRef]
67. Choufani, S.; Turinsky, A.L.; Melamed, N.; Greenblatt, E.; Brudno, M.; Bérard, A.; Fraser, W.D.; Weksberg, R.; Trasler, J.; Monnier, P.; et al. Impact of assisted reproduction, infertility, sex and paternal factors on the placental DNA methylome. *Hum. Mol. Genet.* **2018**, *28*, 372–385. [CrossRef]
68. Tierling, S.; Souren, N.Y.; Gries, J.; LoPorto, C.; Groth, M.; Lutsik, P.; Neitzel, H.; Utz-Billing, I.; Gillessen-Kaesbach, G.; Kentenich, H.; et al. Assisted reproductive technologies do not enhance the variability of DNA methylation imprints in human. *J. Med. Genet.* **2009**, *47*, 371–376. [CrossRef]
69. El Hajj, N.; Haertle, L.; Dittrich, M.; Denk, S.; Lehnen, H.; Hahn, T.; Schorsch, M.; Haaf, T. DNA methylation signatures in cord blood of ICSI children. *Hum. Reprod.* **2017**, *32*, 1761–1769. [CrossRef]
70. Choux, C.; Binquet, C.; Carmignac, V.; Bruno, C.; Chapusot, C.; Barberet, J.; LaMotte, M.; Sagot, P.; Bourc'His, D.; Fauque, P. The epigenetic control of transposable elements and imprinted genes in newborns is affected by the mode of conception: ART versus spontaneous conception without underlying infertility. *Hum. Reprod.* **2017**, *33*, 331–340. [CrossRef]
71. Rivera, R.M.; Stein, P.; Weaver, J.R.; Mager, J.; Schultz, R.M.; Bartolomei, M.S. Manipulations of mouse embryos prior to implantation result in aberrant expression of imprinted genes on day 9.5 of development. *Hum. Mol. Genet.* **2007**, *17*, 1–14. [CrossRef]
72. Nelissen, E.C.; Dumoulin, J.C.; Daunay, A.; Evers, J.L.; Tost, J.; van Montfoort, A.P. Placentas from pregnancies conceived by IVF/ICSI have a reduced DNA methylation level at the H19 and MEST differentially methylated regions. *Hum. Reprod.* **2013**, *28*, 1117–1126. [CrossRef] [PubMed]
73. Fortier, A.L.; Lopes, F.L.; Darricarrère, N.; Martel, J.; Trasler, J.M. Superovulation alters the expression of imprinted genes in the midgestation mouse placenta. *Hum. Mol. Genet.* **2008**, *17*, 1653–1665. [CrossRef] [PubMed]
74. De Waal, E.; Mak, W.; Calhoun, S.; Stein, P.; Ord, T.; Krapp, C.; Coutifaris, C.; Schultz, R.M.; Bartolomei, M. In Vitro Culture Increases the Frequency of Stochastic Epigenetic Errors at Imprinted Genes in Placental Tissues from Mouse Concepti Produced Through Assisted Reproductive Technologies1. *Biol. Reprod.* **2014**, *90*, 22. [CrossRef]
75. Yang, H.; Ma, Z.; Peng, L.; Kuhn, C.; Rahmeh, M.; Mahner, S.; Jeschke, U.; von Schönfeldt, V. Comparison of Histone H3K4me3 between IVF and ICSI Technologies and between Boy and Girl Offspring. *Int. J. Mol. Sci.* **2021**, *22*, 8574. [CrossRef]
76. Choux, C.; Petazzi, P.; Sánchez, A.M.; Mora, J.R.H.; Monteagudo, A.; Sagot, P.; Monk, D.; Fauque, P. The hypomethylation of imprinted genes in IVF/ICSI placenta samples is associated with concomitant changes in histone modifications. *Epigenetics* **2020**, *15*, 1386–1395. [CrossRef]
77. Potabattula, R.; Zacchini, F.; Ptak, G.E.; Dittrich, M.; Müller, T.; El Hajj, N.; Hahn, T.; Drummer, C.; Behr, R.; Lucas-Hahn, A.; et al. Increasing methylation of sperm rDNA and other repetitive elements in the aging male mammalian germline. *Aging Cell* **2020**, *19*, e13181. [CrossRef]
78. Potabattula, R.; Dittrich, M.; Böck, J.; Haertle, L.; Müller, T.; Hahn, T.; Schorsch, M.; Hajj, N.E.; Haaf, T. Allele-specific methylation of imprinted genes in fetal cord blood is influenced by cis-acting genetic variants and parental factors. *Epigenomics* **2018**, *10*, 1315–1326. [CrossRef]
79. Mitchell, M.; Strick, R.; Strissel, P.L.; Dittrich, R.; McPherson, N.O.; Lane, M.; Pliushch, G.; Potabattula, R.; Haaf, T.; El Hajj, N. Gene expression and epigenetic aberrations in F1-placentas fathered by obese males. *Mol Reprod Dev.* **2017**, *84*, 316–328. [CrossRef]
80. Potabattula, R.; Dittrich, M.; Schorsch, M.; Hahn, T.; Haaf, T.; El Hajj, N. Male obesity effects on sperm and next-generation cord blood DNA methylation. *PLoS ONE* **2019**, *14*, e0218615. [CrossRef]

81. Bernhardt, L.; Dittrich, M.; El-Merahbi, R.; Saliba, A.E.; Müller, T.; Sumara, G.; Vogel, J.; Nichols-Burns, S.; Mitchell, M.; Haaf, T.; et al. A genome-wide transcriptomic analysis of embryos fathered by obese males in a murine model of diet-induced obesity. *Sci. Rep.* **2021**, *11*, 1979. [CrossRef]
82. Atsem, S.; Reichenbach, J.; Potabattula, R.; Dittrich, M.; Nava, C.; Depienne, C.; Böhm, L.; Rost, S.; Hahn, T.; Schorsch, M.; et al. Paternal age effects on sperm *FOXK1* and *KCNA7* methylation and transmission into the next generation. *Hum. Mol. Genet.* **2016**, *25*, 4996–5005. [CrossRef] [PubMed]
83. Vieweg, M.; Dvorakova-Hortova, K.; Dudkova, B.; Waliszewski, P.; Otte, M.; Oels, B.; Hajimohammad, A.; Turley, H.; Schorsch, M.; Schuppe, H.-C.; et al. Methylation analysis of histone H4K12ac-associated promoters in sperm of healthy donors and subfertile patients. *Clin. Epigenet.* **2015**, *7*, 31. [CrossRef] [PubMed]
84. El Hajj, N.; Zechner, U.; Schneider, E.; Tresch, A.; Gromoll, J.; Hahn, T.; Schorsch, M.; Haaf, T. Methylation status of imprinted genes and repetitive elements in sperm DNA from infertile males. *Sex. Dev.* **2011**, *5*, 60–69. [CrossRef]
85. Schon, S.B.; Luense, L.J.; Wang, X.; Bartolomei, M.S.; Coutifaris, C.; Garcia, B.A.; Berger, S.J. Histone modification sig-natures in human sperm distinguish clinical abnormalities. *J. Assist. Reprod. Genet.* **2019**, *36*, 267–275. [CrossRef] [PubMed]
86. Dang, V.Q.; Vuong, L.N.; Luu, T.M.; Pham, T.D.; Ho, T.M.; Ha, A.N.; Truong, B.T.; Phan, A.K.; Nguyen, D.P.; Pham, T.N.; et al. Intracytoplasmic sperm injection versus conventional in-vitro fertilisation in couples with infertility in whom the male partner has normal total sperm count and motility: An open-label, randomised controlled trial. *Lancet* **2021**, *397*, 1554–1563. [CrossRef]
87. Practice Committees of American Society for Reproductive Medicine and Society for Assisted Reproduction Technology. In-tracytoplasmic sperm injection (ICSI) for non- male factor indications: A committee opinion. *Fertil. Steril.* **2020**, *114*, 239–245. [CrossRef]
88. Huntriss, J.; Picton, H.M. Epigenetic consequences of assisted reproduction and infertility on the human preimplantation embryo. *Hum. Fertil.* **2008**, *11*, 85–94. [CrossRef]
89. Osman, E.; Franasiak, J.; Scott, R. Oocyte and Embryo Manipulation and Epigenetics. *Semin. Reprod. Med.* **2018**, *36*, e1–e9. [CrossRef]
90. Siqueira, L.G.; Silva, M.V.G.; Panetto, J.; Viana, J. Consequences of assisted reproductive technologies for offspring function in cattle. *Reprod. Fertil. Dev.* **2020**, *32*, 82–97. [CrossRef]
91. El Hajj, N.; Haaf, T. Epigenetic disturbances in in vitro cultured gametes and embryos: Implications for human assisted reproduction. *Fertil. Steril.* **2013**, *99*, 632–641. [CrossRef]
92. Market-Velker, B.; Fernandes, A.; Mann, M. Side-by-Side Comparison of Five Commercial Media Systems in a Mouse Model: Suboptimal In Vitro Culture Interferes with Imprint Maintenance1. *Biol. Reprod.* **2010**, *83*, 938–950. [CrossRef]
93. Estill, M.S.; Bolnick, J.M.; Waterland, R.A.; Bolnick, A.D.; Diamond, M.P.; Krawetz, S.A. Assisted reproductive technology alters deoxyribonucleic acid methylation profiles in bloodspots of newborn infants. *Fertil. Steril.* **2016**, *106*, 629–639. [CrossRef] [PubMed]
94. Katari, S.; Turan, N.; Bibikova, M.; Erinle, O.; Chalian, R.; Foster, M.; Gaughan, J.P.; Coutifaris, C.; Sapienza, C. DNA methylation and gene expression differences in children conceived in vitro or in vivo. *Hum. Mol. Genet.* **2009**, *18*, 3769–3778. [CrossRef] [PubMed]
95. Castillo-Fernandez, J.; Loke, Y.J.; Bass-Stringer, S.; Gao, F.; Xia, Y.; Wu, H.; Lu, H.; Liu, Y.; Wang, J.; Spector, T.D.; et al. DNA methylation changes at infertility genes in newborn twins conceived by in vitro fertilisation. *Genome Med.* **2017**, *9*, 28. [CrossRef] [PubMed]
96. Schwarzer, C.; Esteves, T.C.; Araúzo-Bravo, M.J.; Le Gac, S.; Nordhoff, V.; Schlatt, S.; Boiani, M. ART culture conditions change the probability of mouse embryo gestation through defined cellular and molecular responses. *Hum. Reprod.* **2012**, *27*, 2627–2640. [CrossRef] [PubMed]
97. Gad, A.; Schellander, K.; Hoelker, M.; Tesfaye, D. Transcriptome profile of early mammalian embryos in response to culture environment. *Anim. Reprod. Sci.* **2012**, *134*, 76–83. [CrossRef]
98. Kleijkers, S.H.; Eijssen, L.M.; Coonen, E.; Derhaag, J.G.; Mantikou, E.; Jonker, M.J.; Mastenbroek, S.; Repping, S.; Evers, J.L.; Dumoulin, J.C.; et al. Differences in gene expression profiles between human preimplantation embryos cultured in two different IVF culture media. *Hum. Reprod.* **2015**, *30*, 2303–2311. [CrossRef]
99. Mantikou, E.; Jonker, M.J.; Wong, K.M.; van Montfoort, A.P.; De Jong, M.; Breit, T.M.; Repping, S.; Mastenbroek, S. Factors affecting the gene ex-pression of in vitro cultured human preimplantation embryos. *Hum. Reprod.* **2016**, *31*, 298–311.
100. Mulder, C.L.; Wattimury, T.M.; Jongejan, A.; de Winter-Korver, C.M.; van Daalen, S.K.M.; Struijk, R.B.; Borgman, S.C.M.; Wurth, Y.; Consten, D.; van Echten-Arends, J.; et al. Comparison of DNA methylation patterns of parentally imprinted genes in placenta derived from IVF conceptions in two different culture media. *Hum. Reprod.* **2020**, *35*, 516–528. [CrossRef]
101. Fischer, B.; Bavister, B.D. Oxygen tension in the oviduct and uterus of rhesus monkeys, hamsters and rabbits. *J. Reprod. Fertil.* **1993**, *99*, 673–679. [CrossRef]
102. Ng, K.Y.B.; Mingels, R.; Morgan, H.; Macklon, N.; Cheong, Y. In vivo oxygen, temperature and pH dynamics in the female reproductive tract and their importance in human conception: A systematic review. *Hum. Reprod. Update* **2017**, *24*, 15–34. [CrossRef] [PubMed]
103. Gardner, D.K.; Lane, M. Ex vivo early embryo development and effects on gene expression and imprinting. *Reprod. Fertil. Dev.* **2005**, *17*, 361–370. [CrossRef]
104. Sciorio, R.; Smith, G. Embryo culture at a reduced oxygen concentration of 5%: A mini review. *Zygote* **2019**, *27*, 355–361. [CrossRef]

5. Katz-Jaffe, M.G.; Linck, D.W.; Schoolcraft, W.B.; Gardner, D.K. A proteomic analysis of mammalian preimplantation embryonic development. *Reproduction* **2005**, *130*, 899–905. [CrossRef]
6. Rinaudo, P.F.; Giritharan, G.; Talbi, S.; Dobson, A.T.; Schultz, R.M. Effects of oxygen tension on gene expression in pre-implantation mouse embryos. *Fertil. Steril.* **2006**, *86* (Suppl. 4), 1252–1265. [CrossRef] [PubMed]
7. Meintjes, M.; Chantilis, S.J.; Douglas, J.D.; Rodriguez, A.J.; Guerami, A.R.; Bookout, D.M.; Barnett, B.D.; Madden, J.D. A controlled randomized trial evaluating the effect of lowered incubator oxygen tension on live births in a predominantly blas-tocyst transfer program. *Hum. Reprod.* **2009**, *24*, 300–307. [CrossRef] [PubMed]
8. Gardner, D.K.; Kuramoto, T.; Tanaka, M.; Mitzumoto, S.; Montag, M.; Yoshida, A. Prospec-tive randomized multicentre comparison on sibling oocytes comparing G-Series media system with antioxidants versus standard G-Series media system. *Reprod. Biomed. Online* **2020**, *40*, 637–644. [CrossRef]
9. Bontekoe, S.; Mantikou, E.; van Wely, M.; Seshadri, S.; Repping, S.; Mastenbroek, S. Low oxygen concentrations for embryo culture in assisted reproductive technologies. *Cochrane Database Syst. Rev.* **2012**, CD008950. [CrossRef]
10. Painter, R.C.; de Rooij, S.R.; Bossuyt, P.M.; Simmers, T.A.; Osmond, C.; Barker, D.J.; Bleker, O.P.; Roseboom, T.J. Early onset of coronary artery disease after prenatal exposure to the Dutch famine. *Am. J. Clin. Nutr.* **2006**, *84*, 322–327. [CrossRef]
11. Dumoulin, J.C.; Land, J.A.; Van Montfoort, A.P.; Nelissen, E.C.; Coonen, E.; Derhaag, J.G.; Schreurs, I.L.; Dunselman, G.A.; Kester, A.D.; Geraedts, J.P.; et al. Effect of in vitro culture of human embryos on birthweight of newborns. *Hum. Reprod.* **2010**, *25*, 605–612. [CrossRef]
12. Nelissen, E.C.; van Montfoort, A.; Coonen, E.; Derhaag, J.G.; Geraedts, J.P.; Smits, L.J.; Land, J.A.; Evers, J.; Dumoulin, J.C. Further evidence that culture media affect perinatal outcome: Findings after transfer of fresh and cryopreserved embryos. *Hum. Reprod.* **2012**, *27*, 1966–1976. [CrossRef] [PubMed]
13. Vergouw, C.G.; Kostelijk, E.H.; Doejaaren, E.; Hompes, P.G.; Lambalk, C.B.; Schats, R. The influence of the type of embryo culture medium on neonatal birthweight after single embryo transfer in IVF. *Hum. Reprod.* **2012**, *27*, 2619–2626. [CrossRef] [PubMed]
14. Roberts, S.A.; Vail, A. On the appropriate interpretation of evidence: The example of culture media and birth weight. *Hum. Reprod.* **2017**, *32*, 1151–1154. [CrossRef] [PubMed]
15. Kleijkers, S.H.; Mantikou, E.; Slappendel, E.; Consten, D.; Van Echten-Arends, J.; Wetzels, A.M.; van Wely, M.; Smits, L.J.; van Montfoort, A.; Repping, S.; et al. Influence of embryo culture medium (G5 and HTF) on pregnancy and perinatal outcome after IVF: A multicenter RCT. *Hum. Reprod.* **2016**, *31*, 2219–2230. [CrossRef]
16. Kleijkers, S.H.; van Montfoort, A.; Smits, L.J.M.; Viechtbauer, W.; Roseboom, T.J.; Nelissen, E.C.; Coonen, E.; Derhaag, J.G.; Bastings, L.; Schreurs, I.E.; et al. IVF culture medium affects post-natal weight in humans during the first 2 years of life. *Hum. Reprod.* **2014**, *29*, 661–669. [CrossRef]
17. Lin, S.; Li, M.; Lian, Y.; Chen, L.; Liu, P. No effect of embryo culture media on birthweight and length of newborns. *Hum. Reprod.* **2013**, *28*, 1762–1767. [CrossRef]
18. De Vos, A.; Janssens, R.; Van De Velde, H.; Haentjens, P.; Bonduelle, M.; Tournaye, H.; Verheyen, G. The type of culture medium and the duration of in vitro culture do not influence birthweight of ART singletons. *Hum. Reprod.* **2015**, *30*, 20–27. [CrossRef]
19. Eskild, A.; Monkerud, L.; Tanbo, T. Birthweight and placental weight; do changes in culture media used for IVF matter? Comparisons with spontaneous pregnancies in the corresponding time periods. *Hum. Reprod.* **2013**, *28*, 3207–3214. [CrossRef]
20. Kleijkers, S.H.; van Montfoort, A.P.; Smits, L.J.M.; Coonen, E.; Derhaag, J.G.; Evers, J.L.; Dumoulin, J.C. Age of G-1 PLUS v5 embryo culture medium is inversely associated with birthweight of the newborn. *Hum. Reprod.* **2015**, *30*, 1352–1357. [CrossRef]
21. Zhu, J.; Li, M.; Chen, L.; Liu, P.; Qiao, J. The protein source in embryo culture media influences birthweight: A comparative study between G1 v5 and G1-PLUS v5. *Hum. Reprod.* **2014**, *29*, 1387–1392. [CrossRef]
22. Zhu, J.; Lin, S.; Li, M.; Chen, L.; Lian, Y.; Liu, P.; Qiao, J. Effect of in vitro culture period on birthweight of singleton newborns. *Hum. Reprod.* **2014**, *29*, 448–454. [CrossRef] [PubMed]
23. Zandstra, H.; Van Montfoort, A.P.; Dumoulin, J.C. Does the type of culture medium used influence birthweight of children born after IVF? *Hum. Reprod.* **2015**, *30*, 530–542. [CrossRef] [PubMed]
24. Litzky, J.F.; Boulet, S.; Esfandiari, N.; Zhang, Y.; Kissin, D.M.; Theiler, R.; Marsit, C.J. Effect of frozen/thawed embryo transfer on birthweight, macrosomia, and low birthweight rates in US singleton infants. *Am. J. Obstet. Gynecol.* **2017**, *218*, 433.e1–433.e10. [CrossRef] [PubMed]
25. Cetin, I.; Cozzi, V.; Antonazzo, P. Fetal development after assisted reproduction–a review. *Placenta* **2003**, *24*, S104–S113. [CrossRef]
26. Källén, B.; Finnström, O.; Lindam, A.; Nilsson, E.; Nygren, K.G.; Otterblad, P.O. Congenital malformations in infants born after in vitro fertilization in Sweden. *Birth Defects Res. A Clin. Mol. Teratol.* **2010**, *88*, 137–143.
27. Hart, R.; Norman, R.J. The longer-term health outcomes for children born as a result of IVF treatment: Part I–General health outcomes. *Hum. Reprod. Update* **2013**, *19*, 232–243. [CrossRef]
28. Scherrer, U.; Rimoldi, S.F.; Rexhaj, E.; Stuber, T.; Duplain, H.; Garcin, S.; de Marchi, S.F.; Nicod, P.; Germond, M.; Allemann, Y.; et al. Systemic and pulmonary vascular dys-function in children conceived by assisted reproductive technologies. *Circulation* **2012**, *125*, 1890–1896. [CrossRef]
29. Von Arx, R.; Allemann, Y.; Sartori, C.; Rexhaj, E.; Cerny, D.; De Marchi, S.F.; Soria, R.; Germond, M.; Scherrer, U.; Rimoldi, S.F. Right ventricular dysfunction in children and adolescents conceived by assisted reproductive technologies. *J. Appl. Physiol.* **2015**, *118*, 1200–1206. [CrossRef]

130. Valenzuela-Alcaraz, B.; Cruz-Lemini, M.; Rodriguez-Lopez, M.; Goncé, A.; García-Otero, L.; Ayuso, H.; Sitges, M.; Bijnens, B.; Balasch, J.; Gratacós, E.; et al. Fetal cardiac remodeling in twin pregnancy conceived by assisted reproductive technology. *Ultrasound Obstet. Gynecol.* **2017**, *51*, 94–100. [CrossRef]
131. Sakka, S.D.; Loutradis, D.; Kanaka-Gantenbein, C.; Margeli, A.; Papastamataki, M.; Papassotiriou, I.; Chrousos, G.P. Absence of insulin resistance and low-grade inflammation despite early metabolic syndrome manifestations in children born after in vitro fertilization. *Fertil. Steril.* **2010**, *94*, 1693–1699. [CrossRef]
132. Ceelen, M.; van Weissenbruch, M.M.; Roos, J.C.; Vermeiden, J.P.; van Leeuwen, F.E.; Delemarre-van de Waal, H.A. Body composition in children and adolescents born after in vitro fertilization or spontaneous conception. *J. Clin. Endocrinol. Metab.* **2007**, *92*, 3417–3423. [CrossRef] [PubMed]
133. Ceelen, M.; van Weissenbruch, M.M.; Vermeiden, J.P.; van Leeuwen, F.E.; Delemarre-van de Waal, H.A. Cardiometabolic differences in children born after in vitro fertilization: Follow-up study. *J. Clin. Endocrinol. Metab.* **2008**, *93*, 1682–1688. [CrossRef] [PubMed]
134. Bi, W.; Xiao, Y.; Wang, X.; Cui, L.; Song, G.; Yang, Z.; Zhang, Y.; Ren, W. The association between assisted reproductive technology and cardiac remodeling in fetuses and early infants: A prospective cohort study. *BMC Med.* **2022**, *20*, 104. [CrossRef]
135. Huang, J.Y.; Cai, S.; Huang, Z.; Tint, M.T.; Yuan, W.L.; Aris, I.M.; Godfrey, K.M.; Karnani, N.; Lee, Y.S.; Chan, J.K.Y.; et al. Analyses of child cardiometabolic phenotype following assisted reproductive technologies using a pragmatic trial emulation approach. *Nat. Commun.* **2021**, *12*, 5613. [CrossRef]
136. Halliday, J.; Lewis, S.; Kennedy, J.; Burgner, D.P.; Juonala, M.; Hammarberg, K.; Amor, D.J.; Doyle, L.W.; Saffery, R.; Ranganathan, S.; et al. Health of adults aged 22 to 35 years con-ceived by assisted reproductive technology. *Fertil. Steril.* **2019**, *112*, 130–139. [CrossRef]
137. Novakovic, B.; Lewis, S.; Halliday, J.; Kennedy, J.; Burgner, D.P.; Czajko, A.; Kim, B.; Sexton-Oates, A.; Juonala, M.; Hammarberg, K.; et al. Assisted reproductive technologies are associated with limited epigenetic variation at birth that largely resolves by adulthood. *Nat. Commun.* **2019**, *10*, 3922. [CrossRef] [PubMed]
138. Denomme, M.M.; Mann, M.R. Genomic imprints as a model for the analysis of epigenetic stability during ARTs. *Reproduction* **2012**, *144*, 393–409. [CrossRef]
139. Zechner, U.; Pliushch, G.; Schneider, E.; El Hajj, N.; Tresch, A.; Shufaro, Y.; Seidmann, L.; Coerdt, W.; Müller, A.M.; Haaf, T. Quantitative methylation analysis of developmentally important genes in human pregnancy losses after ART and spontaneous conception. *Mol. Hum. Reprod.* **2009**, *16*, 704–713. [CrossRef]
140. Sciorio, R.; Dattilo, M. PGT-A preimplantation genetic testing for aneuploidies and embryo selection in routine ART cycles: Time to step back? *Clin. Genet.* **2020**, *98*, 107–115. [CrossRef]
141. Dokras, A.; Sargent, I.; Ross, C.; Gardner, R.; Barlow, D. Trophectoderm biopsy in human blastocysts. *Hum. Reprod.* **1990**, *5*, 821–825. [CrossRef]
142. Honguntikar, S.D.; Salian, S.R.; D'Souza, F.; Uppangala, S.; Kalthur, G.; Adiga, S.K. Epigenetic changes in preimplan-tation embryos subjected to laser manipulation. *Lasers Med. Sci.* **2017**, *32*, 2081–2087. [CrossRef] [PubMed]
143. Glujovsky, D.; Farquhar, C.; Quinteiro Retamar, A.M.; Alvarez Sedo, C.R.; Blake, D. Cleavage stage versus blastocyst stage embryo transfer in assisted reproductive technology (Review). *Cochrane Database Syst. Rev.* **2016**, *30*, CD002118.
144. Salilew-Wondim, D.; Saeed-Zidane, M.; Hoelker, M.; Gebremedhn, S.; Poirier, M.; Pandey, H.O.; Tholen, E.; Neuhoff, C.; Held, E.; Besenfelder, U.; et al. Genome-wide DNA methylation patterns of bovine blastocysts derived from in vivo embryos subjected to in vitro culture before, during or after embryonic genome activation. *BMC Genom.* **2018**, *19*, 424. [CrossRef] [PubMed]
145. Beyer, C.; Osianlis, T.; Boekel, K.; Osborne, E.; Rombauts, L.; Catt, J.; Kralevski, V.; Aali, B.; Gras, L. Preimplantation genetic screening outcomes are associated with culture conditions. *Hum. Reprod.* **2009**, *24*, 1212–1220. [CrossRef] [PubMed]
146. Picton, H.M.; Elder, K.; Houghton, F.D.; Hawkhead, J.A.; Rutherford, A.J.; Hogg, J.E.; Leese, H.J.; Harris, S.E. Association between amino acid turnover and chromosome aneuploidy during human preimplantation embryo development in vitro. *Mol. Hum. Reprod.* **2010**, *16*, 557–569. [CrossRef] [PubMed]

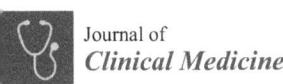

Review

PCOS Physiopathology and Vitamin D Deficiency: Biological Insights and Perspectives for Treatment

Giuseppe Morgante [†], Ilenia Darino [†], Amelia Spanò, Stefano Luisi, Alice Luddi, Paola Piomboni, Laura Governini * and Vincenzo De Leo

Department of Molecular and Developmental Medicine, University of Siena, 53100 Siena, Italy; giuseppe.morgante@unisi.it (G.M.); ileniadarino@hotmail.it (I.D.); ameliaspano94@gmail.com (A.S.); stefano.luisi@unisi.it (S.L.); alice.luddi@unisi.it (A.L.); paola.piomboni@unisi.it (P.P.); vincenzo.deleo@unisi.it (V.D.L.)
* Correspondence: laura.governini@unisi.it; Tel.: +39-0577-586810
† The first two authors should be regarded as joint first authors.

Abstract: Recent literature has stressed the importance of vitamin D (VD) in polycystic ovary syndrome (PCOS). Women with PCOS are deficient in VD, particularly those with a higher weight. Hypovitaminosis is a risk factor for glucose intolerance, and reduced levels of VD is associated with insulin resistance and increased diabetes risk. Since women with PCOS and hirsutism seem to have lower levels of VD than women with PCOS without hirsutism, a correlation between VD deficiency and hyperandrogenism may be suggested. Interestingly, VD is crucial for many human physiological functions, including to counteract inflammation and oxidative stress. Some studies evaluated effects of VD supplementation on glucose homeostasis variables, hormonal status, lipid concentrations, and biomarkers of inflammation and oxidative stress among VD-deficient women. Moreover, VD has been shown to play a role in egg quality and fertility. This review aims to show the relationship between VD and the endocrine and metabolic profile of PCOS patients, as well as its implications for their fertility. The supplement of VD to the common therapy can lead to an improvement of the insulin resistance and lipid metabolism, a reduction of circulating androgens, as well as a better response to the induction of ovulation in PCOS women.

Keywords: polycystic ovary syndrome (PCOS); vitamin D; insulin resistance; oxidative stress; fertility; supplementation

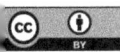

1. Introduction

Polycystic ovary syndrome (PCOS) constitutes the most frequent endocrine disorder in women of reproductive age. PCOS affects up to one-sixth of women with a prevalence that may reach or even exceed 10–15%, depending on the diagnostic criteria applied and the populations studied in different geographical areas [1,2]. It is a multisystem disorder characterized by oligo or anovulation, and consequently oligo or amenorrhea, and the development of hyperandrogenism, resulting from circulating luteinizing hormone (LH) levels and the altered ratio of LH to follicle stimulating hormone (FSH) [3]. Morphologically, the ovaries may appear polycystic (polycystic ovarian morphology, PCOM). PCOS is also associated with hyperinsulinemia, impaired glucose tolerance, and sometimes even type 2 diabetes mellitus (T2DM) [4]. Factors such as insulin resistance (IR) dyslipidemia, endothelial connection, and systemic inflammation are other elements that add to this set of signs and symptoms and predispose patients to a higher risk of cardiovascular disease than women without PCOS [5,6]. Probably, the reduced insulin sensitivity leads to an inevitable compensatory hyperinsulinemia, and this contributes to the development of hyperandrogenism through a chronic stimulus directed toward the cells of the ovarian theca. Evidence has suggested a correlation between IR pathogenesis and vitamin D (VD) deficiency, placing hypovitaminosis as a causal factor for the metabolic syndrome in PCOS women [7]. The vitamin D receptor (VDR) is almost ubiquitously expressed, regulating at about 3% of human genome, counting the genes coding for glucose metabolism as well [8]. This suggests the role and the correlation of VD deficiency with PCOS symptoms such as T2DM, IR, and cardiovascular diseases. A meta-analysis provided evidence regarding the correlation of VD receptor polymorphisms and PCOS, identifying some susceptibility markers as well. To date, the use of metformin in PCOS patients represents a milestone in therapy for these patients [9,10]. Supplementation with natural molecules, such as VD, may help overcome PCOS-related symptoms [11]. This review, analyzing data from the published literature on PubMed, identifies the different possible contribution of VD deficiency in the physiopathology of PCOS, and aims to show how VD supplementation to common therapy results in improved IR, reduced circulating androgens, and improved response to ovulation induction in women with PCOS.

The Pathophysiology of PCOS

The 2003 Rotterdam workshop consensus, in accordance with the recommendations of the European Society of Human Reproduction and Embryology (ESHRE) [12], established criteria for diagnosis based on the association of at least two of three clinical features: (i) clinical or biochemical signs of androgen excess, such as acne, alopecia, and hirsutism; (ii) ovarian dysfunction with oligo-/anovulation; and (iii) polycystic ovaries on ultrasound examination.

These criteria were utilized to classify patients into four different phenotypes [13]: (i) phenotype A, the most prevalent, which is characterized by clinical and/or biochemical hyperandrogenism, menstrual dysfunction (oligo/amenorrhea), and ultrasonographic evidence of polycystic ovaries; (ii) phenotype B, characterized by hyperandrogenism, and menstrual dysfunction (oligo/amenorrhea); (iii) phenotype C is characterized by hyperandrogenism, and polycystic ovarian morphology; (iv) phenotype D, defined by oligomenorrhea, polycystic ovarian morphology, and normal androgens.

The exact etiology of PCOS remains poorly understood to date. The pathophysiological picture of PCOS is complex and involves several elements: the ovary, the hypothalamus, and genetic susceptibility and metabolic syndrome. Recently, IR and hyperandrogenism have assumed the role of key factors in the genesis of this disease [14]. Certainly, the first deficit is functional ovarian hyperandrogenism (FOH), caused by steroidogenic hyperactivity, which disrupts ovarian synthesis of both androgens and estrogens [15]. The main cause of FOH can be attributed to increased secretion by the hypothalamus of GnRH and subsequent release of LH by the pituitary gland. This improper secretion is manifested by an elevated LH/FSH ratio. Consequently, there will be increased thecal secretion of androgens, which is manifested by the presence of small and numerous growing antral follicles. These follicles are found to be more resistant to the hormonal activity of FSH and, consequently, the increased concentration of LH will inhibit the proliferation of granulosa cells, causing their premature luteinization. This abnormality associated with reduced sensitivity to FSH leads to blockage of follicular maturation, resulting in oligo-/anovulation [16]. Overstimulation of theca cells by LH is exacerbated by insulin, which acts directly through the insulin receptor or indirectly through the growth factor 1 (IGF-1) receptor [17].

2. Vitamin D

VD regulates calcium metabolism and bone mineralization. VD exists in two forms: ergocalciferol (VD2) and cholecalciferol (VD3). VD3 is of animal origin and is synthesized endogenously in the human body. Ultraviolet radiation from the sun's rays acts on the skin and converts 7-dehydrocholesterol to a pre-vitamin form that is subsequently converted to VDFor VD activation, two different hydroxylations are required: the first occurs in the liver where the enzyme 25-hydroxylase metabolizes VD to 25-hydroxyvitamin D (25-OH-D). Subsequently, 25-OH-D is transported to the kidneys where it undergoes the second hydroxylation; thus 1,25-dihydroxyvitamin D (1,25-OH-D) or calcitriol, the biologically active form of VD, is formed [18].

It is estimated that there are 1 billion people who are VD-deficient or VD-insufficient in the world. The Endocrine Society of North America has defined VD deficiency as 25-OH-D levels < 20 ng/mL and insufficiency as 20–30 ng/mL. Numerous studies state with certainty that deficiency of this hormone is linked to IR, impaired glucose and lipid metabolism, and ultimately infertility—scenarios commonly seen in women with PCOS [19,20].

VDR is a transcription factor that, by eliciting the genomic actions of VD, is able to regulate several endocrine and cell functions including calcium metabolism. Both VD and calcium are known to be associated with endocrine dysfunctions, insulin resistance, and type 2 diabetes in PCOS [3].

All of this information, along with the reported key role of VDR in the regulation more than 3% of the human genome, prompted researchers to examine the real contribution of the VDR gene polymorphisms in metabolic and endocrine disturbance of PCOS [21,22]. Despite some evidence pointing to an influence of VDR gene variants in PCOS features, it is difficult to definitively establish a clear association of VDR polymorphisms with the development of PCOS [23].

2.1. Vitamin D Deficiency and PCOS Phenotypes

Interestingly, it has been shown that low VD levels may worsen PCOS symptoms, so that an inverse correlation has been reported between serum VD level and metabolic and hormonal disturbances of PCOS [7,20,24].

Few studies investigated the relationship between VD deficiency and PCOS phenotypes. Davis et al. analyzed PCOS women, grouped into three diagnostic phenotypes according to the Rotterdam criteria: (i) group 1, women with ovulatory dysfunction and polycystic ovaries; (ii) group 2, women with ovulatory dysfunction and androgen excess; (iii) group 3, women with ovulatory dysfunction associated with polycystic ovaries and androgen excess. According to this study, a higher prevalence of VD deficiency in PCOS cases with androgen excess may be demonstrated [25].

Maktabi et al. performed a placebo-controlled trial on VD-deficient (serum concentrations < 20 ng/mL) women with phenotype B-PCOS according to the Rotterdam criteria. After the 12-week intervention, VD supplementation significantly decreased fasting plasma glucose, insulin, HOMA-IR index, and increased quantitative insulin sensitivity [26].

The main mechanisms described in this review that have a key role in the direct and indirect activity of VD on female fertility are plotted in Figure 1.

2.2. Vitamin D, Hypothalamic–Pituitary–Gonadal Axis, and Androgen Levels

Despite numerous studies investigating the effects of VD on reproductive function and gonadal hormone production, our knowledge about the mechanism by which VD affects reproductive physiology is still limited.

Regarding to the impact of VD on the hypothalamic–pituitary–gonadal (HPG) axis, an interesting insight comes from mini-puberty, the period of time within the first few months of life during which a transient activation of the HPG axis correlates to a brief activation of gonadal hormone production [27].

This HPG activation is important for future gonadal function. According to Kılınç et al., there is an association between 25-OH-D levels and gonadal hormones at mini-puberty. Total testosterone level was higher and inhibin B was lower in 25OH-D deficient than sufficient girls, while a modest effect of 25OH-D was identified on total testosterone and inhibin B. Therefore, the 25OH-D seems to have an effect on gonadal function during early life [28].

In regard to androgen levels, a study demonstrated a positive relationship between serum VD level and total testosterone and free androgen index. Therefore, this finding lets us hypothesize that VD may improve female fertility by modulating androgenic activity [29]. This is not surprising, since VD is able to affect the expression and activities of some of the enzymes involved in the production of sex hormones [24,30,31] (see *Vitamin D, Ovarian Physiology and Oxidative Stress Section*).

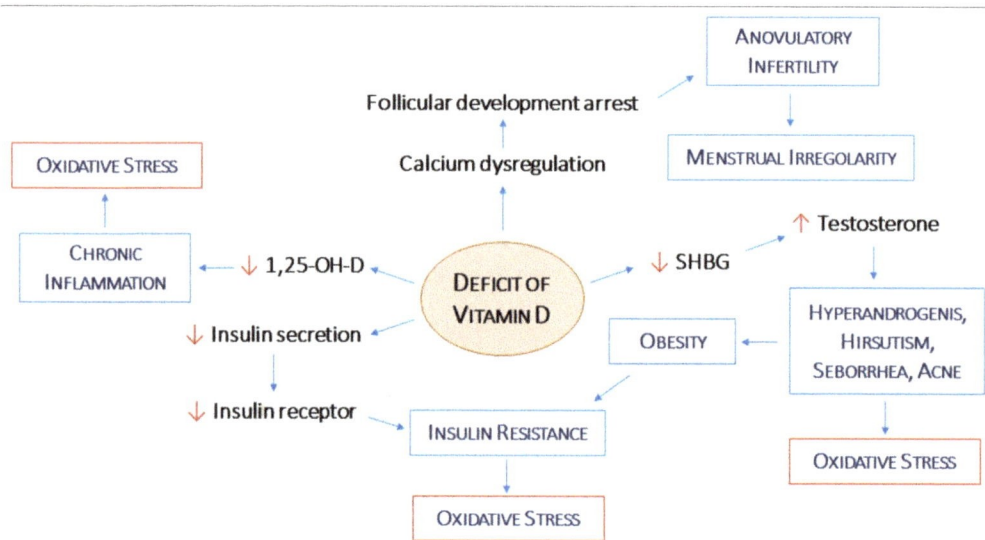

Figure 1. Relationship of vitamin D deficiency with the pathogenesis of insulin resistance and the metabolic syndrome in PCOS, hormonal alteration, and infertility. (1,25-OH-D: 1,25-hydroxyvitamin D; SHBG: Sex Hormone Binding Globulin).

Confirming this, numerous studies associated VD deficiency with an alteration in serum levels of dehydroepiandrosterone, testosterone, sex hormone binding globulin (SHBG), and free androgen. In particular, testosterone is reported to be significantly higher in patients with PCOS compared to non-PCOS controls. The effect of VD supplementation on regulating testosterone unbalance is reported by a pilot study [32], conducted on overweight women with PCOS and VD deficiency that have been supplemented with high doses of this vitamin and calcium daily. This treatment induced, after 3 months, a significant reduction in the total level of testosterone and androstenedione. This is a proof of concept of the direct effects of VD and calcium supplementation on the steroidogenesis pathway (ovarian and/or adrenal). Therefore, all these data suggest potential therapeutic benefits of VD and calcium supplementation in ameliorating hormonal milieu and PCOS related sequelae in women deficient in VD.

2.3. Vitamin D, Ovarian Physiology, and Oxidative Stress

Many studies have demonstrated that VD can alter anti-Mullerian hormone (AMH) signaling, follicle stimulating hormone (FSH) sensitivity, and progesterone (P) production and release in human granulosa cells, indicating a possible physiologic role for VD in ovarian follicular development and luteinization [33,34]. Indeed, in human luteinized granulosa cells, VD decreases the expression of both the AMH receptor and FSH receptor. Following follicular selection in a women's late follicular phase, the follicle becomes less dependent on FSH and more dependent on LH, followed by terminal maturation and ovulation. AMH and FSH receptor expression in granulosa cells has been found to be the highest in small immature follicles and to diminishes gradually with the progression of the maturation of oocytes [35,36].

On the other hand, animal models have shown that VD stimulates ovarian steroidogenesis by inducing the expression of both dehydroepiandrosterone sulfotransferase (DHEAS), an enzyme that mediates sulfo-conjugation of endogenous hydroxysteroids, and of aromatase [37–39]. Moreover, VD has been also reported to increase in vitro 3β-hydroxysteroid dehydrogenase (3β-HSD) RNA levels, possibly reflecting a state of granulosa cells luteinization [39,40]. Finally, it has been reported that VD may change the expression of the aromatase, the enzyme catalyzing the biosynthesis of estrogen, which is an androgen precursor [29,41,42].

PCOS women show elevated levels of advanced glycation end products (AGEs), a pro-inflammatory molecule family. AGEs and their receptors may contribute to the pathogenesis of PCOS, with negative consequences on metabolic and reproductive fields. Data from the literature indicate that VD might improve the PCOS phenotype and could alleviate the detrimental effects of AGEs [43]. According to these data, VD may play a pivotal role in enhancing key steroidogenic enzymes, thus potentiating granulosa cell luteinization and providing a better ovarian environment [44].

VD is an essential antioxidant because of its ability to control systemic inflammation, oxidative stress, and mitochondrial respiratory function in humans [45]. Interestingly, various studies reported the presence of oxidative stress in PCOS patients. Indeed, key oxidative stress markers such as malondialdehyde (MDA), nitric oxide (NO) advanced glycosylated end products (AGEs), and xanthine oxidase are increased in PCOS patients [46]. Moreover, mitochondrial dysfunction, along with the correlated increased ROS production, explains the oxidative status in PCOS patients, even if it should be mentioned that the oxidative status varied between individuals because of changes in lifestyle, diet, and antioxidant uptake.

In this context, the well described antioxidant activity of VD seems to play a pivotal role. In the presence of physiologic concentration of VD, nuclear factor-E2-related factor 2 (Nrf2) transcription is activated through VDRE, and then Nrf2 translocates from the cytoplasm to the nucleus, thus activating the expression of several genes with antioxidant activity [45]. Therefore, low levels of VD are correlated to decreased Nrf2 transcription and, in turn, to increased risks from oxidative stress-related tissue damage.

2.4. Vitamin D, Insulin Resistance, and Obesity

Insulin resistance (IR) is one of the more specific traits of PCOS, and is mainly marked in obese women, suggesting that PCOS and obesity have a synergistic effect on the magnitude of the insulin disorder, leading to increased insulin secretion by pancreatic β-cells and compensatory hyperinsulinemia [47]. IR and related hyperinsulinemia have been linked to all symptoms of the syndrome, such as reproductive disorders, hyperandrogenism, acne, hirsutism, and metabolic disturbances. Finally, insulin resistance in PCOS may be considered a risk factor for gestational diabetes [48]. To this regard, one theory relies on the regulatory effect of VD on the intracellular and extracellular calcium level that is essential for insulin-mediated intracellular processes and may have impact on insulin secretion [49–52]. Another hypothesis involves the stimulatory effect of VD on the expression of insulin receptors leading to the increase of insulin sensitivity. Indeed, VD activates the transcription of the VD response element (VDRE) of the human insulin gene [53].

In the clinical practice, many studies stressed that serum 25OH-D is negatively correlated with body mass index (BMI) [54–57]. In women with type 2 diabetes mellitus, an association between low levels of VD and increased insulin resistance was found [58].

There is some proof suggesting that VD deficiency might be involved in the pathogenesis of insulin resistance in PCOS [59,60]. VD deficiency is a contributing factor to IR, obesity, and metabolic syndrome, all of which are commonly associated with ovulatory dysfunction; indeed, a VD supplement implies a better and healthier ovarian physiology [61–63].

In any case, what may be the mechanisms underlying the association of low 25OH-D levels and insulin resistance is still a matter of debate. It is of note that the association of obesity with VD deficiency warrants more discussion, since it is not well understood if VD deficiency comes from obesity (e.g., VD may be trapped in fat tissues) and/or if obesity is due to VD insufficiency [64].

Ott et al. investigated the correlation between serum 25OH-D concentrations and metabolic parameters in obese and non-obese women with PCOS [65]. The serum 25OH-D mean levels were lower in obese PCOS patients. There was an association of increased

HOMA-IR, BMI, triglycerides, and total testosterone, with decreased 25OH-D concentrations in obese PCOS patients.

Gallea et al. evaluated the role of body weight on the serum VD levels in women with or without PCOS. Results show that VD levels were lower in obese PCOS, and VD serum levels were comparable between normoinsulinemic lean PCOS women and controls. In conclusion, weight and hyperinsulinemia had a significant influence on these values [66].

More recently, one study has showed that VD supplement in obese female and deficient adolescents was associated with significant rising in insulin sensitivity [63]. After 6 months, although there were no significant differences between groups in BMI, serum inflammatory markers, and plasma glucose concentrations, women supplemented with VD had increased serum 25OH-D concentrations and significantly reduced HOMA-IR (marker of insulin resistance) and fasting plasma insulin. According to these results, the association of low VD levels with insulin resistance might, at least in part, be mediated by obesity.

However, the association of VD deficiency with insulin resistance may also be explained by mechanisms other than obesity. First of all, it has been reported that VD may improve insulin activity by stimulating VDR gene expression. Indeed, it is known that VDR is present in the promoter of the human insulin gene [67], and that 1,25OH-D3 is able to induce the transcription of the human insulin gene [53]. Moreover, VD may affect insulin-responsiveness through calcium, since insulin secretion is a calcium-dependent process [51]. Finally, by means of its immunomodulatory effect [68], low levels of VD may induce an inflammatory response, which is again associated with insulin resistance [69].

3. Relevance of Supplementation

3.1. Impact of Vitamin D Supplementation on Biomarkers of Oxidative Stress in PCOS

The effectiveness of VD supplementation on the reduction of biomarkers of inflammation and oxidative stress among women with polycystic ovary syndrome is controversial (Figure 2).

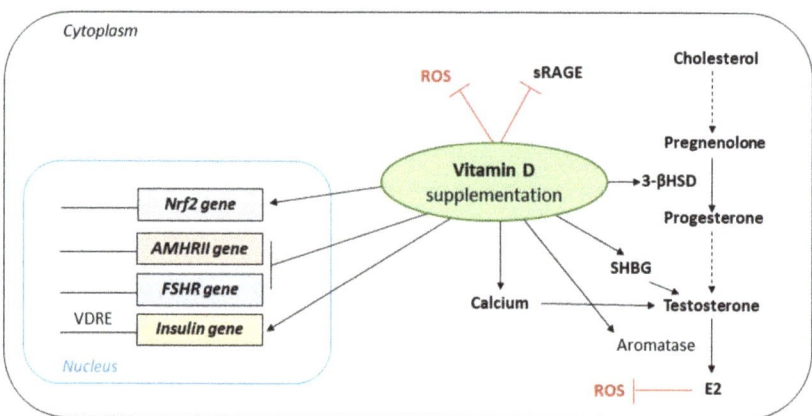

Figure 2. Impact of vitamin D supplementation on ovarian cells physiology. (Nrf2: Nuclear factor erythroid 2-related factor 2; AMHRII: Anti-Müllerian Hormone Receptor type 2; FSHR: Follicle Stimulating Hormone Receptor; VDRE: Vitamin D Response Element; ROS: Reactive Oxygen Species; sRAGE: Soluble Form of the Receptor for Advanced Glycation Endproduct; 3-βHSD: 3β-Hydroxysteroid dehydrogenase; SHBG: Sex Hormone Binding Globulin; E2: Estradiol).

A recent systematic review and meta-analysis of randomized controlled trials provided evidence for a significant improvement in high-sensitivity C-reactive protein, MDA, and total antioxidant capacity in women with PCOS receiving a VD supplementation, while no effects were reported for both nitric oxide (NO) and glutathione (GSH) levels [70].

Others studies have reported that VD showed benefit in improving oxidative stress [26,71]. A randomized double-blind placebo-controlled clinical trial involving 104 overweight VD-deficient PCOS women were randomly supplemented with 1000 mg calcium daily and/or 50,000 IU VD weekly for 8 weeks. The combined calcium plus VD supplements had greater decreases in plasma MDA concentrations, and significant increases in plasma total antioxidant capacity and GSH levels compared with calcium alone, VD alone, and placebo groups, suggesting that calcium plus VD co-supplementation had beneficial effects on inflammatory factors and biomarkers of oxidative stress [71]. Interestingly, the co-administration of VD and probiotic for 12 weeks to women with PCOS was demonstrated to significantly improve the serum levels of high-sensitivity C-reactive protein, plasma total antioxidant capacity, GSH, and MDA [72].

Despite these findings, others studies did not observe a beneficial effect from VD supplementation [73]. Further studies are needed to define the effects of only VD on biomarkers of inflammation and oxidative stress.

3.2. Vitamin D Supplementation and Fertility Outcomes in PCOS Women

In PCOS women, VD is related to menstrual irregularity, altered follicular development, ovulatory dysfunction, metabolic alterations, and decreased pregnancy rate [34,74–76].

In a prospective cohort study, the parathyroid hormone (PTH), the active form 1,25-hydroxy vitamin D3 (1,25OH-D3), and testosterone were measured in infertile women with PCOS undergoing clomiphene citrate stimulation [65]. This study demonstrated that high PTH hormone levels correlated with low serum calcium and low 1,25OH-D3, whereas high PTH was associated with high body mass index and with higher testosterone serum levels. When comparing women who had developed a follicle with those who were resistant after stimulation with 50 mg of clomiphene citrate, lower 1,25OH-D3 serum levels were detected in resistant ones. Moreover, significantly improved pregnancy rate was highlighted in women with higher BMI and lower 1,25OH-D3 serum levels. Finally, the significant correlation between lower 1,25OH-D3 serum levels and lower follicle development after stimulation with 50 mg of clomiphene citrate may be ascribed to the well reported role of 1,25OH-D3 in ovarian activity.

The effects of calcium-VD and metformin supplementation on the menstrual cycle and ovulation of patients with PCOS was investigated in a randomized clinical trial, enrolling 60 infertile PCOS patients [74]. Menstrual regularity and the number of dominant follicles (≥ 14 mm) during the 2–3 months of follow-up was higher in the calcium-vitamin D plus metformin group than in either of the other two groups.

Fang et al. evaluated the effect of VD supplementation on patients with PCOS. According to this review, VD supplementation significantly improves follicular development with a higher number of dominant follicles. Moreover, the combined supplementation with metformin plus VD improves the regularity of the menstrual cycles [77].

There is evidence suggesting that 25OH-D may also play an important role during pregnancy, but data regarding VD deficiency during gestation in PCOS patients and its association with perinatal outcome is limited. It is already well known that vitamin supplementation is safe and improves VD and calcium status; also, during pregnancy, sufficient 25(OH)D supplementation can prevent neonatal hypocalcemia, which may result in the softening of bones. VD supplementation decreased the risk of babies being small for gestational age and increased birth weight [78]. Therefore, these observations enable us to hypothesize the beneficial effects of VD supplementation in patients with PCOS seeking a pregnancy.

It is of note that a relationship exists between VD and markers of ovarian reserve. AMH is a glycoprotein produced by granulosa cells of primary follicles in the ovaries and then secreted in the blood and is considered to be one of the best ovarian reserve markers [33,79]; its expression and serum levels are altered by environmental factors, such as VD deficiency and obesity. The non-significant fluctuation of AMH during the menstrual cycle represents a strength over the other ovarian reserve markers (such as day 3 FSH), making it clinically useful and convenient. Investigators identified a functional VDRE in the promoter region of the human AMH gene, which demonstrates a potential direct effect of VD on AMH expression [80].

In the serum, 25OH-D is positively correlated with AMH, and appropriate VD supplementation in VD-depleted women can suppress the seasonal changes that occur in serum AMH. In VD-deficient women with PCOS, VD supplementation lowers the abnormally elevated serum AMH levels, possibly indicating a mechanism by which VD improves folliculogenesis [33,81].

The huge number of observational studies described in the following paragraphs of this review, shedding light on the association between VD status with PCOS, are summarized in Table 1.

Table 1. Summary of observational studies.

Issue	References	Main Outcomes
Vitamin D deficienc and PCOS phenotypes	[7,20,24]	VD low levels may worsen PCOS symptoms; an inverse correlation has been reported between serum VD level and metabolic and hormonal disturbances in different PCOS phenotypes.
	[25,26]	A higher prevalence of VD deficiency in PCOS cases with androgen excess may be demonstrated. In the B-PCOS phenotype, VD supplementation significantly decreased fasting plasma glucose, insulin, HOMA-IR index, and increased quantitative insulin sensitivity.
Vitamin D, PG axis, and androgen levels	[29]	VD may improve female fertility by modulating androgenic activity.
	[28]	Association between 25-OH-D levels and gonadal hormones at mini-puberty.
	[30,31]	VD is able to affect the expression and activities of some of the enzymes involved in the production of sex hormones.
	[32]	Effect of VD supplementation on regulating testosterone unbalance.
Vitamin D, ovarian physiology, and oxidative stress	[46]	Oxidative stress markers are increased in PCOS patients.
	[45]	Low levels of VD are correlated to decreased Nrf2 transcription and increased risks from oxidative stress-related tissue damage.
	[33,34]	VD shows a possible physiologic role in ovarian follicular development and luteinization, and VD supplement can contribute to these processes.
	[35,36]	In human luteinized granulosa cells, VD decreases the expression of both the AMH receptor and FSH receptor.
	[37,39]	VD stimulates ovarian steroidogenesis by inducing the expression of DHEAS and aromatase.
	[39,40]	VD increases the 3β-HSD RNA levels in vitro, possibly reflecting a state of granulosa cell luteinization.
	[29,41,42]	VD may change the expression of the aromatase, the enzyme catalyzing the biosynthesis of estrogen, which is an androgen precursor.

Table 1. *Cont.*

Issue	References	Main Outcomes
Vitamin D, insulin resistance, and obesity	[61–63]	VD deficiency is a contributing factor to IR, obesity, and metabolic syndrome, all of which are commonly associated with ovulatory dysfunction: a VD supplement implies a better and healthier ovarian physiology.
	[64]	Association between concentration of VD and obesity has been strongly demonstrated both in adults and in adolescents: adipose tissue decreases circulating 25OH-D by trapping it.
	[65]	Association of increased HOMA-IR, BMI, triglycerides, and total testosterone, with decreased 25OH-D concentrations in the obese PCOS patients.
	[66]	Weight and hyperinsulinemia had a significant influence on these values: VD levels were lower in obese PCOS women, and VD serum levels were comparable between normoinsulinemic PCOS women and controls.
	[53,67]	VD may improve insulin activity by stimulating VDR gene expression. VDR is present in the promoter of the human insulin gene and 1,25OH-D3 is able to induce the transcription of the human insulin gene.
	[51]	VD may affect insulin-responsiveness through calcium, since insulin secretion is a calcium-dependent process.
	[68,69]	VD shows an immunomodulatory effect: low levels of VD may induce an inflammatory response, which is associated with insulin resistance.
Vitamin D supplementation and oxidative stress in PCOS	[70]	Significant improvement in high-sensitivity C-reactive protein, MDA, and total antioxidant capacity in women with PCOS receiving VD supplementation, while no effects were reported for NO and GSH levels.
	[71]	The combined calcium plus VD supplements had greater decreases in plasma MDA concentrations, and significant increases in plasma total antioxidant capacity and GSH levels compared with calcium alone, VD alone, and placebo groups.
	[72]	Co-administration of VD and probiotic to women with PCOS significantly improved the serum levels of high-sensitivity C-reactive protein, plasma total antioxidant capacity, GSH, and MDA.
	[73]	Beneficial effects from VD supplementation were not observed.
Vitamin D and fertility outcomes in PCOS women	[74,76]	VD is related to menstrual irregularity, altered follicular development, ovulatory dysfunction, metabolic alterations, and decreased pregnancy rate.
	[82]	Significant improvement in regulating menstrual abnormalities and follicle maturation in women receiving calcium and VD supplementation.
	[77]	The combined supplementation with metformin plus VD improves the regularity of the menstrual cycles.
	[33,79]	Relationship between VD and AMH: its expression and serum levels are altered by environmental factors, such as VD deficiency and obesity. In the serum, 25OH-D is positively correlated with AMH, and appropriate VD supplementation in VD-depleted women can suppress the seasonal changes that occur in serum AMH. In VD-deficient women with PCOS, VD supplementation lowers the abnormally elevated serum AMH levels, possibly indicating a mechanism by which VD improves folliculogenesis.

4. Conclusions

VD has protective effects on the cardiovascular system and on chronic and autoimmune diseases, regulates the expression of genes involved in glucose and lipid metabolism, and plays a key role in the reproductive system of women [6,45,83]. VD deficiency has been shown to be associated with many of the signs present in PCOS: ovulatory dysfunction, hyperandrogenism, insulin resistance, diabetes and dyslipidemia, adiposity indices, and systemic proinflammatory environments [25,64,84].

In general, PCOS women have lower 25-OH-D levels compared to healthy controls, even if the mechanisms involved in this dysfunction are still debated. In addition, association exists between VD levels and obesity. Moreover, despite conflicting results, this review highlighted an increased oxidative stress level in women with PCOS.

The in-depth knowledge of these mechanisms might potentially lead to this oral, rather safe and cost-effective vitamin becoming an adjunct treatment in therapies for PCOS patients. To this regard, in the clinical management of PCOS patients, the measurement of VD serum levels, along with other endocrine markers and the patient's phospho-calcium metabolism, should be always recommended. This will lead the clinician to evaluate the oral VD dose necessary, in association with other more specific therapies. This approach may be an effective weapon in obese women and in the treatment of PCOS patients with insulin-resistance. Excluding kidney, liver, or internistic disease that modifies absorption, after evaluation of VD3 dose requirement, data from the literature suggest that the dose of 1000 IU per day corresponding to 25 mcg seems to be the most effective at raising 25-OH-D levels to sufficient amounts, during three months of therapy in PCOS women with VD deficiency [85].

Future contributions of VD should have broad significance to increase natural conception in women with PCOS with an aim to decrease costs related to in vitro fertilization procedures. In conclusion, based on these data, we suggest that VD administration in PCOS women can represent a safe strategy to improve their symptoms without adverse effects.

Author Contributions: Conceptualization, G.M., S.L. and V.D.L.; investigation, L.G., A.L., A.S. and I.D.; writing—original draft preparation, L.G., A.L. and I.D.; writing—review and editing, P.P., V.D.L. and G.M.; supervision, G.M. All authors have read and agreed to the published version of the manuscript.

Funding: This research received no external funding.

Institutional Review Board Statement: Not applicable.

Informed Consent Statement: Not applicable.

Data Availability Statement: Not applicable.

Conflicts of Interest: The authors declare no conflict of interest.

References

1. Azziz, R. Introduction: Determinants of Polycystic Ovary Syndrome. *Fertil. Steril.* **2016**, *106*, 4–5. [CrossRef] [PubMed]
2. Bozdag, G.; Mumusoglu, S.; Zengin, D.; Karabulut, E.; Yildiz, B.O. The Prevalence and Phenotypic Features of Polycystic Ovary Syndrome: A Systematic Review and Meta-Analysis. *Hum. Reprod. Oxf. Engl.* **2016**, *31*, 2841–2855. [CrossRef] [PubMed]
3. De Leo, V.; Musacchio, M.C.; Cappelli, V.; Massaro, M.G.; Morgante, G.; Petraglia, F. Genetic, Hormonal and Metabolic Aspects of PCOS: An Update. *Reprod. Biol. Endocrinol. RBE* **2016**, *14*, 38. [CrossRef]
4. Teede, H.; Deeks, A.; Moran, L. Polycystic Ovary Syndrome: A Complex Condition with Psychological, Reproductive and Metabolic Manifestations That Impacts on Health across the Lifespan. *BMC Med.* **2010**, *8*, 41. [CrossRef] [PubMed]
5. De Groot, P.C.M.; Dekkers, O.M.; Romijn, J.A.; Dieben, S.W.M.; Helmerhorst, F.M. PCOS, Coronary Heart Disease, Stroke and the Influence of Obesity: A Systematic Review and Meta-Analysis. *Hum. Reprod. Update* **2011**, *17*, 495–500. [CrossRef] [PubMed]
6. Sangaraju, S.L.; Yepez, D.; Grandes, X.A.; Talanki Manjunatha, R.; Habib, S. Cardio-Metabolic Disease and Polycystic Ovarian Syndrome (PCOS): A Narrative Review. *Cureus* **2022**, *14*, e25076. [CrossRef]
7. Wehr, E.; Pilz, S.; Schweighofer, N.; Giuliani, A.; Kopera, D.; Pieber, T.R.; Obermayer-Pietsch, B. Association of Hypovitaminosis D with Metabolic Disturbances in Polycystic Ovary Syndrome. *Eur. J. Endocrinol.* **2009**, *161*, 575–582. [CrossRef]
8. Shi, X.-Y.; Huang, A.-P.; Xie, D.-W.; Yu, X.-L. Association of Vitamin D Receptor Gene Variants with Polycystic Ovary Syndrome: A Meta-Analysis. *BMC Med. Genet.* **2019**, *20*, 32. [CrossRef]

1. Armanini, D.; Boscaro, M.; Bordin, L.; Sabbadin, C. Controversies in the Pathogenesis, Diagnosis and Treatment of PCOS: Focus on Insulin Resistance, Inflammation, and Hyperandrogenism. *Int. J. Mol. Sci.* **2022**, *23*, 4110. [CrossRef]
2. Smirnov, V.V.; Beeraka, N.M.; Butko, D.Y.; Nikolenko, V.N.; Bondarev, S.A.; Achkasov, E.E.; Sinelnikov, M.Y.; Sinelnikov, P.R.H. Updates on Molecular Targets and Epigenetic-Based Therapies for PCOS. *Reprod. Sci. Thousand Oaks Calif* **2022**. *online ahead of print*. [CrossRef] [PubMed]
3. Cappelli, V.; Musacchio, M.C.; Bulfoni, A.; Morgante, G.; De Leo, V. Natural Molecules for the Therapy of Hyperandrogenism and Metabolic Disorders in PCOS. *Eur. Rev. Med. Pharmacol. Sci.* **2017**, *21*, 15–29.
4. Rotterdam ESHRE/ASRM-Sponsored PCOS consensus workshop group Revised 2003 Consensus on Diagnostic Criteria and Long-Term Health Risks Related to Polycystic Ovary Syndrome (PCOS). *Hum. Reprod. Oxf. Engl.* **2004**, *19*, 41–47. [CrossRef] [PubMed]
5. Clark, N.M.; Podolski, A.J.; Brooks, E.D.; Chizen, D.R.; Pierson, R.A.; Lehotay, D.C.; Lujan, M.E. Prevalence of Polycystic Ovary Syndrome Phenotypes Using Updated Criteria for Polycystic Ovarian Morphology. *Reprod. Sci.* **2014**, *21*, 1034–1043. [CrossRef] [PubMed]
6. Zhang, Y.; Hu, M.; Jia, W.; Liu, G.; Zhang, J.; Wang, B.; Li, J.; Cui, P.; Li, X.; Lager, S.; et al. Hyperandrogenism and Insulin Resistance Modulate Gravid Uterine and Placental Ferroptosis in PCOS-like Rats. *J. Endocrinol.* **2020**, *246*, 247–263. [CrossRef]
7. Rosenfield, R.L.; Ehrmann, D.A. The Pathogenesis of Polycystic Ovary Syndrome (PCOS): The Hypothesis of PCOS as Functional Ovarian Hyperandrogenism Revisited. *Endocr. Rev.* **2016**, *37*, 467–520. [CrossRef]
8. Drummond, A.E. The Role of Steroids in Follicular Growth. *Reprod. Biol. Endocrinol.* **2006**, *4*, 16. [CrossRef] [PubMed]
9. Dupont, J.; Scaramuzzi, R.J. Insulin Signalling and Glucose Transport in the Ovary and Ovarian Function during the Ovarian Cycle. *Biochem. J.* **2016**, *473*, 1483. [CrossRef] [PubMed]
10. DeLuca, H.F. The Metabolism and Functions of Vitamin D. *Adv. Exp. Med. Biol.* **1986**, *196*, 361–375. [CrossRef] [PubMed]
11. Bikle, D.D. Vitamin D: Newer Concepts of Its Metabolism and Function at the Basic and Clinical Level. *J. Endocr. Soc.* **2020**, *4*, bvz038. [CrossRef]
12. Grzesiak, M. Vitamin D3 Action within the Ovary-an Updated Review. *Physiol. Res.* **2020**, *69*, 371–378. [CrossRef] [PubMed]
13. Kinuta, K.; Tanaka, H.; Moriwake, T.; Aya, K.; Kato, S.; Seino, Y. Vitamin D Is an Important Factor in Estrogen Biosynthesis of Both Female and Male Gonads. *Endocrinology* **2000**, *141*, 1317–1324. [CrossRef]
14. Mahmoudi, T. Genetic Variation in the Vitamin D Receptor and Polycystic Ovary Syndrome Risk. *Fertil. Steril.* **2009**, *92*, 1381–1383. [CrossRef] [PubMed]
15. Vulcan, T.; Filip, G.A.; Lenghel, L.M.; Suciu, T.; Ilut, P.; Procopciuc, L.M. Polymorphisms of Vitamin D Receptor and the Effect on Metabolic AndEndocrine Abnormalities in Polycystic Ovary Syndrome: A Review. *Horm. Metab. Res.* **2021**, *53*, 645–653. [CrossRef] [PubMed]
16. He, C.; Lin, Z.; Robb, S.W.; Ezeamama, A.E. Serum Vitamin D Levels and Polycystic Ovary Syndrome: A Systematic Review and Meta-Analysis. *Nutrients* **2015**, *7*, 4555–4577. [CrossRef] [PubMed]
17. Davis, E.M.; Peck, J.D.; Hansen, K.R.; Neas, B.R.; Craig, L.B. Associations between Vitamin D Levels and Polycystic Ovary Syndrome Phenotypes. *Minerva Endocrinol.* **2019**, *44*, 176–184. [CrossRef] [PubMed]
18. Maktabi, M.; Chamani, M.; Asemi, Z. The Effects of Vitamin D Supplementation on Metabolic Status of Patients with Polycystic Ovary Syndrome: A Randomized, Double-Blind, Placebo-Controlled Trial. *Horm. Metab. Res.* **2017**, *49*, 493–498. [CrossRef] [PubMed]
19. Kuiri-Hänninen, T.; Sankilampi, U.; Dunkel, L. Activation of the Hypothalamic-Pituitary-Gonadal Axis in Infancy: Minipuberty. *Horm. Res. Paediatr.* **2014**, *82*, 73–80. [CrossRef] [PubMed]
20. Kılınç, S.; Atay, E.; Ceran, Ö.; Atay, Z. Evaluation of Vitamin D Status and Its Correlation with Gonadal Function in Children at Mini-Puberty. *Clin. Endocrinol. (Oxf.)* **2019**, *90*, 122–128. [CrossRef]
21. Chang, E.M.; Kim, Y.S.; Won, H.J.; Yoon, T.K.; Lee, W.S. Association between Sex Steroids, Ovarian Reserve, and Vitamin D Levels in Healthy Nonobese Women. *J. Clin. Endocrinol. Metab.* **2014**, *99*, 2526–2532. [CrossRef] [PubMed]
22. Hahn, S.; Haselhorst, U.; Tan, S.; Quadbeck, B.; Schmidt, M.; Roesler, S.; Kimmig, R.; Mann, K.; Janssen, O.E. Low Serum 25-Hydroxyvitamin D Concentrations Are Associated with Insulin Resistance and Obesity in Women with Polycystic Ovary Syndrome. *Exp. Clin. Endocrinol. Diabetes* **2006**, *114*, 577–583. [CrossRef] [PubMed]
23. Lundqvist, J. Vitamin D as a Regulator of Steroidogenic Enzymes. *F1000Research* **2014**, *3*, 155. [CrossRef]
24. Pal, L.; Berry, A.; Coraluzzi, L.; Kustan, E.; Danton, C.; Shaw, J.; Taylor, H. Therapeutic Implications of Vitamin D and Calcium in Overweight Women with Polycystic Ovary Syndrome. *Gynecol. Endocrinol.* **2012**, *28*, 965–968. [CrossRef]
25. Irani, M.; Merhi, Z. Role of Vitamin D in Ovarian Physiology and Its Implication in Reproduction: A Systematic Review. *Fertil. Steril.* **2014**, *102*, 460–468.e3. [CrossRef] [PubMed]
26. Bianchi, L.; Gagliardi, A.; Landi, C.; Focarelli, R.; De Leo, V.; Luddi, A.; Bini, L.; Piomboni, P. Protein Pathways Working in Human Follicular Fluid: The Future for Tailored IVF? *Expert Rev. Mol. Med.* **2016**, *18*, e9. [CrossRef] [PubMed]
27. Bakhshalizadeh, S.; Amidi, F.; Alleyassin, A.; Soleimani, M.; Shirazi, R.; Shabani Nashtaei, M. Modulation of Steroidogenesis by Vitamin D3 in Granulosa Cells of the Mouse Model of Polycystic Ovarian Syndrome. *Syst. Biol. Reprod. Med.* **2017**, *63*, 150–161. [CrossRef] [PubMed]

36. Yao, X.; Zhang, G.; Guo, Y.; Ei-Samahy, M.; Wang, S.; Wan, Y.; Han, L.; Liu, Z.; Wang, F.; Zhang, Y. Vitamin D Receptor Expression and Potential Role of Vitamin D on Cell Proliferation and Steroidogenesis in Goat Ovarian Granulosa Cells. *Theriogenology* **2017**, *102*, 162–173. [CrossRef]
37. Echchgadda, I.; Song, C.S.; Roy, A.K.; Chatterjee, B. Dehydroepiandrosterone Sulfotransferase Is a Target for Transcriptional Induction by the Vitamin D Receptor. *Mol. Pharmacol.* **2004**, *65*, 720–729. [CrossRef]
38. Baka, S.; Malamitsi-Puchner, A. Novel Follicular Fluid Factors Influencing Oocyte Developmental Potential in IVF: A Review. *Reprod. Biomed. Online* **2006**, *12*, 500–506. [CrossRef]
39. Masjedi, F.; Keshtgar, S.; Zal, F.; Talaei-Khozani, T.; Sameti, S.; Fallahi, S.; Kazeroni, M. Effects of Vitamin D on Steroidogenesis, Reactive Oxygen Species Production, and Enzymatic Antioxidant Defense in Human Granulosa Cells of Normal and Polycystic Ovaries. *J. Steroid Biochem. Mol. Biol.* **2020**, *197*, 105521. [CrossRef]
40. Merhi, Z.; Doswell, A.; Krebs, K.; Cipolla, M. Vitamin D Alters Genes Involved in Follicular Development and Steroidogenesis in Human Cumulus Granulosa Cells. *J. Clin. Endocrinol. Metab.* **2014**, *99*, E1137–E1145. [CrossRef] [PubMed]
41. Usluogullari, B.; Duvan, C.; Usluogullari, C. Use of Aromatase Inhibitors in Practice of Gynecology. *J. Ovarian Res.* **2015**, *8*, 4. [CrossRef] [PubMed]
42. Krishnan, A.V.; Swami, S.; Peng, L.; Wang, J.; Moreno, J.; Feldman, D. Tissue-Selective Regulation of Aromatase Expression by Calcitriol: Implications for Breast Cancer Therapy. *Endocrinology* **2010**, *151*, 32–42. [CrossRef] [PubMed]
43. Merhi, Z. Crosstalk between Advanced Glycation End Products and Vitamin D: A Compelling Paradigm for the Treatment of Ovarian Dysfunction in PCOS. *Mol. Cell. Endocrinol.* **2019**, *479*, 20–26. [CrossRef] [PubMed]
44. Merhi, Z.; Buyuk, E.; Cipolla, M.J. Advanced Glycation End Products Alter Steroidogenic Gene Expression by Granulosa Cells: An Effect Partially Reversible by Vitamin D. *MHR Basic Sci. Reprod. Med.* **2018**, *24*, 318–326. [CrossRef]
45. Wimalawansa, S.J. Vitamin D Deficiency: Effects on Oxidative Stress, Epigenetics, Gene Regulation, and Aging. *Biology* **2019**, *8*, 30. [CrossRef]
46. Mohammadi, M. Oxidative Stress and Polycystic Ovary Syndrome: A Brief Review. *Int. J. Prev. Med.* **2019**, *10*, 86. [CrossRef] [PubMed]
47. Morgante, G.; Massaro, M.G.; Scolaro, V.; Cappelli, V.; Luddi, A.; Troìa, L.; De Leo, V. Metformin Doses and Body Mass Index: Clinical Outcomes in Insulin Resistant Polycystic Ovary Syndrome Women. *Eur. Rev. Med. Pharmacol. Sci.* **2020**, *24*, 8136–8142. [CrossRef] [PubMed]
48. De Leo, V.; Musacchio, M.C.; Morgante, G.; La Marca, A.; Petraglia, F. Polycystic Ovary Syndrome and Type 2 Diabetes Mellitus. *Minerva Ginecol.* **2004**, *56*, 53–62.
49. Lerchbaum, E.; Obermayer-Pietsch, B. Vitamin D and Fertility: A Systematic Review. *Eur. J. Endocrinol.* **2012**, *166*, 765–778. [CrossRef]
50. Pittas, A.G.; Lau, J.; Hu, F.B.; Dawson-Hughes, B. The Role of Vitamin D and Calcium in Type 2 Diabetes. A Systematic Review and Meta-Analysis. *J. Clin. Endocrinol. Metab.* **2007**, *92*, 2017–2029. [CrossRef]
51. Milner, R.D.; Hales, C.N. The Role of Calcium and Magnesium in Insulin Secretion from Rabbit Pancreas Studied in Vitro. *Diabetologia* **1967**, *3*, 47–49. [CrossRef] [PubMed]
52. Lerchbaum, E.; Rabe, T. Vitamin D and Female Fertility. *Curr. Opin. Obstet. Gynecol.* **2014**, *26*, 145–150. [CrossRef]
53. Maestro, B.; Molero, S.; Bajo, S.; Dávila, N.; Calle, C. Transcriptional Activation of the Human Insulin Receptor Gene by 1,25-Dihydroxyvitamin D(3). *Cell Biochem. Funct.* **2002**, *20*, 227–232. [CrossRef] [PubMed]
54. Rajakumar, K.; de las Heras, J.; Chen, T.C.; Lee, S.; Holick, M.F.; Arslanian, S.A. Vitamin D Status, Adiposity, and Lipids in Black American and Caucasian Children. *J. Clin. Endocrinol. Metab.* **2011**, *96*, 1560–1567. [CrossRef] [PubMed]
55. Oliveira, R.M.S.; Novaes, J.F.; Azeredo, L.M.; Azeredo, L.M.; Cândido, A.P.C.; Leite, I.C.G. Association of Vitamin D Insufficiency with Adiposity and Metabolic Disorders in Brazilian Adolescents. *Public Health Nutr.* **2014**, *17*, 787–794. [CrossRef] [PubMed]
56. Guasch, A.; Bulló, M.; Rabassa, A.; Bonada, A.; Del Castillo, D.; Sabench, F.; Salas-Salvadó, J. Plasma Vitamin D and Parathormone Are Associated with Obesity and Atherogenic Dyslipidemia: A Cross-Sectional Study. *Cardiovasc. Diabetol.* **2012**, *11*, 149. [CrossRef]
57. Ganie, M.A.; Marwaha, R.K.; Nisar, S.; Farooqi, K.J.; Jan, R.A.; Wani, S.A.; Gojwari, T.; Shah, Z.A. Impact of Hypovitaminosis D on Clinical, Hormonal and Insulin Sensitivity Parameters in Normal Body Mass Index Polycystic Ovary Syndrome Women. *J. Obstet. Gynaecol. J. Inst. Obstet. Gynaecol.* **2016**, *36*, 508–512. [CrossRef] [PubMed]
58. Alvarez, J.A.; Ashraf, A. Role of Vitamin d in Insulin Secretion and Insulin Sensitivity for Glucose Homeostasis. *Int. J. Endocrinol.* **2010**, *2010*, 351385. [CrossRef]
59. Li, H.W.R.; Brereton, R.E.; Anderson, R.A.; Wallace, A.M.; Ho, C.K.M. Vitamin D Deficiency Is Common and Associated with Metabolic Risk Factors in Patients with Polycystic Ovary Syndrome. *Metabolism.* **2011**, *60*, 1475–1481. [CrossRef]
60. Ngo, D.T.M.; Chan, W.P.; Rajendran, S.; Heresztyn, T.; Amarasekera, A.; Sverdlov, A.L.; O'Loughlin, P.D.; Morris, H.A.; Chirkov, Y.Y.; Norman, R.J.; et al. Determinants of Insulin Responsiveness in Young Women: Impact of Polycystic Ovarian Syndrome, Nitric Oxide, and Vitamin D. *Nitric Oxide Biol. Chem.* **2011**, *25*, 326–330. [CrossRef] [PubMed]
61. Menichini, D.; Facchinetti, F. Effects of Vitamin D Supplementation in Women with Polycystic Ovary Syndrome: A Review. *Gynecol. Endocrinol.* **2020**, *36*, 1–5. [CrossRef] [PubMed]
62. De Leo, V.; Cappelli, V.; Morgante, G.; Di Sabatino, A. The role of vitamin D in assisted reproduction techniques. *Minerva Ginecol.* **2018**, *70*, 268–285. [CrossRef]

63. Belenchia, A.M.; Tosh, A.K.; Hillman, L.S.; Peterson, C.A. Correcting Vitamin D Insufficiency Improves Insulin Sensitivity in Obese Adolescents: A Randomized Controlled Trial. *Am. J. Clin. Nutr.* **2013**, *97*, 774–781. [CrossRef] [PubMed]
64. Yildizhan, R.; Kurdoglu, M.; Adali, E.; Kolusari, A.; Yildizhan, B.; Sahin, H.G.; Kamaci, M. Serum 25-Hydroxyvitamin D Concentrations in Obese and Non-Obese Women with Polycystic Ovary Syndrome. *Arch. Gynecol. Obstet.* **2009**, *280*, 559–563. [CrossRef] [PubMed]
65. Ott, J.; Wattar, L.; Kurz, C.; Seemann, R.; Huber, J.C.; Mayerhofer, K.; Vytiska-Binstorfer, E. Parameters for Calcium Metabolism in Women with Polycystic Ovary Syndrome Who Undergo Clomiphene Citrate Stimulation: A Prospective Cohort Study. *Eur. J. Endocrinol.* **2012**, *166*, 897–902. [CrossRef]
66. Gallea, M.; Granzotto, M.; Azzolini, S.; Faggian, D.; Mozzanega, B.; Vettor, R.; Mioni, R. Insulin and Body Weight but Not Hyperandrogenism Seem Involved in Seasonal Serum 25-OH-Vitamin D3 Levels in Subjects Affected by PCOS. *Gynecol. Endocrinol.* **2014**, *30*, 739–745. [CrossRef]
67. Maestro, B.; Dávila, N.; Carranza, M.C.; Calle, C. Identification of a Vitamin D Response Element in the Human Insulin Receptor Gene Promoter. *J. Steroid Biochem. Mol. Biol.* **2003**, *84*, 223–230. [CrossRef]
68. Bikle, D. Nonclassic Actions of Vitamin D. *J. Clin. Endocrinol. Metab.* **2009**, *94*, 26–34. [CrossRef]
69. Shoelson, S.E.; Herrero, L.; Naaz, A. Obesity, Inflammation, and Insulin Resistance. *Gastroenterology* **2007**, *132*, 2169–2180. [CrossRef]
70. Akbari, M.; Ostadmohammadi, V.; Lankarani, K.B.; Tabrizi, R.; Kolahdooz, F.; Heydari, S.T.; Kavari, S.H.; Mirhosseini, N.; Mafi, A.; Dastorani, M.; et al. The Effects of Vitamin D Supplementation on Biomarkers of Inflammation and Oxidative Stress Among Women with Polycystic Ovary Syndrome: A Systematic Review and Meta-Analysis of Randomized Controlled Trials. *Horm. Metab. Res. Horm. Stoffwechselforschung Horm. Metab.* **2018**, *50*, 271–279. [CrossRef]
71. Foroozanfard, F.; Jamilian, M.; Bahmani, F.; Talaee, R.; Talaee, N.; Hashemi, T.; Nasri, K.; Asemi, Z.; Esmaillzadeh, A. Calcium plus Vitamin D Supplementation Influences Biomarkers of Inflammation and Oxidative Stress in Overweight and Vitamin D-Deficient Women with Polycystic Ovary Syndrome: A Randomized Double-Blind Placebo-Controlled Clinical Trial. *Clin. Endocrinol. (Oxf.)* **2015**, *83*, 888–894. [CrossRef] [PubMed]
72. Ostadmohammadi, V.; Jamilian, M.; Bahmani, F.; Asemi, Z. Vitamin D and Probiotic Co-Supplementation Affects Mental Health, Hormonal, Inflammatory and Oxidative Stress Parameters in Women with Polycystic Ovary Syndrome. *J. Ovarian Res.* **2019**, *12*, 5. [CrossRef] [PubMed]
73. Sepehrmanesh, Z.; Kolahdooz, F.; Abedi, F.; Mazroii, N.; Assarian, A.; Asemi, Z.; Esmaillzadeh, A. Vitamin D Supplementation Affects the Beck Depression Inventory, Insulin Resistance, and Biomarkers of Oxidative Stress in Patients with Major Depressive Disorder: A Randomized, Controlled Clinical Trial. *J. Nutr.* **2016**, *146*, 243–248. [CrossRef] [PubMed]
74. Rashidi, B.; Haghollahi, F.; Shariat, M.; Zayerii, F. The Effects of Calcium-Vitamin D and Metformin on Polycystic Ovary Syndrome: A Pilot Study. *Taiwan. J. Obstet. Gynecol.* **2009**, *48*, 142–147. [CrossRef]
75. Zec, I.; Tislaric-Medenjak, D.; Megla, Z.B.; Kucak, I. Anti-Müllerian Hormone: A Unique Biochemical Marker of Gonadal Development and Fertility in Humans. *Biochem. Medica* **2011**, *21*, 219–230. [CrossRef] [PubMed]
76. Chen, Y.; Zhi, X. Roles of Vitamin D in Reproductive Systems and Assisted Reproductive Technology. *Endocrinology* **2020**, *161*, bqaa023. [CrossRef] [PubMed]
77. Fang, F.; Ni, K.; Cai, Y.; Shang, J.; Zhang, X.; Xiong, C. Effect of Vitamin D Supplementation on Polycystic Ovary Syndrome: A Systematic Review and Meta-Analysis of Randomized Controlled Trials. *Complement. Ther. Clin. Pract.* **2017**, *26*, 53–60. [CrossRef] [PubMed]
78. Kollmann, M.; Obermayer-Pietsch, B.; Lerchbaum, E.; Feigl, S.; Hochstätter, R.; Pregartner, G.; Trummer, C.; Klaritsch, P. Vitamin D Concentrations at Term Do Not Differ in Newborns and Their Mothers with and without Polycystic Ovary Syndrome. *J. Clin. Med.* **2021**, *10*, 537. [CrossRef]
79. Dennis, N.A.; Houghton, L.A.; Jones, G.T.; van Rij, A.M.; Morgan, K.; McLennan, I.S. The Level of Serum Anti-Müllerian Hormone Correlates with Vitamin D Status in Men and Women but Not in Boys. *J. Clin. Endocrinol. Metab.* **2012**, *97*, 2450–2455. [CrossRef] [PubMed]
80. Malloy, P.J.; Peng, L.; Wang, J.; Feldman, D. Interaction of the Vitamin D Receptor with a Vitamin D Response Element in the Mullerian-Inhibiting Substance (MIS) Promoter: Regulation of MIS Expression by Calcitriol in Prostate Cancer Cells. *Endocrinology* **2009**, *150*, 1580–1587. [CrossRef] [PubMed]
81. Holzer, I.; Parry, J.P.; Beitl, K.; Pozderovic, B.; Marculescu, R.; Ott, J. Parameters for Calcium Metabolism in Women with Polycystic Ovary Syndrome Who Undergo Stimulation with Letrozole: A Prospective Cohort Study. *J. Clin. Med.* **2022**, *11*, 2597. [CrossRef] [PubMed]
82. Dehghani Firouzabadi, R.; Aflatoonian, A.; Modarresi, S.; Sekhavat, L.; MohammadTaheri, S. Therapeutic Effects of Calcium & Vitamin D Supplementation in Women with PCOS. *Complement. Ther. Clin. Pract.* **2012**, *18*, 85–88. [CrossRef]
83. Conway, G.; Dewailly, D.; Diamanti-Kandarakis, E.; Escobar-Morreale, H.F.; Franks, S.; Gambineri, A.; Kelestimur, F.; Macut, D.; Micic, D.; Pasquali, R.; et al. The Polycystic Ovary Syndrome: A Position Statement from the European Society of Endocrinology. *Eur. J. Endocrinol.* **2014**, *171*, P1–P29. [CrossRef] [PubMed]

84. Wild, R.A.; Rizzo, M.; Clifton, S.; Carmina, E. Lipid Levels in Polycystic Ovary Syndrome: Systematic Review and Meta-Analysis. *Fertil. Steril.* **2011**, *95*, 1073–1079.e11. [CrossRef] [PubMed]
85. Bacha, D.S.; Rahme, M.; Al-Shaar, L.; Baddoura, R.; Halaby, G.; Singh, R.J.; Mahfoud, Z.R.; Habib, R.; Arabi, A.; El-Hajj Fuleihan, G. Vitamin D3 Dose Requirement That Raises 25-Hydroxyvitamin D to Desirable Level in Overweight and Obese Elderly. *J. Clin. Endocrinol. Metab.* **2021**, *106*, e3644–e3654. [CrossRef] [PubMed]

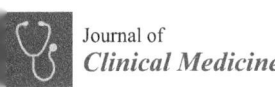

Systematic Review

DNA Methylation in Offspring Conceived after Assisted Reproductive Techniques: A Systematic Review and Meta-Analysis

Rossella Cannarella [1,*], Andrea Crafa [1], Laura M. Mongioì [1], Loredana Leggio [2], Nunzio Iraci [2], Sandro La Vignera [1], Rosita A. Condorelli [1] and Aldo E. Calogero [1]

1. Department of Clinical and Experimental Medicine, University of Catania, 95123 Catania, Italy
2. Department of Biomedical and Biotechnological Sciences (BIOMETEC), University of Catania, Torre Biologica, 95125 Catania, Italy
* Correspondence: rossella.cannarella@phd.unict.it

Abstract: Background: In the last 40 years, assisted reproductive techniques (ARTs) have emerged as potentially resolving procedures for couple infertility. This study aims to evaluate whether ART is associated with epigenetic dysregulation in the offspring. **Methods**. To accomplish this, we collected all available data on methylation patterns in offspring conceived after ART and in spontaneously conceived (SC) offspring. **Results**. We extracted 949 records. Of these, 50 were considered eligible; 12 were included in the quantitative synthesis. Methylation levels of *H19* CCCTC-binding factor 3 (CTCF3) were significantly lower in the ART group compared to controls (SMD −0.81 (−1.53; −0.09), I^2 = 89%, *p* = 0.03). In contrast, *H19* CCCTC-binding factor 6 (CTCF6), *Potassium Voltage-Gated Channel Subfamily Q Member 1* (*KCNQ1OT1*), *Paternally-expressed gene 3* (*PEG3*), and *Small Nuclear Ribonucleoprotein Polypeptide N* (*SNRPN*) were not differently methylated in ART vs. SC offspring. **Conclusion**: The methylation pattern of the offspring conceived after ART may be different compared to spontaneous conception. Due to the lack of studies and the heterogeneity of the data, further prospective and well-sized population studies are needed to evaluate the impact of ART on the epigenome of the offspring.

Keywords: DNA methylation; assisted reproductive technique; ART; offspring; epigenetics

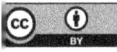

1. Introduction

Couple infertility represents a relevant public problem, burdening psychological health, economic, and social aspects of couples looking for children. The last report of the World Health Organization (WHO) on 277 health surveys concluded that 48 million couples suffered from infertility in 2010 [1]. Nowadays, the global prevalence of infertility is, very likely, even higher.

For the past 40 years, assisted reproductive techniques (ARTs) have emerged as potentially resolving procedures for couple infertility. They mainly include ovarian stimulation, fertilization (which can be achieved by in vitro fertilization (IVF) or by intracytoplasmic sperm injection (ICSI)), embryo culture, and embryo transfer. The first IVF baby was Louise Joy Brown who was born on 25 July 1978 [2]. Since then, ART has been broadly suggested to couples, even without being preceded by the attempt to identify and treat the etiological factors responsible for couple infertility [3]. The use of ICSI has increased from 36.4% in 1996 to 76.2% in 2012; although, the number of male-infertility cases did not change over time [4]. Moreover, some data indicate no real benefit from the use of ICSI (instead of IVF) in couples without male infertility, as the live birth rate seems 10% lower with ICSI than with IVF [5]. This may appear as an unjustified (or even blinded) use of ICSI [3].

In recent times, some data questioned the safety of ARTs. A retrospective longitudinal cohort study carried out on 797,657 children born in 2008–2019 reported a 1.23 times higher risk of hospitalization for any reason, 1.25 times higher risk of hospitalization for infection, and 1.25 times higher risk of hospitalization for allergy, in children conceived after ART compared to the spontaneously conceived (SC) siblings. These findings were not confirmed when a cohort of discordant siblings was used as a control [6]. Evidence from systematic reviews and meta-analyses suggested a trend towards a significantly increased risk of asthma (RR 1.31 (1.03–1.65)), but not allergies [7], a higher risk of autism [8] and of urogenital tract malformations (OR 1.42, (0.99–2.04)) [9] in offspring conceived after ART compared to controls. On the other hand, two recent longitudinal studies with a limited sample size failed in finding any difference in cardiometabolic profile and thyroid function between the ART and the non-ART cohort [10,11].

It has been speculated that the higher risk for adverse outcomes in the offspring conceived after ART could be due to epigenetic dysregulation [12,13]. In fact, the timing of ART procedures (ovarian stimulation, IVF/ICSI, embryo culture, and embryo transfer) coincides with crucial steps of embryo DNA methylation. DNA methylation takes place in the CpG islets, which are regions of the genome characterized by a large number of CpG dinucleotide repeats, and localized within the gene promoters. These regions are usually unmethylated and in specific circumstances (e.g., X-inactivation, genomic imprinting) undergo methylation to regulate gene expression. Indeed, hypermethylation generally interferes with chromatin accessibility, leading to gene silencing. In humans, more than 100 imprinted genes have been identified. They are clustered in differently methylated regions (DMR), which allow monoallelic gene expression [14]. During preimplantation development (day 1st to 5th), the embryo undergoes genome-wide demethylation and subsequent de novo methylation. The pattern of methylation of imprinted genes is not altered by this wave of reprogramming, thus ensuring their parent-specific expression [15].

An active debate is currently underway regarding the impact of ART on epigenetic reprogramming and imprinting in gametes and early embryos. In particular, there is no consensus on the possible effect of endogenous (gametes and embryo quality) and exogenous (e.g., light, cryopreservation, oxygen concentration, pH, temperature, culture media, mineral oil, humidity, centrifugation, etc.) factors in the ART setting responsible for increased reactive oxygen species (ROS) generation, which can lead to embryo epigenetic damage [16]. Furthermore, an abnormal methylation pattern has been reported in sperm from infertile men [17]. In turn, an altered methylation of imprinted genes at the sperm levels correlates with a poor ART outcome [18]. Whether the epigenetic risk of the ART-conceived offspring is due to the ART manipulation or to the epigenetic dysregulation of the gametes is still unknown.

To assess whether ART is associated with an epigenetic dysregulation in the offspring, we performed a systematic review and meta-analysis, and gathered all the available data on methylation patterns in the offspring conceived after ART and in SC offspring. In line with a recently published systematic review and meta-analysis [19], data were grouped based on the examined tissue (placenta, cord blood, buccal smear, and peripheral blood).

2. Methods

The articles were selected through extensive searches in the PubMed and Scopus databases from their establishment until May 2022. The search strategy included the combination of the following Medical Subjects Headings (MeSH) terms and keywords: "assisted reproductive techn*", "intracytoplasmic sperm injection", "ICSI", "in vitro fertilization", and "epigenetic".

The following search string was used to search the Scopus database: TITLE-ABS-KEY ((assisted AND reproductive AND techn*) OR (in AND vitro AND fertilization) OR (icsi) OR (intracytoplasmic AND sperm AND injection)) AND TITLE-ABS-KEY (epigenetic) AND (LIMIT-TO (DOCTYPE, "ar")) AND (EXCLUDE (EXACT KEY WORD, "Animals")) AND (EXCLUDE (SUBJAREA, "VETE")) AND (EXCLUDE (LANGUAGE, "French") OR EXCLUDE (LANGUAGE, "Russian") OR EXCLUDE (LANGUAGE, "German") OR EXCLUDE (LANGUAGE, "Chinese")). The search was limited to human studies and only English articles were selected. The above-mentioned search strategy belongs to an unregistered protocol.

Studies were first evaluated for inclusion by reading their abstracts. When the abstract did not help to decide whether the study contained data relevant to our meta-analysis, the full text was read carefully. The identification of eligible studies was carried out independently by two different researchers (A.C. and R.C.). Any disagreements were resolved by a third author (A.E.C.). Others articles were manually extracted by searching the reference lists of the articles selected by the above keywords.

The inclusion criteria are listed in Table 1. We considered for inclusion all studies that evaluated DNA methylation of offspring conceived using ARTs. Case reports, comments, letters to the editor, systematic or narrative reviews, and those studies that did not allow for extracting the outcomes of interest were excluded from the analysis. Two investigators (A.C. and R.C.) independently assessed the full text of the studies selected for eligibility. In case of disagreement, a third author (R.A.C. or A.E.C) decided against inclusion or exclusion after discussion.

Table 1. Inclusion criteria.

	Inclusion	Exclusion
Population	Human offspring	/
Intervention	ART (including IVF, ICSI, IUI, FET, ET, COS, OI)	/
Comparison	SC	/
Outcome	Methylation statuses of both imprinted and non-imprinted genes, global DNA methylation, evaluated in any kind of tissue and at any age	Aborted embryos
Study type	Observational, cohort, cross-sectional, and case-control	Case reports, comments, letters to the editor, systematic or narrative reviews, in vitro studies, studies on animals

Abbreviations. ART, assisted reproductive techniques; COS, controlled ovarian stimulation; ET, embryo transfer; FET, frozen embryo transfer; ICSI, intracytoplasmic sperm injection; IUI, intrauterine insemination; IVF, in vitro fertilization; OI, ovulation induction; SC, spontaneous conception.

The quality assessment of the articles included in this systematic review and meta-analysis was performed using the "Cambridge Quality Checklists" [20]. In detail, three domains are designed to identify high-quality studies of correlates, risk factors, and causal risk factors. The checklist for correlates consists of five items. Each item can be given a score of 0 or 1 for a total score of 5. This checklist evaluates the appropriateness of the sample size and the quality of the outcome measurements. The checklist for risk factors consists of three items; the selection of one of the 3 excludes the other two, with a maximum score of 3 points. This checklist assigns high-quality scores only to those studies with appropriate time-ordered data. Finally, there is the checklist for causal risk factors that evaluates the type of study design, assigning the highest score to randomized clinical trials (RCTs) and the lowest score to cross-sectional studies without a control group. The maximum score is seven. To draw confident conclusions about correlates, the correlate score must be high. This means that the sample size must be large and the outcome assessment must be adequate and reproducible. To draw confident conclusions about risk factors, both the checklists for correlates and risk factor scores must be high. Thus, the studies that allow the most reliable conclusions to be drawn are prospective studies. To draw confident conclusions about causal risk factors, all three-checklist scores must be high. Thus, in the absence of randomized clinical trials, confident conclusions can be drawn from studies with adequately controlled samples. Subgroup analyzes were performed based on the tissue in which methylation values were analyzed. Statistical heterogeneity was assessed by Cochran-Q and I^2 statistics. For $I^2 \leq 50\%$, the variation in the studies was considered homogenous and the fixed effect model was adopted. The random-effect model was used for $I^2 > 50\%$, underlying significant heterogeneity between studies. All p values ≤ 0.05 were considered statistically significant. The analysis was performed using RevMan software v. 5.3 (Cochrane Collaboration, Oxford, UK). The standard mean difference (SMD) with the 95% confidential interval (CI) was calculated for each outcome.

3. Results

Using the above-mentioned search strategy, we extracted 949 records. After the exclusion of 114 duplicates, the remaining 835 articles were assessed for inclusion in the systematic review. Of these, 167 were judged not pertinent after reading their title and abstract, 600 were excluded because they were reviews (n = 388), systematic reviews and meta-analyses (n = 4), and animal studies (n = 208). The remaining 68 articles were carefully read. Based on the inclusion and exclusion criteria, 15 articles were excluded because of the inability to extract the data required, and 3 were excluded because used miscarriage embryos [21–23]. Finally, 50 articles met our inclusion criteria and, therefore, were included in this meta-analysis (Figure 1).

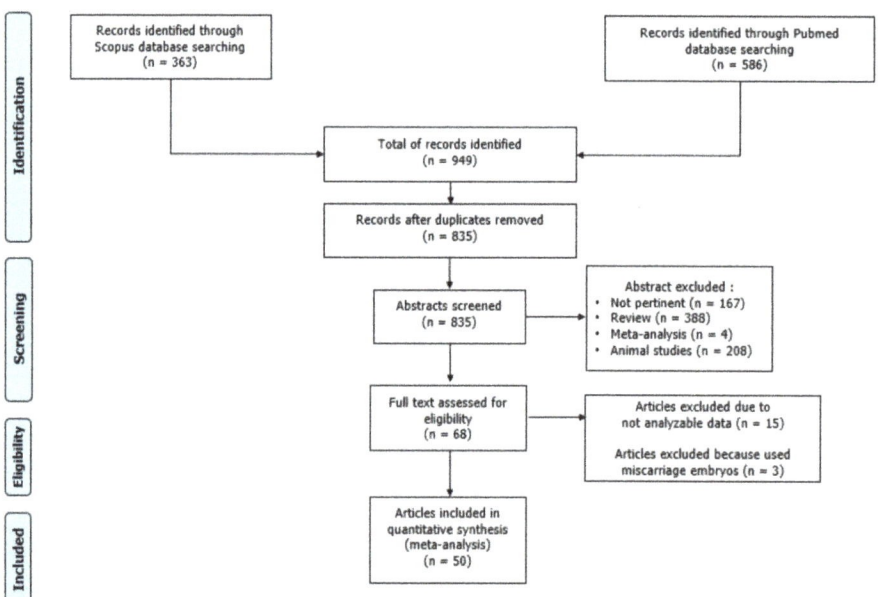

Figure 1. Flowchart of the included studies.

Information on the design of the studies, the type of population and sample analyzed, the methodology for assessing DNA methylation, and the outcomes analyzed are summarized in Table 2. Analysis of study quality showed that all studies had a low to medium risk of bias (Table 3).

Table 2. Main features of the included studies.

Author and Year	Study Design	Etiology of Infertility (M/F)	Paternal/Maternal Age (y)	Tissue	Timing	ART Group	SC Group (Parents' Fertility Status)	Outcome Assessed	Methylation Evaluation Method
Argyraki et al., 2021 [24]	Cross-sectional	NR	NR/35.2 ± 3.12	Cord blood	Birth	10	30 (10 delivered naturally, 10 by cesarean section in head position, 10 by cesarean section in breech position) (NS)	IGF2, MEST, PEG10	Methylation-specific PCR
Barberet et al., 2021 [25]	Cross-sectional	NR	NR	Buccal smear	Childhood	37 (16 IVF, 21 ICSI)	21 (fertile)	H19, SNURF, PEG3 KCNQ1, LINE1, AluYa5	Pyrosequencing and EPIC array
Barberet et al., 2021 [26]	Cross-sectional	NR	NR/ICSI-ET: 33.1 ± 3.9; ICSI-FET: 31.3 ± 5.1; SC: 29.1 ± 3.6	Placenta Cord blood	Pregnancy Birth	118 (66 IVF/ICSI-ET, 52 IVF/ICSI-FET)	84 (fertile)	H19/IGF2, KCNQ1OT1, SNURF, LINE1, HERV-FRD	Pyrosequencing
Camprubi et al., 2013 [27]	Cross-sectional	NR	NR/ART: 36.2 ± 5.0; SC: 33.3 ± 5.4	Placenta Cord blood	Birth	73	121 (NS)	LINE1, AluYb1, α-satellite repeats, and the promoters of SLC2A3, PLA2G2A, and VEGFA	Illumina Goldengate methylation array and pyrosequencing
Caramaschi et al., 2011 [28]	Cross-sectional	NR	29.65 ± 4.41; SC: 28.84 ± 4.83	Placenta	Birth	205	2439 (NS)	Global DNA methylation	Illumina Methylation 450k BeadChip Array
Castillo-Fernandez et al., 2017 [29]	Cross-sectional	NR	NR/NR in total sample	Cord blood	Birth	47	60 (NS)	Global DNA methylation	MeDIP-sequencing
Chen et al., 2013 [30]	Cross-sectional	NR	NR/ART: 32.9 ± 3.3; SC: 31.5 ± 4.3	Placenta	Birth	35 (COS-FET)	37 (NS)	CDKN1C, IGF2	Bisulfite sequencing
Chen et al., 2020 [31]	Cross-sectional	NR	NR	Cord blood	Birth	NR	NR	Global DNA methylation	RRBs for DNA methylome and CHIP for histone modifications
Choufani et al., 2018 [32]	Cross-sectional	M in 12/40 F in 6/40	ART: 34.5 ± 4.3; SC: 33.0 ± 3.8/ART: 34.7 ± 7.0; SC: 36.0 ± 5.3	Placenta	Birth	23 (18 ICSI, 5 IVF), 11 IUI, 10 (more than one technique)	44 (fertile)	Global DNA methylation	Illumina Human Methylation 450 BeadChip array and pyrosequencing
Choux et al., 2018 [33]	Cross-sectional	NR	ART: 33.7 ± 5.7; SC: 31.9 ± 5.2/ART: 31.1 ± 5.3; SC: 29.4 ± 4.0	Placenta Cord blood	Birth	51	48 (fertile)	ERVFRD1, ERVW1, LINE1, AluYa5	Bisulfite pyrosequencing
DeBaun et al., 2003 [34]	Observational uncontrolled	NR	NR	Peripheral blood	Children	6 (ICSI)	/	LIT1, H19	Southern blot
El Haj et al., 2017 [35]	Cross-sectional	NR	NR/IVF: 34.3 ± 4.5; ICSI: 34.0 ± 3.9; SC: 30.2 ± 5.9	Cord blood	Birth	48	46 (NS)	Global DNA methylation	Illumina 450 k Methylation Array and pyrosequencing
Estill et al., 2016 [36]	Cross-sectional	NR	NR	Peripheral blood	Children	76 (38 ICSI-ET, 38 ICSI-FET, 18 IUI	43 (NS)	Global DNA Methylation	Illumina Infinium Human Methylation 450 BeadChip Array

Table 2. Cont.

Author and Year	Study Design	Etiology of Infertility (M/F)	Paternal/Maternal Age (y)	Tissue	Timing	ART Group	SC Group (Parents' Fertility Status)	Outcome Assessed	Methylation Evaluation Method
Feng et al., 2011 [37]	Cross-sectional	NR	NR/IVF: 31.0 ± 3.7; ICSI: 29.1 ± 3.6; SC: 29.7 ± 4.2	Cord blood	Birth	60 (30 IVF, 30 ICSI)	60 (NS)	L3MBTL	Bisulfite sequencing
Ghosh et al., 2017 [38]	Cross-sectional	NR	ART: 36.9 ± 5.7; SC: 33.3 ± 5.2/ART: 34.7 ± 3.6; SC: 32.2 ± 4.8	Placenta	Birth	182	77 (NS)	LINE 1	Pyrosequencing for LINE1 and
Gomes et al., 2009 [39]	Cross-sectional	M = 7, F = 7, M + F = 4	NR/ART: 32.3 ± 4.27	CSV, cord blood, placenta, peripheral blood	Birth, children	12, 6	8, 22, 3 (NS)	KvDMR1	Methylation-specific PCR
Ji et al., 2018 [40]	Cross-sectional	NR	NR/Total: 30.1 ± 3.2; IVF-ET-D3: 31.6 ± 3.5; IVF-FET-D3: 30.7 ± 4.6; IVF-FET-D5: 29.7 ± 0.6; ICSI-ET-D3: 28 ± 3.6; ICSI-FET-D3: 31.3 ± 4.7; COS: 29.33 ± 1.5	Fetal fraction	Pregnancy	3 (IVF fresh D3), 3 (IVF frozen D3), 3 (IVF frozen D5), 3 (ICSI fresh D3), 3 (ICSI frozen D3), 3 (COS)	/	H19, IGF2, SNRPN	Methylation-specific PCR and pyrosequencing
Jiang et al., 2022 [41]	Cross-sectional	NR	NR/ART: 32.7 ± 3.35; SC: 33.8 ± 3.05	Cord blood	Birth	21	22 (NS)	MEG3	Pyrosequencing
Katari et al., 2009 [42]	Cross-sectional	F = 4; M = 2; M + F = 1; Unexp: 3	ART 38.3 ± 5.85; SC: 33.4 ± 7.6/ART: 33.5 ± 7.6; SC: 32.5 ± 4.5	Cord blood Placenta	Birth	10	13 (fertile)	Global DNA methylation	Golden Gate Array
Li et al., 2011 [43]	Cross-sectional	NR	NR/ART: 31.7 ± 3.93; SC:28.9 ± 3.75	Cord blood	Birth	29	30 (NS)	KvDMR1, PEG1, H19/IGF2	DNA bisulfite sequencing
Lim et al., 2009 [44]	Cross-sectional	NR	41.8/36.7	Peripheral blood	Children	25 (11 IVF, 13 ICSI)	87 (NS)	KvDMR1, ZAC, PEG1, SNRPN, DLK1	Methylation-specific PCR, bisulfite sequencing, pyrosequencing
Litzky et al., 2017 [45]	Cross-sectional	NR	NR/31.5 ± 4.81	Placenta	Birth	18 IVF	158 (NS)	Differences in DNA methylation among groups at the level of 108 imprinted genes	Illumina Infinium Human Methylation 450 array
Liu et al., 2021b [46]	Cross-sectional	NR	NR for al sample/ART: 32.3 ± 5.5; SC: 27.7 ± 2.5	Cord blood	Birth	12 (IVF-ET)	12 (NS)	Global DNA methylation	Human Methylation 450k BeadChip array and bisulfite sequencing

Table 2. Cont.

Author and Year	Study Design	Etiology of Infertility (M/F)	Paternal/Maternal Age (y)	Tissue	Timing	ART Group	SC Group (Parents' Fertility Status)	Outcome Assessed	Methylation Evaluation Method
Loke et al., 2015 [47]	Cross-sectional	NR	NR/IVF: 36.9 ± 4.9; SC: 32.2 ± 4.9	Buccal smear	Children	34	174 (fertile)	LINE1, AluYa5, H19/IGF2, H19	Mass Array EpiTYPER
Lou et al., 2018 [48]	Cross-sectional	NR	NR	Fetal fraction	Pregnancy	42 COS, 36 IVF, 20 ICSI	/	H19, IGF2, SNRPN	Methylation-specific PCR and pyrosequencing
Marti et al., 2018 [49]	Cross-sectional	NR	35.0–40.5/33.0–36.7	Placenta	Birth	35	35 (NS)	Global DNA methylation	Illumina MethylationEPIC BeadChip array and validation with pyrosequencing
Manning et al., 2000 [50]	Prospective uncontrolled	M	NR	Peripheral blood	Children	92 (ICSI)	/	DNA methylation at 15q11-q13 region (PWS/AS region)	Methyl-specific PCR
Melamed et al., 2015 [51]	Cross-sectional	NR	NR/ART: 38.2 ± 2.8; SC: 36.4 ± 2.3	Cord blood	Birth	10	8 (NS)	Global DNA Methylation	Infinium Illumina Methylation 27 Array; pyrosequencing for HOP gene
Nelissen et al., 2013 [52]	Cross-sectional	M = 28 F = 3 Unexpl = 4	NR	Placenta	Birth	35 (5 IVF, 30 ICSI)	35 (fertile)	IGF2, H19, MEG3, MEST α and β, PEG3, SNRPN, KCNQ1OT1	Pyrosequencing
Nelissen et al., 2014 [53]	Cross-sectional	NR	ART: 36.3 ± 5.8; SC: 33.5 ± 5.1 / ART: 33.9 ± 4.1; SC: 31.1 ± 4.6	Placenta	Birth	81 (IVF/ICSI + ET)	105 (fertile)	H19, IGF2, MEST α and β, PHLDA2, CDKN1C	Pyrosequencing
Novakovic et al., 2019 [54]	Cross-sectional	NR	NR	Peripheral blood	Children/Adults	149 infants + 158 adults	58 infants + 75 adults (NS)	Global DNA methylation	Infinium Illumina Methylation Epic Bead Chip array
Oliver et al., 2012 [55]	Cross-sectional	NR	NR	Peripheral blood	Children	66 (34 IVF, 32 ICSI)	69 (NS)	H19, KCNQ1OT1, SNRPN, IGF2, INSL5, ARHGAP24, STK19, NCRNA00282, IPH4, SYP, BEX1	MSO-PCR; Bisulfite Sequencing; MeDIP and promoter array; Sequenom MassARRAY EpyTIPER
Penova-Veselinovic et al., 2021 [56]	Cross-sectional	M = 32.47% F = 43.29% Unexpl = 18.18%	NR/ART: 33.9 ± 3.9 SC: 28.5 ± 5.8	Peripheral blood	Adults	231	1188 (NS)	Global DNA methylation	In the ART group evaluated by and in the SC group by Illumina INfinium Human Methylation BeadChip Array
Pliushch et al., 2015 [57]	Cross-sectional	NR	IVM + ART: 36 ± 4; ART: 36.5 ± 4.5/IVM+ART: 32.0 ± 1.5; ART: 35.0 ± 4.0	CVS, cord blood	Birth	30 (11 IVM + IVF/ICSI, 19 IVF/ICSI)	/	LIT1, MEST, MEG3, NESPas, PEG3, SNRPN, APC, ATM, BRCA1, RAD51C, TP53, NANOG, OCT4, LEP, NR3C1, LINE1, ALU	Bisulfite pyrosequencing
Puumala et al., 2012 [58]	Cross-sectional	M = 17.28% F = 21.34% M and F = 16.26% Unexpl. = 6.10%	NR/ART: 34.1 ± 3.9; SC: 29.6 ± 4.3	Buccal smear	Children	67 (IVF/ICSI)	31 (fertile)	IGF2, H19, IGF2R, KvDMR	Pyrosequencing

Table 2. Cont.

Author and Year	Study Design	Etiology of Infertility (M/F)	Paternal/Maternal Age (y)	Tissue	Timing	ART Group	SC Group (Parents' Fertility Status)	Outcome Assessed	Methylation Evaluation Method
Rancourt et al., 2012 [59]	Cross-sectional	NR	NR/IVF: 36.5 ± 4.5; OI: 34.5 ± 4.6; SC: 35.5 ± 4.7	Placenta, cord blood	Children	86 (27 OI, 59 IVF)	61 (NS)	MEST, GRB10, KCNQ1, SNRPN, H19, IGF2	Pyrosequencing
Rossignol et al., 2006 [60]	Cross-sectional	NR	NR	Peripheral blood	Children	11	29 (NS)	H19, IGF2, SNRPN, PEG1/MEST	Southern blot Bisulfite sequencing
Sakian et al., 2015 [61]	Cross-sectional	NR	NR/IVF: 35.3 ± 3.9; ICSI: 34.1 ± 2.9; SC: 32.4 ± 8.7	Placenta	Birth	97 (56 IVF, 41 ICSI)	22 (fertile)	H19	Pyrosequencing
Santos et al., 2010 [62]	Cross-sectional	NR	NR	Embryo, blasts	/	138 (75 IVF, 63 ICSI), 27 (14 IVF, 13 ICSI)	/	Global DNA methylation	Anti-5-methyl cytosine antibodies
Shi et al., 2014 [63]	Observational uncontrolled	M = 3/23 F = 20/23	NR	Embryo	/	254	/	H19, PEG1, KvDMR	Bisulfite PCR and pyrosequencing
Song et al., 2015 [64]	Cross-sectional	NR	ART: 36.2 ± 5.3; SC: 34.9 ± 5.7/ART: 35.3 ± 3.7; SC: 34.5 ± 5.0	Placenta	Birth	88	49 (fertile)	DNA methylation of 37 CpG in 16 different genes (CCDC62, CRTAM, FLJ10260, FLJ90650, GRB10, GRIN2C, H19, IL5, LYST, MEST, NDN, PCDHGB7, PTPN20B, SNRPN, TCF2, TTR)	Bisulfite DNA and pyrosequencing
Tang et al., 2017 [65]	Cross-sectional	M	NR	Cord blood	Birth	13 ICSI	30 (fertile)	H19, SNRPN, KCQ1OT1	Pyrosequencing
Tierling et al., 2010 [66]	Cross-sectional	NR	NR/IVF: 34.8 ± 4; ICSI: 35.3 ± 4.3; SC: 31.7 ± 5.7	Peripheral blood	Children	112 (35 IVF, 77 ICSI)	73 (NS)	KvDMR1, H19, SNRPN, MEST, GRB10, DLK1/MEG	Bisulfite techniques (SNuPE assay with SIRPH, Homoduplex separation, pyrosequencing)
Turan et al., 2010 [67]	Cross-sectional	NR	NR/ART: 36 ± 4; SC: 31 ± 6	Placenta, cord blood	Children	45	56 (fertile)	IGF2/H19	Pyrosequencing
Vincent et al., 2016 [68]	Cross-sectional	NR	NR/NR in total sample	CVS, cord blood	Birth	150 (68 ICSI, 82 IVF)	66 (NS)	PLAGL1, KvDMR1, PEG10, LINE1	Bisulfite assay and pyrosequencing
White et al., 2015 [69]	Cross-sectional	NR	NR	Embryo, blasts	/	24 + 29	/	SNRPN, KCNQ1OT1, H19	Bisulfite clonal sequencing
Whitelaw et al., 2014 [70]	Retrospective cohort	NR	NR/ART: 34.6 ± 3.3; SC: 34.1 ± 3.4	Buccal smear	Children	69 (49 IVF-ET, 20 ICSI-ET)	89 (fertile)	LINE1, SNRPN, PEG3, INS, IGF2	Pyrosequencing
Wong et al., 2010 [71]	Cross-sectional	NR	NR/ART: 36.4 ± 3.1; ICSI: 35.0 ± 4.8; SC: 33.0 ± 4.9	Placenta, cord blood	Children	77 (32 IVF, 45 ICSI)	12 (NS)	H19	MS-SNuPE

Table 2. Cont.

Author and Year	Study Design	Etiology of Infertility (M/F)	Paternal/Maternal Age (y)	Tissue	Timing	ART Group	SC Group (Parents' Fertility Status)	Outcome Assessed	Methylation Evaluation Method
Yoshada et al., 2013 [72]	Cross-sectional	NR	NR	Placenta, cord blood	Children	8 IVM + IVF	/	H19, GTL2, ZdbJ2, PEG1, PEG3, LIT1, ZAC, SNRPN	Imprinted methylation Assay
Zhang et al., 2019 [73]	Cross-sectional	NR	NR	Cord blood	Birth	33	43 (NS)	AGTR1	Bisulfite sequencing

Abbreviations. ART, assisted reproductive technique; COS, controlled ovarian stimulation; CVS, chorionic villus sampling; ET, embryo transfer; FET, frozen embryo transfer; ICSI, intracytoplasmic sperm injection; IUI, intrauterine insemination; IVF, in vitro fertilization; OI, ovulation induction; SC, spontaneous conception, NR, not reported. **Genes:** APC, Adenomatous Polyposis Coli; AGTR1, angiotensin II receptor type 1; ALU, Arthrobacter luteus; ARHGAP24, Rho GTPase Activating Protein 24; ATM, Ataxia-Telangiectasia Mutated; BEX1, Brain Expressed X-Linked 1; BRCA1, BReast CAncer gene 1; CCDC62, Coiled-Coil Domain Containing 62; CDKN1C, Cyclin-dependent kinase inhibitor 1C; CRTAM, Cytotoxic And Regulatory T Cell Molecule; DLK1, Delta Like Non-Canonical Notch Ligand 1; ERVFRD1, Endogenous Retrovirus Group FRD Member 1; ERW1, Endogenous Retrovirus Group W Member 1; FLJ10260, Schlafen Family Member gene; FLJ90650, Lacevrin gene; GRB10, Growth Factor Receptor Bound Protein 10; GRIN2C, Glutamate Ionotropic Receptor NMDA Type Subunit 2C; GTL2, gene trap locus2; HERV-FRD, Human Endogenous Retrovirus FRD; IGF2, insuline-like growth factor 2; IL5, Interleukin 5; INSL5, insulin like 5; JPH4, Junctophilin 4; KCNQ1, Potassium Voltage-Gated Channel Subfamily Q Member 1; KCNQ1OT1, KCNQ1 Opposite Strand/Antisense Transcript 1; KvDMR1, Potassium Voltage Differentially Methylated Region 1; L3MBTL, Lethal(3) Malignant Brain Tumor-Like protein; LEP, Leptin gene; LINE1, Long Interspersed Nuclear Elements 1; LIT1, Long QT Intronic Transcript 1; LYST, Lysosomal Trafficking Regulator; MEG3, Maternally Expressed Gene 3; MEST, Mesoderm Specific Transcript; NANOG, Homeobox protein Nanog; NDN, Necdin; NESPas, GNAS antisense; NCRNA00282, Non-Coding Ribonucleic Acid 00282; NR3C1, Nuclear Receptor Subfamily 3 Group C Member 1; OCT4, octamer-binding transcription factor 4; PCDHGB7, Protocadherin Gamma Subfamily B 7; PEG1, Paternally expressed gene 1; PEG3, Paternally expressed gene 3; PEG10, Paternally expressed gene 10; PHLDA2, Pleckstrin Homology Like Domain Family A Member 2; PLA2GA2, phospholipase A2 group IIA; PTPN20B, protein tyrosine phosphatase non-receptor type 20B; RAD51C, Rad recombinase 51 paralog C; SNRPN, Small Nuclear Ribonucleoprotein Polypeptide N; SNURF, SNRPN Upstream Open Reading Frame; SLC2A3, Solute Carrier Family 2 Member 3; STK19, Serine/threonine-protein kinase 19; SYP, Synaptophysin; TCF2, Transcription factor 2 gene; TP53, Tumor Protein 53; TTR, Transthyretin; VEGFA, Vascular endothelial growth factor A; ZAC, Zinc-Activated ion Channel; ZDBF2, Zinc Finger DBF-Type Containing 2. NS, non-specified.

Table 3. Evaluation of study quality using "The Cambridge Quality Checklists".

Author and Year of Publication	Checklist for Correlates	Checklist for Risk Factors	Checklist for Causal Risk Factors	Total
Argyraki et al., 2021 [24]	2	1	2	5/15
Barberet et al., 2021 [25]	3	1	2	6/15
Barberet et al., 2021 [26]	2	1	2	5/15
Camprubì et al., 2013 [27]	3	1	2	6/15
Caramaschi et al., 2011 [28]	3	1	2	6/15
Castillo-Fernandez et al., 2017 [29]	2	1	2	5/15
Chen et al., 2018 [30]	2	1	2	5/15
Chen et al., 2020 [31]	3	1	2	6/15
Choufani et al., 2018 [32]	3	1	5	9/15
Choux et al., 2018 [33]	2	1	2	5/15
DeBaun et al., 2003 [34]	2	1	1	4/15
El Hajj et al., 2017 [35]	2	1	2	5/15
Estill et al., 2016 [36]	3	1	2	6/15
Feng et al., 2011 [37]	2	1	2	5/15
Ghosh et al., 2017 [38]	2	1	2	5/15
Gomes et al., 2009 [39]	1	1	2	4/15
Ji et al., 2018 [40]	2	1	1	4/15
Jiang et al., 2022 [41]	2	1	2	5/15
Katari et al., 2009 [42]	2	1	2	5/15
Li et al., 2011 [43]	2	1	2	5/15
Lim et al., 2009 [44]	2	1	2	5/15
Litzky et al., 2017 [45]	2	1	5	8/15
Liu et al., 2021b [46]	2	1	2	5/15
Loke et al., 2015 [47]	1	1	2	4/15
Lou et al., 2018 [48]	3	1	1	5/10
Mani et al., 2018 [49]	3	1	5	9/15
Manning et al., 2000 [50]	2	3	1	6/15
Melamed et al., 2015 [51]	3	1	2	6/15
Nelissen et al., 2013 [52]	2	1	2	5/15
Nelissen et al., 2014 [53]	3	1	2	6/15
Novakovic et al., 2019 [54]	3	1	2	6/15
Oliver et al., 2012 [55]	3	1	2	6/15
Penova-Vaselinovic et al., 2021 [56]	3	1	2	6/15
Pliushch et al., 2015 [57]	3	1	1	5/15
Puumala et al., 2012 [58]	2	1	2	5/15
Rancourt et al., 2012 [59]	2	1	2	5/15

Table 3. Cont.

Author and Year of Publication	Checklist for Correlates	Checklist for Risk Factors	Checklist for Causal Risk Factors	Total
Rossignol et al., 2006 [60]	3	1	2	6/15
Sakian et al., 2015 [61]	2	1	2	6/15
Santos et al., 2010 [62]	2	1	1	4/15
Shi et al., 2014 [63]	1	1	1	3/15
Song et al., 2015 [64]	1	1	2	4/15
Tang et al., 2017 [65]	2	1	2	5/15
Tierling et al., 2010 [66]	3	1	2	6/15
Turan et al., 2010 [67]	2	1	2	5/15
Vincent et al., 2016 [68]	2	1	2	5/15
White et al., 2015 [69]	2	1	1	4/15
Whitelaw et al., 2014 [70]	2	2	5	9/15
Wong et al., 2010 [71]	1	1	2	4/15
Yoshida et al., 2013 [72]	1	1	1	3/15
Zhang et al., 2019 [73]	2	1	2	5/15

3.1. Qualitative Synthesis

All the results and limits of the studies included are summarized in Supplementary Table S1.

3.1.1. Global Methylation

Since methylation at the level of transposable elements (TEs) occurs in around 50% of the human genome with a regulatory function for nearby genes, these can be used as an indirect marker of global methylation status [74]. With this premise, in the analysis of studies evaluating the impact of ART on global methylation of the DNA of the offspring, we included both studies assessing global DNA methylation and studies assessing methylation at the levels of TEs. Concerning this outcome, the studies showed considerable discordance. Indeed, in seven studies, variations were observed in the ART group compared to the group of SC offspring [25,26,33,38,42,47,51]. In detail, the studies generally showed the presence of hypomethylation in both global DNA and at the level of TEs in the group conceived by ART compared with that in the group of SC offspring [25,26,33,47,51]. In one study, hypermethylation at the level of cord blood and hypomethylation at the level of the placenta was observed in the ART group compared to the SC group [42]. In another study, hypermethylation was observed in the LUMA assay and hypomethylation in the *LINE1* assessment in the ART group compared to the SC group [38]. However, in other eight studies, no difference was observed between global methylation rates in the ART and control groups [27,31,32,35,46,49,54,56].

3.1.2. Methylation of Imprinted Genes

With regard to the involvement of imprinted genes, 10 studies showed no alteration in the imprinted genes analyzed [24,43,45,53,55,58,61,65,66,71], while another 11 studies showed alterations in at least one of the imprinted genes [25,26,30,39,41,47,52,59,67,68,70]. In particular, among the main genes evaluated in the various studies, we encounter *H19*, *Insulin-like growth factor 2 (IGF2)*, *Small Nuclear Ribonucleoprotein Polypeptide N (SNRPN)*, *Mesoderm Specific Transcript (MEST)*, the *Potassium Voltage Differentially Methylated Region 1 (KvDMR1)* region of the *Potassium Voltage-Gated Channel Subfamily Q Member 1 Opposite Strand/Antisense Transcript 1 (KCNQ1OT1)* gene, and *Maternally Expressed Gene (MEG3)*. For the *H19* gene, five studies showed hypomethylation in the differentially methylated regions (DMRs) of this gene in the ART group compared to the SC group [25,26,47,52,59].

Instead, one study showed hypermethylation [30], and another do not specify the type of aberration [67]. In contrast, eight studies observed no difference [43,55,58,61,65,66,71]. As for the DMRs of its complementary gene, *IGF2*, four studies showed no difference in methylation between the ART and the SC control group [24,55,58,70]. As for the *MEST* gene, two studies showed no difference in methylation levels between the ART group and SC controls [24,66], while two studies found it was hypomethylated in the ART group than SC group [52,59]. For the *SNRPN* gene, three studies showed no difference in its methylation in the ART-conceived offspring compared to SC controls [55,65,66], while two studies found hypermethylation in the ART group compared to SC controls [59,70]. Regarding methylation of KvDMR1 or other regions of the *KCNQ1OT1* gene, three studies found an abnormal methylation of this gene in the ART vs. the spontaneously-conceived offspring [30,39,59]. In detail, two studies found it hypomethylated in the ART group compared with the SC group [30,59], while 1 study found it hypermethylated [39]. On the contrary, five studies did not find any difference between the two groups [43,55,58,65,66]. Similar heterogeneity in results was also observed for other genes, such as MEG3 [41,52].

3.1.3. Role of ART Protocol and Technique

Since numerous protocols of ART (controlled ovarian stimulation (COS), fresh vs. frozen embryo transfer (ET), in vitro fertilization (IVF) vs. intracytoplasmic sperm injection (ICSI), embryo transfer day, and culture medium used [16]) have been implicated in epigenetic changes, we analyzed the results of the studies evaluating the impact of the individual ART processes on DNA methylation.

Regarding the studies that have evaluated the role of COS, four studies concluded it could play a predominant role in causing epigenetic changes [30,40,41,59], while three conclude that COS is not responsible for these alterations [32,48,72].

As for fresh vs. frozen ET, most of the studies that analyzed the difference in methylation between the two methods concluded that fresh ET correlates with major alterations compared to the frozen one [26,36,38], two studies concluded that there is no difference between the two methods [40,54] and one study instead found that cryopreservation could be associated with a greater carcinogenic risk [31]. All studies that analyzed the difference in global methylation of DNA or imprinted genes according to the day of ET found no association [38,40,69].

Only two studies evaluated the impact of the culture medium, with conflicting results [54,55].

Finally, as regards the difference between the various techniques used in ART, only five studies found that ICSI is associated with greater alterations than IVF [26,29,47,70] or intrauterine insemination (IUI) [31], while three studies concluded that IVF is associated with a greater DNA methylation aberration than ICSI [25,48,68]. However, in most of the studies, this difference was not evaluated and no difference was found between the two methods [54,62].

The results of the qualitative analysis are shown in Supplementary Table S1.

3.1.4. Role of Parental Age

Because parental age can also influence gamete quality and thus promote the occurrence of epigenetic abnormalities that can then be transmitted via ART [75], we evaluated the number of studies that reported parental age and performed an adjusted analysis taking it into consideration. We found that only nine studies reported paternal age [32,33,38,42,44,49,53,57,64]. However, three of them did not perform an adjusted analysis by paternal age [33,42,44]. On the other hand, with regard to maternal age, 14 of the 50 included studies did not report the maternal age and, therefore, did not consider it in the adjusted analysis [25,34,36,48,50,54,55,60,62,63,65,69,72,73]. However, in four other studies, although reported, the analysis would not appear to be corrected by parental age [44,46,66,67].

3.1.5. Role of the Etiology of Infertility

Among all the included studies, only 13 corrected the analysis by excluding the male factor or directly analyzed the role of infertility [31,32,35,37,45,50,55,56,63–65,69] with conflicting results in this case as well. In detail, Chen and colleagues showed that both ART methods and infertility per se could lead to alterations in DNA methylation [31]. Another study also showed that, by correcting the analysis taking into account the father's sperm concentration, the ART group still had significant differences in methylation levels compared to the group of SC children [35]. Likewise, White and colleagues observed that two embryos generated by ICSI with donor sperm, therefore healthy, also had methylation aberrations [69]. Finally, Song and colleagues comparing a group of children born from ART by infertile fathers and children born from ART with fathers without infertility identified very similar methylation abnormalities between the two groups that, in turn, differed significantly from those of SC children [64]. These results seem to confirm the role of the methods per se in causing epigenetic alterations regardless of the presence of the underlying paternal infertility. However, other studies have come to the opposite conclusion. Choufani and colleagues showed that the methylation differences in the ICSI/IVF group were seen to be closely related to male infertility and paternal age [32]. In another study, Litzky and colleagues showed that only the group of children conceived by parents with underlying infertility (one or both parents) had methylation alterations, compared to the IVF and SC groups. Therefore, the alterations in methylation observed in children conceived by ART could also be partly attributed to underlying infertility and, therefore, to the alteration of the gametes used for the technique [45].

3.2. Quantitative Synthesis

A total of 12 studies [19,33,39,52,55,58,59,61,63,65,66,71] were included in the quantitative analysis. Methylation levels of the following genes could be meta-analyzed: *H19* CCCTC-binding factor 3 (CTCF3), *H19* CTCF6, *KCNQ1OT1*, Paternally Expressed Gene 3 (*PEG3*), and *SNRPN*. Moreover, also methylation levels of the Arthrobacter luteus (Alu), *Long Interspersed Nuclear Elements* (*LINE*) (most investigated TEs) could be meta-analyzed.

H19 CTCF3 methylation levels were significantly lower in the ART group compared to controls (SMD -0.81 (-1.53; -0.09), $I^2 = 89\%$, $p = 0.03$). Subgroup analysis showed a significantly lower methylation in placenta (-0.53 (-0.83, -0.22), $I^2 = 0\%$, $p < 0.05$) and buccal smear (1.61 (-3.09, -0.12), $I^2 = 92\%$, $p = 0.03$) (Figure 2). In contrast, *H19* CTCF6 methylation was not significantly different between ART and controls (0.02 (-0.23, 0.26), $I^2 = 66\%$, $p = 0.89$). Furthermore, the subgroup analysis showed no difference in the methylation levels of each tissue (Figure 3). Similarly, *KCNQ1OT1* (-0.15 (-0.38, 0.09), $I^2 = 71\%$, $p = 0.22$) (Figure 4), *PEG3* (-0.15 (-0.38, 0.09), $I^2 = 71\%$, $p = 0.59$) (Figure 5), *SNRPN* (-0.02 (-0.19, 0.15), $I^2 = 37\%$, $p = 0.82$) (Figure 6), were not differently methylated in ART vs. SC control offspring.

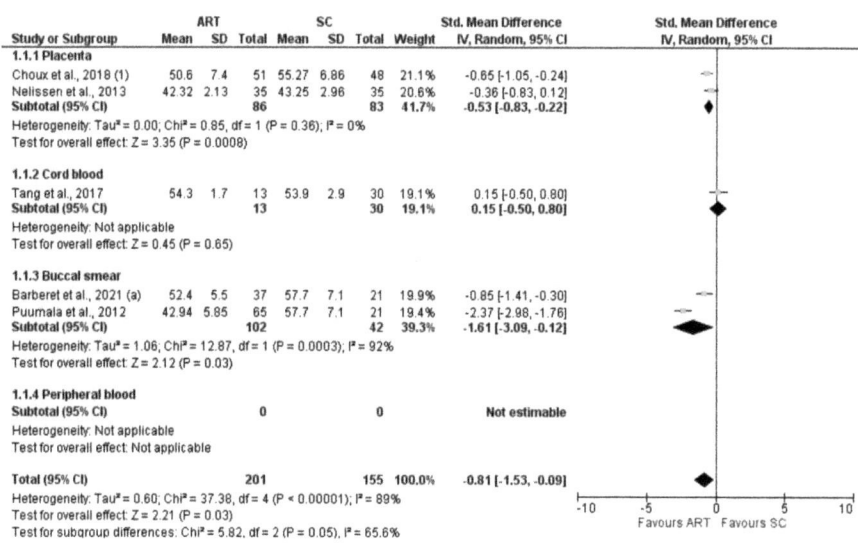

Figure 2. Methylation levels of *H19* CTCF3 [25,33,52,58,65]. ART, assisted reproductive technique; SC, spontaneous conception.

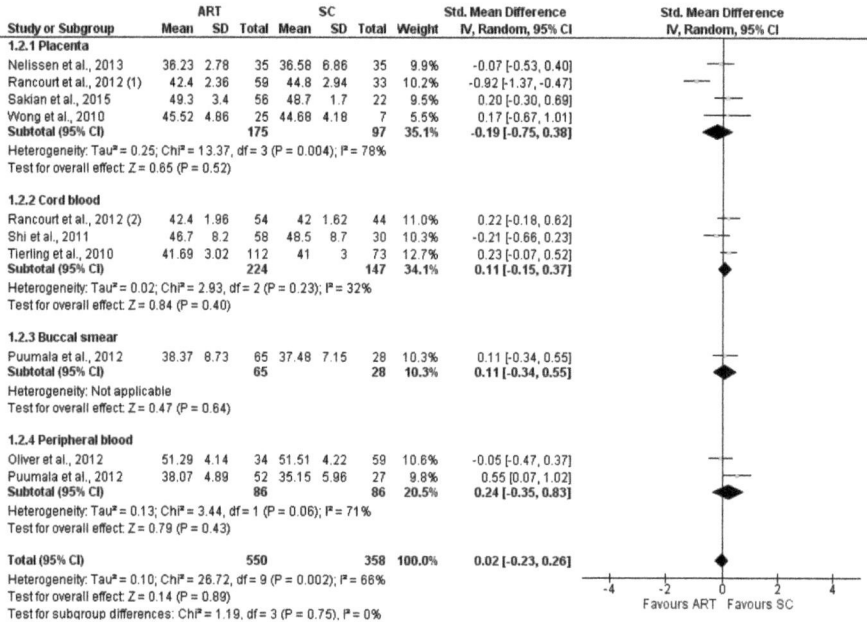

Figure 3. Methylation levels of *H19* CTCF6 [52,55,58,59,61,63,66,71]. ART, assisted reproductive technique; SC, spontaneous conception.

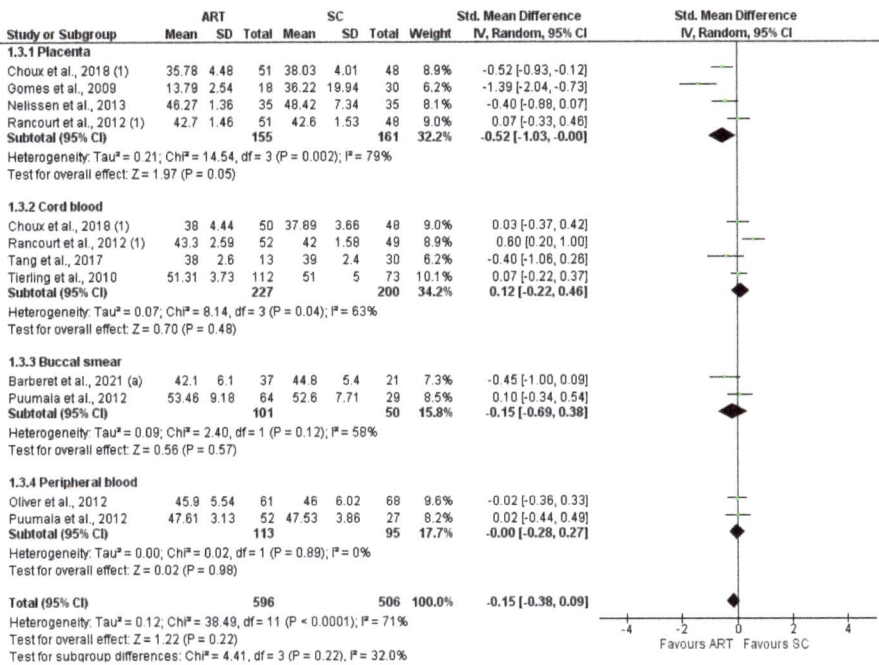

Figure 4. Methylation levels of *KCNQ1OT1* [25,33,39,52,55,58,59,65,66]. ART, assisted reproductive technique; SC, spontaneous conception.

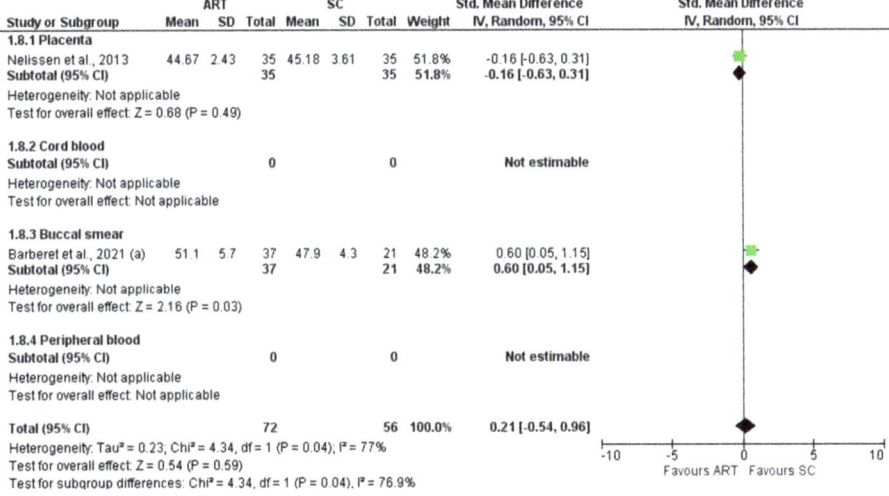

Figure 5. Methylation levels of *PEG3* [25,52]. ART, assisted reproductive technique; SC, spontaneous conception.

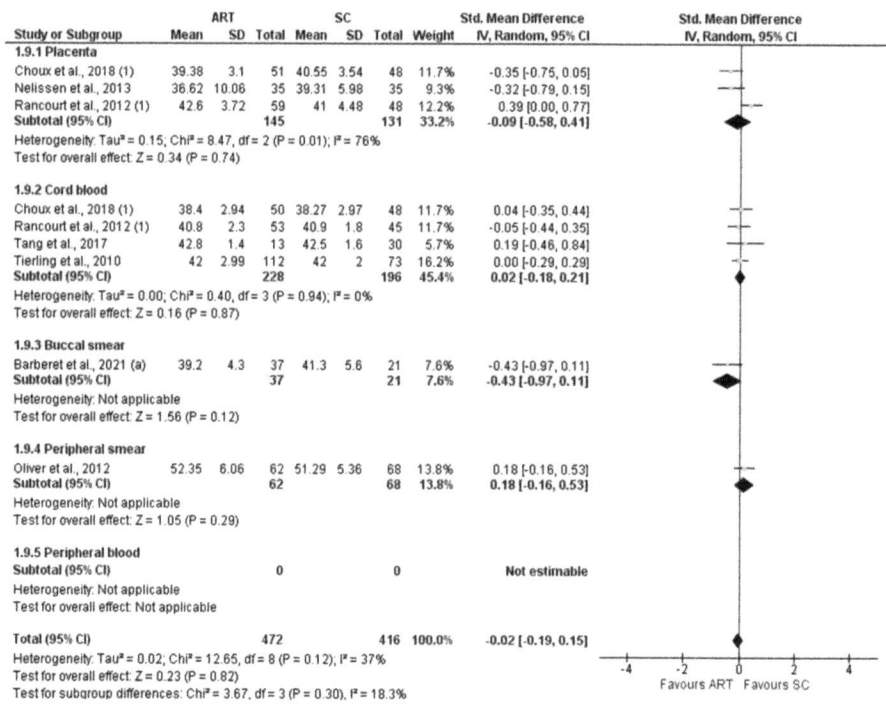

Figure 6. Methylation levels of *SNRPN* [25,33,52,55,59,65,66]. ART, assisted reproductive technique; SC, spontaneous conception.

4. Discussion

The development of ART was a huge step forward in the treatment of couple infertility, leading to the birth of numerous newborns. Every year, more than 200,000 children are born through ART worldwide [76]. However, Barker's theory of Developmental Origins of Health and Disease (DOHaD), according to which alterations in the microenvironment of conception can cause long-term damage, particularly cardiovascular and metabolic diseases, has raised concerns that the techniques used may alter the imprinting and, therefore, lead to long-term disorders [77].

DNA methylation reprogramming occurs in two different moments. The first reprogramming concerns the gametes. The genome of primordial germ cells is completely demethylated as they enter the genital crest, and then undergo sex-specific de novo methylation with the establishment of specific methylation patterns for imprinted genes. The second wave of genome-wide demethylation and subsequent de novo methylation occurs during preimplantation development. Only the methylation pattern of imprinted genes is not altered by this second wave of reprogramming, which ensures their parent-specific expression and activity throughout development [15]. The latter occurs when ART procedures are carried out (Figure 7).

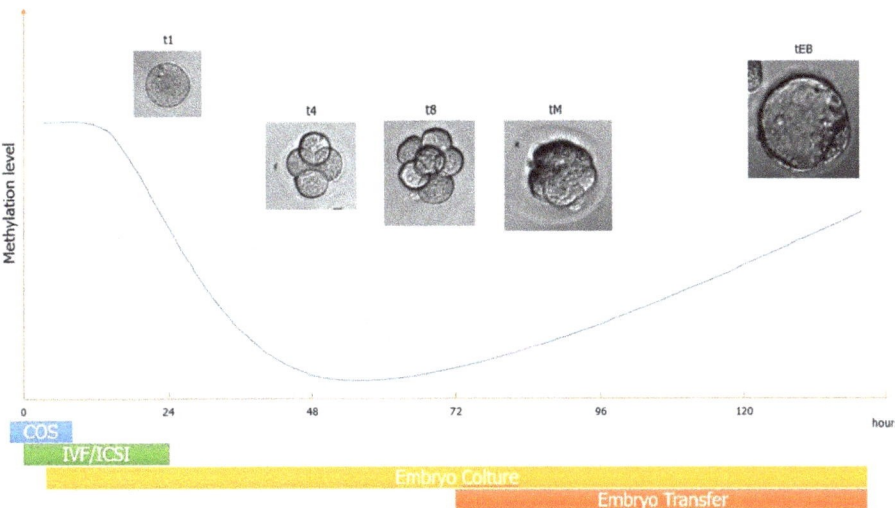

Figure 7. Timing of the methylation pattern of paternal and maternal alleles during human embryogenesis. After fertilization, the embryo undergoes the first wave of global demethylation, followed by de novo methylation. Only the imprinted genes escape epigenetic reprogramming. The timing of these events is concomitant with that of in vitro fertilization (IVF), intracytoplasmic sperm injection (ICSI), embryo culture, and embryo transfer. COS controlled ovarian stimulation.

Several studies have shown a higher prevalence of disorders associated with altered imprinting, such as Beckwith–Wiedemann syndrome (BWS) and Silver–Russell Syndrome (SRS), in ART-born children [78,79]. In this context, some studies have evaluated the effects of ART on DNA methylation. In particular, ART could influence the methylation and, therefore, the expression of imprinted and non-imprinted genes that may be involved in insulin signaling pathways and adipocyte differentiation, suggesting a role of these procedures in the development of diabetes and future obesity [42].

Furthermore, ART can alter the expression of genes involved: (i) in the development of the nervous and immune systems [21]; (ii) in the susceptibility of cancer development [28]; and (iii) also in future fertility, such as *Spermatogenesis* and *Centriole Associated 1 Like* (*SPATC1L*) gene, which encodes for speriolin [36]. The altered methylation of some genes could also be associated with a worsening of short-term fetal outcomes (e.g., birth weight) and gestational complications. In this regard, it has been shown that ART may increase the risk of preeclampsia due to hypomethylation of the *Angiotensin II Receptor Type 1* (*AGTR1*) gene, which results in an upregulation of its levels. In turn, this altered methylation pattern could be due to reduced expression of the DNA methyltransferase 3a (*DNMT3a*) gene, which is responsible for de novo DNA methylation. All of this makes the umbilical veins more sensitive to the effects of angiotensin II, since AGTR1 is the main mediator of vasoconstriction [73]. In addition, ART may be associated with reduced methylation of the promoter of the *MEG3* gene. This leads to the higher expression of *endothelin 1* and *endothelial nitric oxide synthase* (*eNOS*), which increase vasoconstriction. This would explain the increased blood pressure that some studies have found in children born from ART [41]. Finally, the hypomethylation of the *KvDMR* gene, in turn, associated with an increase in *Cyclin Dependent Kinase Inhibitor 1C* (*CDKN1C*), impairs growth. Likewise, alterations in the methylation of H19/IGF2 DMRs or other genes such as *MEST*, can alter fetal growth and increase the prevalence of low birth weight in children born by ART [30].

This systematic review aims to analyze the evidence presented to date in the literature on the effects of ART procedures on the methylation of global DNA and specific imprinted genes. Our quantitative synthesis showed a significantly reduced methylation of *H19*

CTCF3 in the offspring conceived after ART compared to SC. However, there was an inter-study heterogeneity, which could be partly explained by the different samples used for the analysis (placenta, cord blood, or peripheral blood), the different methods to evaluate DNA methylation, and the different sample sizes. For imprinted genes, another reason for heterogeneity is the difference in the region of the gene analyzed for methylation. Furthermore, as suggested by the study of Turan and colleagues, given the extreme variability not only inter- but also intra-individual in DNA methylation, a role in the heterogeneity of the results could also be given by the region in which the placenta biopsy was performed [67]. Finally, there is often a lack of standardization regarding the ART process used. About the latter point, very few studies have specifically examined the impact of the various steps of ART on DNA methylation.

The most investigated aspect is the COS. Several studies have attributed the DNA methylation abnormalities found to the high estrogen levels achieved during COS [59]. Indeed, Jiang and colleagues found that the expression levels of the *MEG3* and *endothelin 1* genes directly correlated to estrogen levels [41]. Similarly, incubation of human trophoblast 8 (*HTR8*) cells with high estrogen levels resulted in hypomethylation of the *KvDMR1* gene after 24 h of incubation and hypermethylation of H19 DMR after 48 h [30]. Other studies that have evaluated the impact of various ART methods, including those where no major manipulation of embryos and gametes was made (e.g., IUI and gamete intra-fallopian transfer (GIFT)), found no difference [40,54]. However, a difference in methylation profiles was found when comparing the ART group in general with that of SC infants [54]. Finally, comparative studies between fresh ET and frozen ET would also seem to confirm a prominent role of COS, since, in fresh ET the higher estrogen levels reached would cause a dysregulation of the endometrial microenvironment, which according to the DOHaD theory would then be responsible for the long-term damage on the embryo [26,36,38]. However, although there is a lot of evidence in favor of COS's role, some studies have disproved this hypothesis. For example, Luo and colleagues compared a group of children conceived by IVF and ICSI with a group of children conceived only by COS, showing that only the former was associated with hypomethylation of *H19* and hypermethylation of *IGF2* DMR2 and *SNRPN* DMR [48]. Another study showed no effect of in vitro maturation (IVM) and COS on the methylation of specific imprinted genes [72]. Finally, another study comparing methylation alterations in a group of children conceived by IUI/COS and a group by IVF/ICSI showed that there was different DNA methylation in the IVF/ICSI group, suggesting that COS, common to both groups, is not the real culprit behind the observed differences. Therefore, the difference could relate to the greater manipulation of gametes and embryos with the more invasive techniques [32].

Another major bias present in most studies is the absence of correction of the analysis for the paternal factor of infertility. Accordingly, only 12 corrected the analysis by excluding the male factor or directly analyzed the role of infertility [31,32,35,37,45,50,55,56,63,64,69], with conflicting results in this case as well. Similarly, many articles did not even consider paternal age, which has instead been seen to correlate with offspring well-being through three basic mechanisms: genetic mutations, telomere length, and epigenetic changes in DNA, and protein expression [75].

Finally, another important limitation of the included studies is that almost all of them and the data analysis are cross-sectional. There are no data to predict whether the methylation changes found in newborns are associated with the development of abnormalities in these children in the long term. The only study with longitudinal data showed a higher prevalence of *SNRPN* DMR hypermethylation in children conceived by ICSI that does not change after 7 years of age, suggesting that these changes may be stable and perpetuate over time [70].

To the best of our knowledge, this is the second meta-analysis evaluating the methylation differences in offspring conceived after ART vs. SC. A recent systematic review and meta-analysis of 51 studies found no difference in *H19* methylation. In contrast, they found different methylation in the *Paternally Expressed Gene 1 (PEG1)/MEST* region. However, the data were analyzed separately for each tissue, thus limiting the amount of data for each gene evaluated [19]. The evidence coming from our systematic review and meta-analysis suggests that *H19* CTCF3 methylation levels are significantly lower in the ART offspring compared to controls. In contrast, *H19* CTCF6, *KCNQ1OT1*, *PEG 3*, and *SNRPN* were not differently methylated in ART than vs. SC.

5. Conclusions

Nowadays, ART is widely used for male and female infertility. Emerging evidence indicates a higher health risk in ART than in SC offspring. Despite this, the exact link between ART and the increased risk of epigenetic abnormalities predisposing to the development of diseases is unclear. The debate is still ongoing as some studies found a different global DNA methylation and the methylation of genes imprinted in ART-conceived offspring compared to controls. However, other studies have not confirmed this evidence, suggesting the absence of any epigenetic aberration. Using a defined search strategy, we extracted 949 records. Among them, 50 were considered eligible. We found that *H19* CTCF3 methylation levels were significantly lower in the ART group compared to controls, in the presence of significant inter-study heterogeneity (SMD -0.81 (-1.53; -0.09), $I^2 = 89\%$, $p = 0.03$). In contrast, *H19* CTCF6, *KCNQ1OT1*, *PEG3*, and *SNRPN* were not differently methylated in ART vs. SC offspring. The heterogeneity of the results could be due to the lack of correction of the data for parental (male or female) infertility, the limited sample size, the retrospective design of almost all studies, the different methods used to analyze the methylation rate (including the different DMRs studied) and, finally, also the different regions where the placenta biopsy was performed. Therefore, further prospective and well-sized population studies are needed to evaluate the impact of ART on the epigenome of the offspring. Furthermore, it is necessary to clarify the contribution of the different protocols and techniques used during ART to the etiology of epigenetic aberrations. Finally, the weight of the presence of maternal and/or paternal infertility in causing alterations in methylation deserves to be further explored.

Supplementary Materials: The following supporting information can be downloaded at: https://www.mdpi.com/article/10.3390/jcm11175056/s1, Table S1: Findings of the included studies.

Author Contributions: Conceptualization, R.C. and A.E.C.; methodology, A.C.; software, R.C.; validation, N.I. and L.L.; formal analysis, A.C. and L.M.M.; investigation, A.C.; data curation, A.C.; writing—original draft preparation, R.C. and A.C.; writing—review and editing, A.E.C.; visualization, R.A.C. and S.L.V.; supervision, R.C. and A.E.C.; project administration, R.C. and A.E.C. All authors have read and agreed to the published version of the manuscript.

Funding: This research received no external funding.

Institutional Review Board Statement: Not applicable.

Informed Consent Statement: Not applicable.

Data Availability Statement: Not applicable.

Conflicts of Interest: The authors declare no conflict of interest.

References

1. Mascarenhas, M.N.; Flaxman, S.R.; Boerma, T.; Vanderpoel, S.; Stevens, G.A. National, regional, and global trends in infertility prevalence since 1990: A systematic analysis of 277 health surveys. *PLoS Med.* **2012**, *9*, e1001356. [CrossRef]
2. Lui Yovich, J. Founding pioneers of IVF update: Innovative researchers generating livebirths by 1982. *Reprod. Biol.* **2020**, *20*, 111–113. [CrossRef] [PubMed]
3. Esteves, S.C. Who cares about oligozoospermia when we have ICSI. *Reprod. Biomed. Online* **2022**, *44*, 769–775. [CrossRef] [PubMed]
4. Boulet, S.L.; Mehta, A.; Kissin, D.M.; Warner, L.; Kawwass, J.F.; Jamieson, J.D. Trends in use of and reproductive outcomes associated with intracytoplasmic sperm injection. *JAMA* **2015**, *313*, 255–263. [CrossRef] [PubMed]

5. Chambers, G.M.; Wand, H.; Macaldowie, A.; Chapman, M.G.; Farquhar, C.M.; Bowman, M.; Molloy, D.; Ledger, W. Population trends and live birth rates associated with common ART treatment strategies. *Hum. Reprod.* **2016**, *31*, 2632–2641. [CrossRef] [PubMed]
6. Wei, S.Q.; Luu, T.M.; Bilodeau-Bertrand, M.; Auger, N. Assisted reproductive technology and childhood morbidity: A longitudinal cohort study. *Fertil. Steril.* **2022**, *118*, 360–368. [CrossRef]
7. Wijs, L.A.; Fusco, M.R.; Doherty, D.A.; Keelan, J.A.; Hart, R.J. Asthma and allergies in offspring conceived by ART: A systematic review and meta-analysis. *Hum. Reprod. Update* **2021**, *28*, 132–148. [CrossRef]
8. Andreadou, M.T.; Katsaras, G.N.; Talimtzi, P.; Doxani, C.; Zintzaras, E.; Stefanidis, I. Association of assisted reproductive technology with autism spectrum disorder in the offspring: An updated systematic review and meta-analysis. *Eur. J. Pediatr.* **2021**, *180*, 2741–2755. [CrossRef]
9. Zhang, Z.; Liu, X.; Wei, C.; Luo, J.; Shi, Y.; Lin, T.; He, D.; Wei, G. Assisted reproductive technologies and the risk of congenital urogenital tract malformations: A systematic review and meta-analysis. *J. Pediatr. Urol.* **2021**, *17*, 9–20. [CrossRef]
10. Wijs, L.A.; Doherty, D.A.; Keelan, J.A.; Burton, P.; Yovich, J.L.; Beilin, L.; Mori, T.A.; Huang, R.C.; Adams, L.A.; Olynyk, J.K.; et al. Comparison of the cardiometabolic profiles of adolescents conceived through ART with those of a non-ART cohort. *Hum. Reprod.* **2022**, *37*, 1880–1895. [CrossRef]
11. Wijs, L.A.; Doherty, D.A.; Keelan, J.A.; Panicker, V.; Burton, P.; Yovich, J.L.; Hart, R.J. Offspring conceived through ART have normal thyroid function in adolescence and as young adults. *Hum. Reprod.* **2022**, *37*, 1572–1580. [CrossRef]
12. Argyraki, M.; Damdimopoulou, P.; Chatzimeletiou, K.; Grimbizis, G.F.; Tarlatzis, B.C.; Syrrou, M.; Lambropoulos, A. In-utero stress and mode of conception: Impact on regulation of imprinted genes, fetal development and future health. *Hum. Reprod. Update* **2019**, *25*, 777–801. [CrossRef]
13. Sciorio, R.; Esteves, S.C. Contemporary Use of ICSI and Epigenetic Risks to Future Generations. *J. Clin. Med.* **2022**, *11*, 2135. [CrossRef]
14. Monk, D.; Mackay, D.J.G.; Eggermann, T.; Maher, E.R.; Riccio, A. Genomic imprinting disorders: Lessons on how genome, epigenome and environment interact. *Nat. Rev. Genet.* **2019**, *20*, 235–248. [CrossRef]
15. Morgan, H.D.; Santos, F.; Green, K.; Dean, W.; Reik, W. Epigenetic reprogramming in mammals. *Hum. Mol. Genet.* **2005**, *14*, R47–R58. [CrossRef]
16. Agarwal, A.; Maldonado Rosas, I.; Anagnostopoulou, C.; Cannarella, R.; Boitrelle, F.; Munoz, L.V.; Finelli, R.; Durairajanayagam, D.; Henkel, R.; Saleh, R. Oxidative Stress and Assisted Reproduction: A Comprehensive Review of Its Pathophysiological Role and Strategies for Optimizing Embryo Culture Environment. *Antioxidants* **2022**, *11*, 477. [CrossRef]
17. Santi, D.; De Vincentis, S.; Magnani, E.; Spaggiari, G. Impairment of sperm DNA methylation in male infertility: A meta-analytic study. *Andrology* **2017**, *5*, 695–703. [CrossRef]
18. Cannarella, R.; Crafa, A.; Condorelli, R.A.; Mongioì, L.M.; La Vignera, S.; Calogero, A.E. Relevance of sperm imprinted gene methylation on assisted reproductive technique outcomes and pregnancy loss: A systematic review. *Syst. Biol. Reprod. Med.* **2021**, *67*, 251–259. [CrossRef]
19. Barberet, J.; Ducreux, B.; Guilleman, M.; Simon, E.; Bruno, C.; Fauque, P. DNA methylation profiles after ART during human lifespan: A systematic review and meta-analysis. *Hum. Reprod. Update* **2022**, dmac010. [CrossRef]
20. Murray, J.; Farrington, D.P.; Eisner, M.P. Drawing conclusions about causes from systematic reviews of risk factors: The Cambridge Quality Checklists. *J. Exp. Criminol.* **2009**, *5*, 1–23. [CrossRef]
21. Liu, Y.; Li, X.; Chen, S.; Wang, L.; Tan, Y.; Li, X.; Tang, L.; Zhang, J.; Wu, D.; Wu, Y.; et al. Comparison of Genome-Wide DNA Methylation Profiles of Human Fetal Tissues Conceived by in vitro Fertilization and Natural Conception. *Front. Cell Dev. Biol.* **2021**, *9*, 694769. [CrossRef] [PubMed]
22. Zechner, U.; Pliushch, G.; Schneider, E.; El Hajj, N.; Tresch, A.; Shufaro, Y.; Seidmann, L.; Coerdt, W.; Müller, A.M.; Haaf, T. Quantitative methylation analysis of developmentally important genes in human pregnancy losses after ART and spontaneous conception. *Mol. Hum. Reprod.* **2010**, *16*, 704–713. [CrossRef] [PubMed]
23. Zheng, H.Y.; Shi, X.Y.; Wu, F.R.; Wu, Y.Q.; Wang, L.L.; Chen, S.L. Assisted reproductive technologies do not increase risk of abnormal methylation of PEG1/MEST in human early pregnancy loss. *Fertil. Steril.* **2011**, *96*, 84–89.e2. [CrossRef] [PubMed]
24. Argyraki, M.; Katafigiotis, S.; Vavilis, T.; Papadopoulou, Z.; Tzimagiorgis, G.; Haidich, A.B.; Chatzimeletiou, K.; Grimbizis, G.; Tarlatzis, B.; Syrrou, M.; et al. Influence of conception and delivery mode on stress response marker Oct4B1 and imprinted gene expression related to embryo development: A cohort study. *Int. J. Reprod. Biomed.* **2021**, *19*, 217–226. [CrossRef]
25. Barberet, J.; Binquet, C.; Guilleman, M.; Doukani, A.; Choux, C.; Bruno, C.; Bourredjem, A.; Chapusot, C.; Bourc'his, D.; Duffourd, Y.; et al. Do assisted reproductive technologies and in vitro embryo culture influence the epigenetic control of imprinted genes and transposable elements in children? *Hum. Reprod.* **2021**, *36*, 479–492. [CrossRef]
26. Barberet, J.; Romain, G.; Binquet, C.; Guilleman, M.; Bruno, C.; Ginod, P.; Chapusot, C.; Choux, C.; Fauque, P. Do frozen embryo transfers modify the epigenetic control of imprinted genes and transposable elements in newborns compared with fresh embryo transfers and natural conceptions? *Fertil. Steril.* **2021**, *116*, 1468–1480. [CrossRef]
27. Camprubí, C.; Iglesias-Platas, I.; Martin-Trujillo, A.; Salvador-Alarcon, C.; Rodriguez, M.A.; Barredo, D.R.; Court, F.; Monk, D. Stability of genomic imprinting and gestational-age dynamic methylation in complicated pregnancies conceived following assisted reproductive technologies. *Biol. Reprod.* **2013**, *89*, 50. [CrossRef]

28. Caramaschi, D.; Jungius, J.; Page, C.M.; Novakovic, B.; Saffery, R.; Halliday, J.; Lewis, S.; Magnus, M.C.; London, S.J.; Håberg, S.E.; et al. Association of medically assisted reproduction with offspring cord blood DNA methylation across cohorts. *Hum. Reprod.* **2021**, *36*, 2403–2413. [CrossRef]
29. Castillo-Fernandez, J.E.; Loke, Y.J.; Bass-Stringer, S.; Gao, F.; Xia, Y.; Wu, H.; Lu, H.; Liu, Y.; Wang, J.; Spector, T.D.; et al. DNA methylation changes at infertility genes in newborn twins conceived by in vitro fertilisation. *Genome Med.* **2017**, *9*, 28. [CrossRef]
30. Chen, X.J.; Chen, F.; Lv, P.P.; Zhang, D.; Ding, G.L.; Hu, X.L.; Feng, C.; Sheng, J.Z.; Huang, H.F. Maternal high estradiol exposure alters CDKN1C and IGF2 expression in human placenta. *Placenta* **2018**, *61*, 72–79. [CrossRef]
31. Chen, W.; Peng, Y.; Ma, X.; Kong, S.; Tan, S.; Wei, Y.; Zhao, Y.; Zhang, W.; Wang, Y.; Yan, L.; et al. Integrated multi-omics reveal epigenomic disturbance of assisted reproductive technologies in human offspring. *EBioMedicine* **2020**, *61*, 103076. [CrossRef]
32. Choufani, S.; Turinsky, A.L.; Melamed, N.; Greenblatt, E.; Brudno, M.; Bérard, A.; Fraser, W.D.; Weksberg, R.; Trasler, J.; Monnier, P. 3D cohort study group. Impact of assisted reproduction, infertility, sex and paternal factors on the placental DNA methylome. *Hum. Mol. Genet.* **2019**, *28*, 372–385. [CrossRef]
33. Choux, C.; Binquet, C.; Carmignac, V.; Bruno, C.; Chapusot, C.; Barberet, J.; Lamotte, M.; Sagot, P.; Bourc'his, D.; Fauque, P. The epigenetic control of transposable elements and imprinted genes in newborns is affected by the mode of conception: ART versus spontaneous conception without underlying infertility. *Hum. Reprod.* **2018**, *33*, 331–340. [CrossRef]
34. DeBaun, M.R.; Niemitz, E.L.; Feinberg, A.P. Association of in vitro fertilization with Beckwith-Wiedemann syndrome and epigenetic alterations of LIT1 and H19. *Am. J. Hum. Genet.* **2003**, *72*, 156–160. [CrossRef]
35. El Hajj, N.; Haertle, L.; Dittrich, M.; Denk, S.; Lehnen, H.; Hahn, T.; Schorsch, M.; Haaf, T. DNA methylation signatures in cord blood of ICSI children. *Hum. Reprod.* **2017**, *32*, 1761–1769. [CrossRef]
36. Estill, M.S.; Bolnick, J.M.; Waterland, R.A.; Bolnick, A.D.; Diamond, M.P.; Krawetz, S.A. Assisted reproductive technology alters deoxyribonucleic acid methylation profiles in bloodspots of newborn infants. *Fertil. Steril.* **2016**, *106*, 629–639.e10. [CrossRef]
37. Feng, C.; Tian, S.; Zhang, Y.; He, J.; Zhu, X.M.; Zhang, D.; Sheng, J.Z.; Huang, H.F. General imprinting status is stable in assisted reproduction-conceived offspring. *Fertil. Steril.* **2011**, *96*, 1417–1423.e9. [CrossRef]
38. Ghosh, J.; Coutifaris, C.; Sapienza, C.; Mainigi, M. Global DNA methylation levels are altered by modifiable clinical manipulations in assisted reproductive technologies. *Clin. Epigenetics* **2017**, *9*, 14. [CrossRef]
39. Gomes, M.V.; Huber, J.; Ferriani, R.A.; Amaral Neto, A.M.; Ramos, E.S. Abnormal methylation at the KvDMR1 imprinting control region in clinically normal children conceived by assisted reproductive technologies. *Mol. Hum. Reprod.* **2009**, *15*, 471–477. [CrossRef]
40. Ji, M.; Wang, X.; Wu, W.; Guan, Y.; Liu, J.; Wang, J.; Liu, W.; Shen, C. ART manipulation after controlled ovarian stimulation may not increase the risk of abnormal expression and DNA methylation at some CpG sites of H19, IGF2 and SNRPN in foetuses: A pilot study. *Reprod. Biol. Endocrinol.* **2018**, *16*, 63. [CrossRef]
41. Jiang, Y.; Zhu, H.; Chen, H.; Yu, Y.C.; Xu, Y.T.; Liu, F.; He, S.N.; Sagnelli, M.; Zhu, Y.M.; Luo, Q. Elevated Expression of lncRNA MEG3 Induces Endothelial Dysfunction on HUVECs of IVF Born Offspring via Epigenetic Regulation. *Front. Cardiovasc. Med.* **2022**, *8*, 717729. [CrossRef] [PubMed]
42. Katari, S.; Turan, N.; Bibikova, M.; Erinle, O.; Chalian, R.; Foster, M.; Gaughan, J.P.; Coutifaris, C.; Sapienza, C. DNA methylation and gene expression differences in children conceived in vitro or in vivo. *Hum. Mol. Genet.* **2009**, *18*, 3769–3778. [CrossRef] [PubMed]
43. Li, L.; Wang, L.; Le, F.; Liu, X.; Yu, P.; Sheng, J.; Huang, H.; Jin, F. Evaluation of DNA methylation status at differentially methylated regions in IVF-conceived newborn twins. *Fertil. Steril.* **2011**, *95*, 1975–1979. [CrossRef] [PubMed]
44. Lim, D.; Bowdin, S.C.; Tee, L.; Kirby, G.A.; Blair, E.; Fryer, A.; Lam, W.; Oley, C.; Cole, T.; Brueton, L.A.; et al. Clinical and molecular genetic features of Beckwith-Wiedemann syndrome associated with assisted reproductive technologies. *Hum. Reprod.* **2009**, *24*, 741–747. [CrossRef]
45. Litzky, J.F.; Deyssenroth, M.A.; Everson, T.M.; Armstrong, D.A.; Lambertini, L.; Chen, J.; Marsit, C.J. Placental imprinting variation associated with assisted reproductive technologies and subfertility. *Epigenetics* **2017**, *12*, 653–661. [CrossRef]
46. Liu, Z.; Chen, W.; Zhang, Z.; Wang, J.; Yang, Y.K.; Hai, L.; Wei, Y.; Qiao, J.; Sun, Y. Whole-Genome Methylation Analysis Revealed ART-Specific DNA Methylation Pattern of Neuro- and Immune-System Pathways in Chinese Human Neonates. *Front. Genet.* **2021**, *12*, 696840. [CrossRef]
47. Loke, Y.J.; Galati, J.C.; Saffery, R.; Craig, J.M. Association of in vitro fertilization with global and IGF2/H19 methylation variation in newborn twins. *J. Dev. Orig. Health Dis.* **2015**, *6*, 115–124. [CrossRef]
48. Lou, H.; Le, F.; Hu, M.; Yang, X.; Li, L.; Wang, L.; Wang, N.; Gao, H.; Jin, F. Aberrant DNA Methylation of IGF2-H19 Locus in Human Fetus and in Spermatozoa from Assisted Reproductive Technologies. *Reprod. Sci.* **2019**, *26*, 997–1004. [CrossRef]
49. Mani, S.; Ghosh, J.; Lan, Y.; Senapati, S.; Ord, T.; Sapienza, C.; Coutifaris, C.; Mainigi, M. Epigenetic changes in preterm birth placenta suggest a role for ADAMTS genes in spontaneous preterm birth. *Hum. Mol. Genet.* **2019**, *28*, 84–95. [CrossRef]
50. Manning, M.; Lissens, W.; Bonduelle, M.; Camus, M.; De Rijcke, M.; Liebaers, I.; Van Steirteghem, A. Study of DNA-methylation patterns at chromosome 15q11-q13 in children born after ICSI reveals no imprinting defects. *Mol. Hum. Reprod.* **2000**, *6*, 1049–1053. [CrossRef]
51. Melamed, N.; Choufani, S.; Wilkins-Haug, L.E.; Koren, G.; Weksberg, R. Comparison of genome-wide and gene-specific DNA methylation between ART and naturally conceived pregnancies. *Epigenetics* **2015**, *10*, 474–483. [CrossRef]

52. Nelissen, E.C.; Dumoulin, J.C.; Daunay, A.; Evers, J.L.; Tost, J.; van Montfoort, A.P. Placentas from pregnancies conceived by IVF/ICSI have a reduced DNA methylation level at the H19 and MEST differentially methylated regions. *Hum. Reprod.* **2013**, *28*, 1117–1126. [CrossRef]
53. Nelissen, E.C.; Dumoulin, J.C.; Busato, F.; Ponger, L.; Eijssen, L.M.; Evers, J.L.; Tost, J.; van Montfoort, A.P. Altered gene expression in human placentas after IVF/ICSI. *Hum Reprod.* **2014**, *29*, 2821–2831. [CrossRef]
54. Novakovic, B.; Lewis, S.; Halliday, J.; Kennedy, J.; Burgner, D.P.; Czajko, A.; Kim, B.; Sexton-Oates, A.; Juonala, M.; Hammarberg, K.; et al. Assisted reproductive technologies are associated with limited epigenetic variation at birth that largely resolves by adulthood. *Nat. Commun.* **2019**, *10*, 3922. [CrossRef]
55. Oliver, V.F.; Miles, H.L.; Cutfield, W.S.; Hofman, P.L.; Ludgate, J.L.; Morison, I.M. Defects in imprinting and genome-wide DNA methylation are not common in the in vitro fertilization population. *Fertil. Steril.* **2012**, *97*, 147–153.e7. [CrossRef]
56. Penova-Vaselinovic, B.; Melton, P.E.; Huang, R.C.; Yovich, J.L.; Burton, P.; Wijs, L.A.; Hart, R.J. DNA methylation patterns within whole blood of adolescents born from assisted reproductive technology are not different from adolescents born from natural conception. *Hum. Reprod.* **2021**, *36*, 2035–2049. [CrossRef]
57. Pliushch, G.; Schneider, E.; Schneider, T.; El Hajj, N.; Rösner, S.; Strowitzki, T.; Haaf, T. In vitro maturation of oocytes is not associated with altered deoxyribonucleic acid methylation patterns in children from in vitro fertilization or intracytoplasmic sperm injection. *Fertil. Steril.* **2015**, *103*, 720–727.e1. [CrossRef]
58. Puumala, S.E.; Nelson, H.H.; Ross, J.A.; Nguyen, R.H.; Damario, M.A.; Spector, L.G. Similar DNA methylation levels in specific imprinting control regions in children conceived with and without assisted reproductive technology: A cross-sectional study. *BMC Pediatr.* **2012**, *12*, 33. [CrossRef]
59. Rancourt, R.C.; Harris, H.R.; Michels, K.B. Methylation levels at imprinting control regions are not altered with ovulation induction or in vitro fertilization in a birth cohort. *Hum. Reprod.* **2012**, *27*, 2208–2216. [CrossRef]
60. Rossignol, S.; Steunou, V.; Chalas, C.; Kerjean, A.; Rigolet, M.; Viegas-Pequignot, E.; Jouannet, P.; Le Bouc, Y.; Gicquel, C. The epigenetic imprinting defect of patients with Beckwith-Wiedemann syndrome born after assisted reproductive technology is not restricted to the 11p15 region. *J. Med. Genet.* **2006**, *43*, 902–907. [CrossRef]
61. Sakian, S.; Louie, K.; Wong, E.C.; Havelock, J.; Kashyap, S.; Rowe, T.; Taylor, B.; Ma, S. Altered gene expression of H19 and IGF2 in placentas from ART pregnancies. *Placenta* **2015**, *36*, 1100–1105. [CrossRef]
62. Santos, F.; Hyslop, L.; Stojkovic, P.; Leary, C.; Murdoch, A.; Reik, W.; Stojkovic, M.; Herbert, M.; Dean, W. Evaluation of epigenetic marks in human embryos derived from IVF and ICSI. *Hum. Reprod.* **2010**, *25*, 2387–2395. [CrossRef]
63. Shi, X.; Chen, S.; Zheng, H.; Wang, L.; Wu, Y. Abnormal DNA Methylation of Imprinted Loci in Human Preimplantation Embryos. *Reprod. Sci.* **2014**, *21*, 978–983. [CrossRef]
64. Song, S.; Ghosh, J.; Mainigi, M.; Turan, N.; Weinerman, R.; Truongcao, M.; Coutifaris, C.; Sapienza, C. DNA methylation differences between in vitro- and in vivo-conceived children are associated with ART procedures rather than infertility. *Clin. Epigenet.* **2015**, *7*, 41. [CrossRef]
65. Tang, L.; Liu, Z.; Zhang, R.; Su, C.; Yang, W.; Yao, Y.; Zhao, S. Imprinting alterations in sperm may not significantly influence ART outcomes and imprinting patterns in the cord blood of offspring. *PLoS ONE.* **2017**, *12*, e0187869. [CrossRef]
66. Tierling, S.; Souren, N.Y.; Gries, J.; Loporto, C.; Groth, M.; Lutsik, P.; Neitzel, H.; Utz-Billing, I.; Gillessen-Kaesbach, G.; Kentenich, H.; et al. Assisted reproductive technologies do not enhance the variability of DNA methylation imprints in human. *J. Med. Genet.* **2010**, *47*, 371–376. [CrossRef]
67. Turan, N.; Katari, S.; Gerson, L.F.; Chalian, R.; Foster, M.W.; Gaughan, J.P.; Coutifaris, C.; Sapienza, C. Inter- and intra-individual variation in allele-specific DNA methylation and gene expression in children conceived using assisted reproductive technology. *PLoS Genet.* **2010**, *6*, e1001033. [CrossRef]
68. Vincent, R.N.; Gooding, L.D.; Louie, K.; Chan Wong, E.; Ma, S. Altered DNA methylation and expression of PLAGL1 in cord blood from assisted reproductive technology pregnancies compared with natural conceptions. *Fertil. Steril.* **2016**, *106*, 739–748.e3. [CrossRef] [PubMed]
69. White, C.R.; Denomme, M.M.; Tekpetey, F.R.; Feyles, V.; Power, S.G.; Mann, M.R. High Frequency of Imprinted Methylation Errors in Human Preimplantation Embryos. *Sci. Rep.* **2015**, *5*, 17311. [CrossRef] [PubMed]
70. Whitelaw, N.; Bhattacharya, S.; Hoad, G.; Horgan, G.W.; Hamilton, M.; Haggarty, P. Epigenetic status in the offspring of spontaneous and assisted conception. *Hum. Reprod.* **2014**, *29*, 1452–1458. [CrossRef] [PubMed]
71. Wong, E.C.; Hatakeyama, C.; Robinson, W.P.; Ma, S. DNA methylation at H19/IGF2 ICR1 in the placenta of pregnancies conceived by in vitro fertilization and intracytoplasmic sperm injection. *Fertil. Steril.* **2011**, *95*, e1–e3. [CrossRef]
72. Yoshida, H.; Abe, H.; Arima, T. Quality evaluation of IVM embryo and imprinting genes of IVM babies. *J. Assist. Reprod. Genet.* **2013**, *30*, 221–225. [CrossRef]
73. Zhang, M.; Lu, L.; Zhang, Y.; Li, X.; Fan, X.; Chen, X.; Tang, J.; Han, B.; Li, M.; Tao, J.; et al. Methylation-reprogrammed AGTR1 results in increased vasoconstriction by angiotensin II in human umbilical cord vessel following in vitro fertilization-embryo transfer. *Life Sci.* **2019**, *234*, 116792. [CrossRef]
74. Hu, T.; Zhu, X.; Pi, W.; Yu, M.; Shi, H.; Tuan, D. Hypermethylated LTR retrotransposon exhibits enhancer activity. *Epigenetics* **2017**, *12*, 226–237. [CrossRef]
75. Xavier, M.J.; Roman, S.D.; Aitken, R.J.; Nixon, B. Transgenerational inheritance: How impacts to the epigenetic and genetic information of parents affect offspring health. *Hum. Reprod. Update* **2019**, *25*, 518–540. [CrossRef]

76. De Mouzon, J.; Lancaster, P.; Nygren, K.G.; Sullivan, E.; Zegers-Hochschild, F.; Mansour, R.; Ishihara, O.; Adamson, D. International Committee for Monitoring Assisted Reproductive Technology. World collaborative report on Assisted Reproductive Technology, 2002. *Hum. Reprod.* **2009**, *24*, 2310–2320. [CrossRef]
77. Barker, D.J. The origins of the developmental origins theory. *J. Intern. Med.* **2007**, *261*, 412–417. [CrossRef]
78. Henningsen, A.A.; Gissler, M.; Rasmussen, S.; Opdahl, S.; Wennerholm, U.B.; Spangsmose, A.L.; Tiitinen, A.; Bergh, C.; Romundstad, L.B.; Laivuori, H.; et al. Imprinting disorders in children born after ART: A Nordic study from the CoNARTaS group. *Hum. Reprod.* **2020**, *35*, 1178–1184. [CrossRef]
79. Uk, A.; Collardeau-Frachon, S.; Scanvion, Q.; Michon, L.; Amar, E. Assisted Reproductive Technologies and imprinting disorders: Results of a study from a French congenital malformations registry. *Eur. J. Med. Genet.* **2018**, *61*, 518–523. [CrossRef]

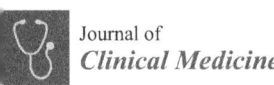

Review

Placental Volume and Uterine Artery Doppler in Pregnancy Following In Vitro Fertilization: A Comprehensive Literature Review

Serena Resta, Gaia Scandella, Ilenia Mappa, Maria Elena Pietrolucci, Pavjola Maqina and Giuseppe Rizzo *

Department of Obstetrics and Gynecology, Fondazione Policlinico Tor Vergata, Università di Roma Tor Vergata, Viale Oxford 81, 00133 Roma, Italy
* Correspondence: giuseppe.rizzo@uniroma2.it

Abstract: The number of pregnancies achieved using in vitro fertilization (IVF) is rapidly increasing around the world. The chance of obtaining a successful pregnancy is also significantly improved due to technological advances and improvement in infertility treatment. Despite this success, there is evidence that pregnancy conceived by IVF has an increased risk of adverse maternal and perinatal outcome mainly represented by the development of hypertensive diseases, pre-eclampsia, and fetal growth restriction. Although different cofactors may play a role in the genesis of these diseases, the development of the placenta has a pivotal function in determining pregnancy outcomes. Advances in ultrasound technology already allows for evaluation in the first trimester, the impedance to flow in the uterine artery, and the placental volume using Doppler and three-dimensional techniques. This review article aims to describe the modification occurring in placental volume and hemodynamics after IVF and to summarize the differences present according to the type of IVF (fresh vs. frozen-thawed embryos).

Keywords: in vitro fertilization; placenta uterine Doppler; fetal growth restriction pre-eclampsia

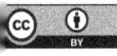

1. Introduction

In the past few years, the percentage of pregnancies obtained from in vitro fertilization (IVF) is dramatically increasing, overall due to an implementation of new technologies and to the relevant percentage of infertile couples in reproductive-age estimated to be between 8 and 12% worldwide and of 15% in Italy [1,2]. An increase in the number of couples that resorted to ART has been registered, going from 77.509 in 2018 to 78.618 in 2019 [2].

An increase in adverse obstetrical outcomes after IVF compared to natural conception has been widely studied, above all placenta-related pregnancy complications such as: placental insertion abnormalities (placenta previa, placental abruptio, placenta accrete) and short-term and long-term placenta-related diseases. The former includes preeclampsia (PE) abnormality in fetal growth causing a small for gestational age (SGA) fetus and fetal growth restriction (FGR) or accelerated resulting in a large for gestational age (LGA) fetus. Short term placental related disease includes preterm birth (PTB) and postpartum hemorrhage [3–5]. Long term placenta-related disease manifests in adulthood and includes cardiovascular disease, metabolic syndrome, diabetes, and obesity [6,7].

The impact of different procedures as elective frozen-thawed embryo transfer (eFET) and fresh embryo transfer (ET) on the pregnancy rate and outcomes was extensively studied and there is evidence that pregnancies from frozen embryos had lower obstetric and perinatal complications when compared those obtained after fresh oocyte cycles in terms of a decreased rate of SGA, and ovarian hyperstimulation (OHSS). No difference in the rate of live birth between the two strategies (eFET and fresh ET) was found, while a higher prevalence of LGA fetuses and maternal hypertension in hormonal treatment cycle eFET was described [8–10]. Thus, the transfer of eFET is nowadays considered a standard procedure in many fertility clinics [8].

Despite these findings, the underlying mechanisms causing higher risk in adverse obstetrical outcomes in pregnancies obtained from IVF are not yet fully clarified. Poor pregnancy outcome has been related to a defective early placentation occurring at different levels, either in the restricted remodeling or in obstructive lesions of the spiral arteries. There are different factors that might cause an impaired trophoblastic invasion and influence placental development such as the impaired endometrium receptivity linked to hormonal therapy, the epigenetic modifications in the embryo related to IVF procedures, maternal immune response, or different cryopreservation procedures [11–13].

In this way, studying the development of placenta in the IVF-pregnancies is becoming a priority in the research agenda. A correct development of the placenta is a prerequisite for the pregnancy progress and studying placental development during pregnancy has become challenging.

The ultrasound has allowed for investigation of the development of the placenta through some variables, such as the evaluation of the placental volume by using three-dimensional (3D) ultrasonography and the evaluation of the impedance to flow in the uterine arteries (UtA) by calculating the pulsatility index (PI) with Doppler. In IVF-pregnancies, the evaluation of these variables promises to be a useful tool for early detection of placenta-related disorders [14,15].

The aim of this review is to provide to readers an update on the impact of IVF on obstetrical and perinatal outcomes in the attempt to clarify if the first trimester ultrasonographic variables may be applied in the prediction of PE and anomalies of fetal growth in such pregnancies. The identification of high-risk pregnancies is of paramount importance as these women could benefit from tighter follow-up and dedicated management to avoid or to reduce maternal and fetal morbidity conditions.

2. Obstetric and Perinatal Outcomes Resulting from Ivf Pregnancies

The placenta must guarantee the maintenance of the pregnancy and the fetal well-being through correct exchange of gases, growth factors, endocrine signals, cytokines, and nutrients. Placenta development starts at approximately 6–10 days post-conception, when trophoblast cells of blastocyst adhere to the decidua [16]. In early gestation, the human placenta is constituted by two layers: an inner one of proliferating cytotrophoblasts, that ensures the exchange of nutrients and oxygen from maternal blood and an outer which assures a correct amount of blood during the pregnancy by invading the endometrial stroma and remodelling the uterine spiral arteries [17]. The placentation process represents a complex and not fully understood process of immunotolerance: during the adhesion and invasion of the myometrium by the blastocyst, an immunomodulation release of pro-angiogenic and endothelial factors happens, which leads to adaptive changes of the uterine spiral arteries [18]. New studies are focusing their attention on the origins of placental mesenchymal cells as they appear to have a pivotal role in establishing and sustaining the development of placental vasculature [16–19]. Despite its importance in the success of reproduction, the development of the human placenta is yet to be fully understood despite an altered placentation could lead to miscarriage, unexplained stillbirth, preterm labor, placental abruption, PE, and fetal growth anomalies [17–22].

Despite the improvement occurring in laboratory technology and clinical management of infertile women requiring IVF, this procedure is still associated with an high rate of adverse perinatal outcomes and overall placenta-related pregnancy complications [23–25].

Recent meta-analysis studies have confirmed how pregnancies obtained from IVF techniques are associated with an increased risk of poor obstetric outcome including: miscarriage, chromosomal abnormalities, PE, PTB, FGR), placenta previa, abruptio placentae, post-partum haemorrhages, as well as peri and postnatal complications, such as neonatal death, low birth weight infants, congenital malformations, musculoskeletal abnormalities and childhood cancers [26,27].

The risk of obstetric complications can be largely increased by many factors: presence of twin pregnancies after multiple embryo transfers, as well as an older pregnant population and gametes quality, previous history of recurrent abortions (RPL) and causes of infertility itself (polycystic ovarian syndrome) [10,28]. Unfortunately, only little data are available on the explanations of such augmented risk. Different mechanisms have been assumed to play a role in the defective early placentation including genetic and epigenetic mechanisms of implantation, alterations in endometrial receptivity, invasion, and growth of the trophoblast, genetic and/or epigenetic alterations of oocyte and/or embryos due to biological manipulations, and immunotolerance in case of egg donor pregnancies [29].

Recent meta-analyses have proved that in singleton IVF pregnancies there is an increased risk of placental abruption (RR 1.83, 95% CI 1.49 to 2.24), placenta previa (RR 3.71, 95% CI 2.67 to 5.16), antepartum (RR 2.11, 95% CI 1.86 to 2.38), and postpartum hemorrhage (RR 1.29, 95% CI 1.06 to 1.57) [27,30]. A higher incidence of gestational hypertension and diabetes, cesarean deliveries, PTB, SGA, and perinatal mortality was also described [30]. Nevertheless, relevant biases were present due to the inclusion in the natural conception group of women who obtained the pregnancy with ovulation induction or intrauterine insemination, leading to an underestimation of the association between ART and adverse outcomes [30]. Consequently, the risk of developing gestational diabetes, placental abruption, PTB, fetal growth defect, and perinatal mortality may be further increased when the control group is constructed excluding these women from the spontaneous conception definition [30] and limit the recalculation of the odds ratio or relative risk of the maternal and perinatal complications occurring in IVF women.

Of interest is the lack of IVF specific pathologies and they resemble the same characteristics of when these diseases are present in a naturally conceived population. In other words, there are no different phenotypes of PE, FGR or placenta accrete spectrum between the 2 groups of women despite the higher prevalence in the IVF group.

2.1. The Role of Ovarian Stimulation

Concerning safety-evaluation in IVF it is necessary to highlight the difficulties in discerning the influence on the outcomes that the underlying causes of infertility might bring versus potential risks related to IVF procedures themselves. IVF are characterized by the ovarian hormonal stimulation followed by the pick-up of the oocytes and their subsequent fertilization. This procedure implies the transfer of a single or fresher or eFET embryos. eFet embryos after thawing may be transferred in the uterus during natural or hormonally artificial induced cycles. In recent years, the number of eFET has increased and so have pregnancy rates, which are now better than those following fresh IVF embryos transfer [31].

It has been suggested that controlled ovarian stimulation (COS) (e.g., subcutaneous gonadotropins) lead inevitably to a change in the maternal hormonal structure, determining changes in the woman's reproductive system, as modifications of the endometrium. Different hormonal treatment strategies used in controlled ovarian stimulation and laboratory IVF techniques can negatively impact endometrial receptivity and gamete status. Hence, it was suggested that performing eFET was better than fresh embryo transfer being associated with decreased ovarian hyperstimulation incidence with improved reproductive outcomes [32]. However, it is still unclear how the different preparation methods of the endometrium can affect the outcomes of eFET pregnancies and the selection of the treatment of choice [33].

2.2. Differences between Fresh and Freeze and Thawed Embryo Transfer

Two recent systematic reviews and meta-analyses demonstrated that singleton pregnancies obtained from eFET show a more favorable maternal and perinatal outcomes than those reached after fresh oocyte transfer including a lower risk of PTB (<37 weeks) (RR 0.84, 95% CI 0.78 to 0.90), SGA (RR 0.45, 95% CI 0.30 to 0.66) and birthweight <2500 g) (RR 0.69, 95%CI 0.62 to 0.76). The incidence of perinatal mortality, antepartum hemorrhage, congenital anomalies, and admission to neonatal units resulted similarly between the two procedures. Conversely, a large, randomized trial demonstrated a higher risk of delivering LGA newborns and the development of hypertensive disorders of pregnancy in the eFET group [31]. Probably, these discoveries suggested that the hyperestrogenism following controlled ovarian stimulation in fresh ET, immediately before embryo implantation, might lead to abnormal endometrial angiogenesis resulting in a reduced implantation and altered placentation. Conversely, hormonal levels in eFET cycle could recreate a more natural uterine environment [34]. However, the underlying mechanisms suggesting a greater incidence of LGA babies in eFET are still to be clarified. Possible explanations should be a better implantation potential, better placentation, and subsequent fetal overgrowth or epigenetic modifications in the early embryonic stages due to freezing and thawing procedures [35].

Unfortunately, there is a heterogeneity among studies, which made their comparability difficult in terms of population sampled, design of the studies, freezing methods (slow freezing or vitrification), embryo stage, natural cycles, or hormone replacement used [9,36]. Furthermore, the results of these meta-analyses were based on observational studies, making them subject to bias.

In contrast with previous Roque M et al. [24] in a recent meta-analyses analyzing 11 randomized controlled studies including 5379 patients showed no difference in rates preterm birth between fresh ET and eFE a result different from that previously reported [9,36]. It also showed a significant increase in live birth rates (LBTs) with eFET solely in hyperresponders patients and in pregnancies undergoing PGT-A. Further, this study confirmed the risk of pre-eclampsia was higher with eFET compared to fresh ET, probably due to endometrial priming with supraphysiological concentrations of estrogen during artificial FET cycles. This conclusion is in agreement with the result of a recent Cochrane review, showing a lower prevalence of ovarian hyperstimulation syndrome in eFET cycle despite no difference in the cumulative life birth ratio between the two strategies [8]. This explains why the transfer of frozen-thawed embryos has become the standard procedure in most fertility clinics. Although this procedure does not seem to reduce IVF success rates, an increased prevalence of PE after eFET technique has been reported [8,37].

2.3. Endometrial Preparation

Endometrial preparation for an embryo transfer (e.g., oral estradiol and luteal phase support) may influence the endocrine uterine environment during the embryo transfer, playing an essential role in vascular adaptation of the mother to pregnancy, increasing the risk of placental development and weight of the offspring.

Endometrial preparation before eFET can occur how ovulatory or programmed cycles. To date, in frozen embryo transfer there is no consensus on the best endometrial preparation method or the duration of hormonal replacement [38]. Emerging data suggests that these differences could have a detrimental impact on adverse obstetrical outcomes in pregnancies from artificial cycles, above all in hypertensive disorders [33].

In 2019 Saito et al. [6] evaluated the pregnancy outcomes of 100,000 patients undergoing FET during natural or hormonal replacement cycles. Pregnancies conceived in a hormone replacement cycle had higher odds of hypertensive disorders of pregnancy (4% vs. 3%, aOR 1.43; 95% CI, 1.14–1.80), placenta accreta (0.9% vs. 0.1%, aOR 6.91; 95% CI, 2.87–16.66) cesarean section (44.5% vs. 33.7%, aOR 1.69; 95% CI, 1.55–1.84) and post term delivery associated with a decreased risk to develop gestational diabetes mellitus (1.5% vs. 3.3%, aOR 0.52; 95% CI, 0.40–0.68) in comparison to natural cycle FET.

In agreement with these results, Ginström Ernstad et al. [39] in a large retrospective study, found an increased risk of hypertensive disorders in pregnancy (10.5 vs. 6.1%, aOR 1.78; 95% CI 1.43–2.21) and postpartum hemorrhage (19.4% vs. 7.9%, aOR 2.63; 95% CI, 2.20–3.13) in hormone replacement cycles when compared to natural cycles. Moreover, higher risks for post-term birth, macrosomia, and cesarean delivery were detected [39].

Given that endometrial preparation is a less physiological condition than a natural cycle, the increased risk of hypertensive disorders may be due to changes in endometrial receptivity modulating placental development. Moreover, it was hypothesized that in patients who have programmed cycles have a decrease of substances produced by the corpus luteum in early pregnancy, particularly the potent vasodilator relaxin and vascular endothelial growth factor levels, lower angiogenic and nonangiogenic circulatory endothelial progenitor cells and a lack of drop in mean arterial pressure during pregnancy [40,41]. It was demonstrated that the CL is implicated in the adaptation of the maternal cardiovascular system in early gestation and its absence in eFET may be associated with reduced aortic compliance and increased risk of PE [40,41]. Anyway, the association between endometrium preparation and adverse obstetric outcomes must be clarified with further studies that include other possible confounders.

Indeed, every single step or procedure carried out during IVF can play an independent and essential role in determining obstetric risks: cryopreservation methods, different hormonal treatment, and laboratory techniques. Vitrification showed higher pregnancy rates than slow-freezing, however perinatal outcomes are similar between the two methods [42,43]. Potential impact of gamete manipulation, as intracytoplasmic sperm injection (ICSI) and in vitro embryo culture were investigated in recent literature. Specific laboratory procedures, such as incubation systems, types of embryos culture used, the duration of the culture, and ICSI could constitute a source of "stress" for the developing embryo. At last, further large studies are required to identify the contribution of each single confounder on pregnancy and obstetrical outcomes after ART.

3. Non-Invasive Parameters in the First Trimester of Placental Development In-Vitro Fertilization Pregnancies

As previously mentioned, the inadequate trophoblastic invasion seems to be the most important etiological factor in the early-onset PE and FGR [44]. Given the increase in the number of pregnancies achieved with IVF, the prediction and possible prevention of adverse outcomes in such women is clinically relevant.

3.1. First Trimester Uterine Doppler

The assessment of placental development during pregnancy is challenging but can be assessed by evaluating some first-trimester non-invasive parameters such as the impedance to flow in the uterine arteries by calculating the UtA-PI and the assessment of first trimester placental volume (PV) and utero-placenta vascular volume (uPVV).

In a spontaneously conceived pregnancy, there is a decline of placental vascular resistance resulting in a progressive decrease of UtA-PI in the three trimesters of pregnancy (Figure 1) [45].

An impaired trophoblastic invasion of the uterine decidua indices an altered remodeling of the spiral arteries determines an increased vascular resistance in the uterine arteries already evident from 11 weeks onwards and it is frequently associated with a later development of PE [46–48]. Therefore, given the potential consequences of a higher incidence of placenta-related adverse outcomes in IVF pregnancies, the evaluation of impedance to flow in the uterine arteries in the context of in vitro fertilization was of particular interest.

Despite the high incidence of PE in IVF women, no difference was found in UtA-PI when compared with natural conceived pregnancies in the first trimester. On this basis there are extensive reports suggesting that the underlying mechanisms behind the increased incidence of PE is not related to an impaired uteroplacental perfusion [49–51]. It might be due to a coexistence of different factors that lead to abnormal placental development, such as different expression in placental gene expression or the presence of an abnormal immune response at the maternal–fetal interface that takes place particularly when the pregnancies are obtained with egg donor [13,52,53].

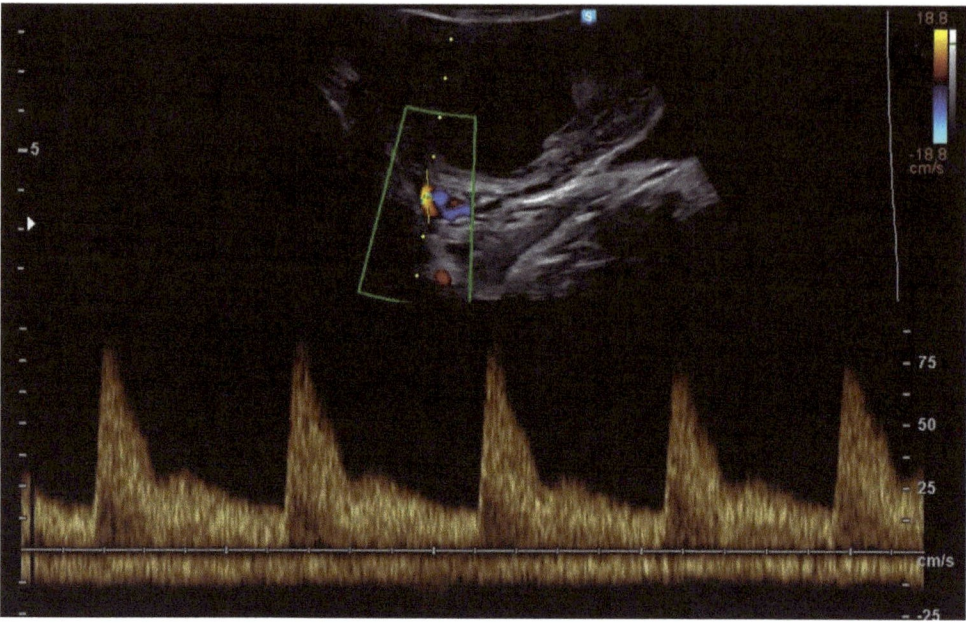

Figure 1. Example of Doppler tracing obtained at 12 weeks from the uterine artery.

Few studies have evaluated UtA-PI in IVF patients comparing between pregnancies conceived from eFET and fresh blastocyst transfer [49–51]. Two studies showed a better uterine perfusion and fetal growth in the frozen blastocyst transfer group compared to those that underwent fresh blastocyst transfer [3,54].

Choux et al. showed that PI was significantly higher in the fresh embryo transfer group (1.86 ± 0.64) than in the naturally conceived (1.52 ± 0.59; $p = 0.001$) and Pi was lower in the eFET group compared to the fresh embryo transfer group ($p = 0.001$) [3]. These results were confirmed by two other studies that observed lower UtA-PI values for the eFET group compared with the fresh-blastocyst-transfer group [54,55].

Differences in maternal characteristics and the IVF procedures used could explain the apparent contradiction of reduced UtA-PI in the eFET group during pregnancy, known to have a higher incidence of early-onset PE [56]. Instead, the higher risk of LGA and the lower risk of SGA could be explained from a lower UtA-PI in eFET.

3.2. First Trimester 3D Placental Volume

A huge advance was made with the introduction of three-dimensional ultrasound, making it easier to measure placental volume. The implementation of three-dimensional (3D) ultrasound allowed for reproducible measurements of placental volume and has been shown to be an indicator of placental insufficiency, predicting the placenta-related pregnancy complications, such as PE (Figure 2) [48,57–59].

In IVF pregnancies, placental volume in ultrasound has been investigated and the results compared with that of the naturally conceived were conflicting [50,51,60–63]. Rifouna et al. [60] analyzed 70 pregnancies and no difference in placental vascular and trophoblastic volume in the first trimester was found between IVF and spontaneous pregnancies Rizzo et al. [51,63] reported significantly reduced placental volume in IVF pregnancies compared to spontaneous pregnancies, particularly in donor oocyte recipients, probably due to different immune responses of the mothers to trophoblast antigens.

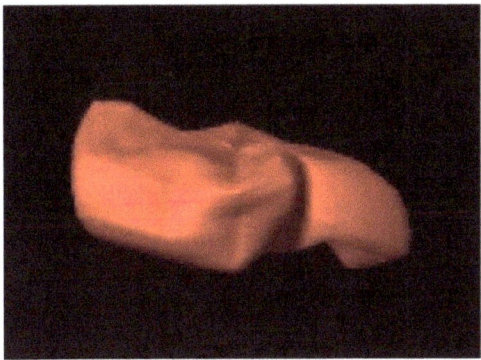 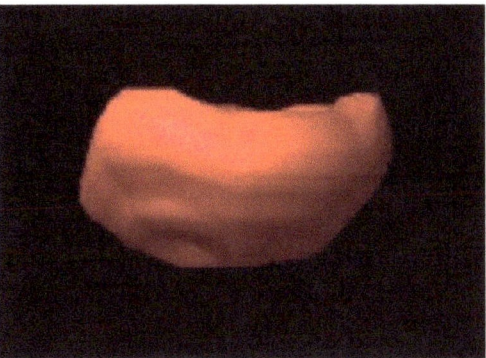

57 ml **36 ml**

Figure 2. Example of 3D reconstruction of the placental volume at 12 weeks in a spontaneously conceived pregnancy and in an IVF with fresh embryo. The volume is significantly reduced in the latter.

These discrepancies may be due to different techniques in performing ultrasounds, the largest samples in Rizzo's study (70 versus 416) and differences among studies in the characteristics of IVF pregnancies [60–63].

To the best of our knowledge, only two studies analyzed placental volume and uterine artery Doppler distinguished IVF after fresh embryo transfer from those after eFET [3,51]. Rizzo et al. [51] found no differences in UtA-PI between frozen-thawed ET, fresh ET, and natural conception in agreement with other authors [49,50]. Furthermore, this study demonstrated the presence of a reduced placental volume in IVF pregnancies compared to those conceived naturally and the IVF pregnancies with fresh embryos showed a significantly lower placental volume than in the frozen-thawed embryos and a higher incidence of PE. It was hypothesized that altered endometrial receptivity due to the use of high-dose gonadotrophin ovarian stimulation in the fresh group could influence the placental development. As with Rizzo's study, Choux et al. [3] found a larger placental volume in pregnancies after eFET compared to pregnancies after fresh embryo transfer. As placental volume correlated to birthweight, this is consistent with the findings of a higher incidence of LGA newborns after frozen-thawed ET [9,35].

A summary of the characteristics and the results obtained in the studies considered is reported in the Supplementary Material.

A possible explanation, as Conrad's theory suggests [40], could be that the role of the corpus luteal is pivotal for a natural maternal hormonal environment during implantation and hemodynamic adaption to pregnancy and in this study, approximately 75% of frozen-thawed ET were performed in a natural cycle, in the presence therefore of a corpus luteal.

Future studies are needed to assess the clinical utility of first trimester vascularization indices and placental volume as a predictor of pre-eclampsia in IVF pregnancies [64].

4. Conclusions

This review confirms that pregnancies obtained with IVF have a higher incidence of maternal and perinatal adverse outcome than naturally conceived pregnancies. Among IVF pregnancies those obtained by eFET showed better obstetric and perinatal outcomes than those obtained after fresh oocyte cycles in term of lower risk of SGA, LBW, and ovarian hyperstimulation. Despite the absence of difference in the cumulative live birth rates between the two conception modes, there is a higher risk of hypertension disorders in hormonal treatment cycle in frozen-thawed ET.

In this review, we were unable to clarify the underling mechanisms causing the maternal and perinatal complications due to the heterogenicity of the available studies on this topic and the impossibility of obtaining direct analysis on human pregnancies. Irrespective of these limitations, the higher risk of PE in eFET contrasts with the discovered that the measurement of placental volume in 3D ultrasound was lower in fresh embryos compared to frozen-thawed embryos. Often the main limitations of these studies were related to a lack of comparability due to a high risk of selection bias, such as the women's characteristics, endometrial preparation, method of cryopreservation, and study populations.

Moreover, the potential clinical benefit should be underlined. Acquisition during the first trimester of uterine Doppler and placental volume allows for the identification of a subgroup of IVF women at a higher risk of developing complications for which a closer surveillance is necessary and in which prophylactic treatment can be applied under prospective multicenter trails

Supplementary Materials: The following supporting information can be downloaded at: https://www.mdpi.com/article/10.3390/jcm11195793/s1.

Author Contributions: Conceptualization G.R. and I.M.; literature search and first draft, S.R., G.S., M.E.P. and P.M.; writing—original draft preparation, S.R. and G.S.; writing—review and editing, G.R. and I.M. All authors have read and agreed to the published version of the manuscript.

Funding: This research received no external funding.

Institutional Review Board Statement: Not applicable.

Informed Consent Statement: Not applicable.

Data Availability Statement: Not applicable.

Conflicts of Interest: The authors declare no conflict of interest.

References

1. Dyer, S.; Chambers, G.M.; de Mouzon, J.; Nygren, K.G.; Zegers-Hochschild, F.; Mansour, R.; Ishihara, O.; Banker, M.; Adamson, G.D. International Committee for Monitoring Assisted Reproductive Technologies World Report: Assisted Reproductive Technology 2008, 2009 and 2010. *Hum. Reprod.* **2016**, *31*, 1588–1609. [CrossRef] [PubMed]
2. Ministero Della Salute: Procreazione Medicalmente Assistita. Available online: https://www.salute.gov.it/portale/donna/dettaglioContenutiDonna.jsp?lingua=italiano&id=4570&area=Salute%20donna&menu=nascita (accessed on 16 September 2022).
3. Choux, C.; Ginod, P.; Barberet, J.; Rousseau, T.; Bruno, C.; Sagot, P.; Astruc, K.; Fauque, P. Placental volume and other first-trimester outcomes: Are there differences between fresh embryo transfer, frozen-thawed embryo transfer and natural conception? *Reprod. Biomed. Online* **2019**, *38*, 538–548. [CrossRef] [PubMed]
4. Jackson, R.A.; Gibson, K.A.; Wu, Y.W.; Croughan, M.S. Perinatal outcomes in singletons following in vitro fertilization: A meta-analysis. *Obstet. Gynecol.* **2004**, *103*, 551–563. [CrossRef]
5. McDonald, S.D.; Han, Z.; Mulla, S.; Murphy, K.E.; Beyene, J.; Ohlsson, A.; Knowledge Synthesis Group. Preterm birth and low birth weight among in vitro fertilization singletons: A systematic review and meta-analyses. *Eur. J. Obstet. Gynecol. Reprod. Biol.* **2009**, *146*, 138–148. [CrossRef]
6. Saito, K.; Kuwahara, A.; Ishikawa, T.; Morisaki, N.; Miyado, M.; Miyado, K.; Fukami, M.; Miyasaka, N.; Ishihara, O.; Irahara, M.; et al. Endometrial preparation methods for frozen-thawed embryo transfer are associated with altered risks of hypertensive disorders of pregnancy, placenta accreta, and gestational diabetes mellitus. *Hum. Reprod.* **2019**, *34*, 1567–1575. [CrossRef] [PubMed]
7. Thomopoulos, C.; Tsioufis, C.; Michalopoulou, H.; Makris, T.; Papademetriou, V.; Stefanadis, C. Assisted reproductive technology and pregnancy-related hypertensive complications: A systematic review. *J. Hum. Hypertens.* **2013**, *27*, 148–157. [CrossRef]
8. Wong, K.M.; Wely, M.; van Mol, F.; Repping, S.; Mastenbroek, S. Fresh versus frozen embryo transfers in assisted reproduction. *Cochrane Libr. Cochrane Rev.* **2017**, *3*, CD011184. [CrossRef]
9. Maheshwari, A.; Pandey, S.; Shetty, A.; Hamilton, M.; Bhattacharya, S. Obstetric and perinatal outcomes in singleton pregnancies resulting from the transfer of frozen thawed versus fresh embryos generated through in vitro fertilization treatment: A systematic review and meta-analysis. *Fertil. Steril.* **2012**, *98*, 368–377. [CrossRef]
10. Sutcliffe, A.G.; Ludwig, M. Outcome of assisted reproduction. *Lancet* **2007**, *370*, 351–359. [CrossRef]
11. Steegers-Theunissen, R.P.; Twigt, J.; Pestinger, V.; Sinclair, K.D. The periconceptional period, reproduction and long-term health of offspring: The importance of one-carbon metabolism. *Hum. Reprod. Update* **2013**, *19*, 640–655. [CrossRef]

12. Choux, C.; Carmignac, V.; Bruno, C.; Sagot, P.; Vaiman, D.; Fauque, P. The placenta: Phenotypic and epigenetic modifications induced by Assisted Reproductive Technologies throughout pregnancy. *Clin. Epigenetics* **2015**, *7*, 87. [CrossRef] [PubMed]
13. van der Hoorn, M.L.; Lashley, E.E.; Bianchi, D.W.; Claas, F.H.; Schonkeren, C.M.; Scherjon, S.A. Clinical and immunologic aspects of egg donation pregnancies: A systematic review. *Hum. Reprod. Update* **2010**, *16*, 704–712. [CrossRef] [PubMed]
14. Effendi, M.; Demers, S.; Giguère, Y.; Forest, J.C.; Brassard, N.; Girard, M.; Gouin, K.; Bujold, E. Association between first-trimester placental volume and birth weight. *Placenta* **2014**, *35*, 99–102. [CrossRef] [PubMed]
15. Plasencia, W.; González-Dávila, E.; González Lorenzo, A.; Armas-González, M.; Padrón, E.; González-González, N.L. First trimester placental volume and vascular indices in pregnancies complicated by preeclampsia. *Prenat. Diagn.* **2015**, *35*, 1247–1254. [CrossRef]
16. Boss, A.L.; Chamley, L.W.; James, J.L. Placental formation in early pregnancy: How is the centre of the placenta made? *Hum. Reprod. Update* **2018**, *24*, 750–760. [CrossRef]
17. Brosens, I. Placental bed & maternal—Fetal disorders. Preface. *Best Pract. Res. Clin. Obstet. Gynaecol.* **2011**, *25*, 247–248.
18. Hanna, J.; Goldman-Wohl, D.; Hamani, Y.; Avraham, I.; Greenfield, C.; Natanson-Yaron, S.; Prus, D.; Cohen-Daniel, L.; Arnon, T.I.; Manaster, I.; et al. Decidual NK cells regulate key developmental processes at the human fetal-maternal interface. *Nat. Med.* **2006**, *12*, 1065–1074. [CrossRef]
19. Turco, M.Y.; Moffett, A. Development of the human placenta. *Development* **2019**, *146*, dev163428. [CrossRef]
20. Smith, G.C. First-trimester determination of complications of late pregnancy. *JAMA* **2010**, *303*, 561–562. [CrossRef]
21. Steegers, E.A.; von Dadelszen, P.; Duvekot, J.J.; Pijnenborg, R. Pre-eclampsia. *Lancet* **2010**, *376*, 631–644. [CrossRef]
22. Reijnders, I.F.; Mulders, A.G.M.G.J.; Koster, M.P.H. Placental development and function in women with a history of placenta-related complications: A systematic review. *Acta Obstet. Et Gynecol. Scand.* **2018**, *97*, 248–257. [CrossRef] [PubMed]
23. Pandey, S.; Shetty, A.; Hamilton, M.; Bhattacharya, S.; Maheshwari, A. Obstetric and perinatal outcomes in singleton pregnancies resulting from IVF/ICSI: A systematic review and meta-analysis. *Hum. Reprod. Update* **2012**, *18*, 485–503. [CrossRef] [PubMed]
24. American College of Obstetricians and Gynecologists Committee on Obstetric Practice Society for Maternal-Fetal Medicine. Committee opinion no 671: Perinatal risks associated with assisted reproductive technology. *Obstet. Gynecol.* **2016**, *128*, e61–e68. [CrossRef] [PubMed]
25. Kawwass, J.F.; Badell, M.L. Maternal and fetal risk associated with assisted reproductive technology. *Obstet. Gynecol.* **2018**, *132*, 763–772. [CrossRef]
26. Woo, I.; Hindoyan, R.; Landay, M.; Ho, J.; Ingles, S.A.; McGinnis, L.K.; Paulson, R.J.; Chung, K. Perinatal outcomes after natural conception versus in vitro fertilization (IVF) in gestational surrogates: A model to evaluate IVF treatment versus maternal effects. *Fertil. Steril.* **2017**, *108*, 993–998. [CrossRef]
27. Palomba, S.; Homburg, R.; Santagni, S.; La Sala, G.B.; Orvieto, R. Risk of adverse pregnancy and perinatal outcomes after high technology infertility treatment: A comprehensive systematic review. *Reprod. Biol. Endocrinol.* **2016**, *14*, 76. [CrossRef]
28. Fitzpatrick, K.E.; Tuffnell, D.; Kurinczuk, J.J.; Knight, M. Pregnancy at very advanced maternal age: A UK population-based cohort study. *BJOG* **2017**, *124*, 1097–1106. [CrossRef]
29. Sandovici, I.; Hoelle, K.; Angiolini, E.; Constância, M. Placental adaptations to the maternal-fetal environment: Implications for fetal growth and developmental programming. *Reprod. Biomed. Online* **2012**, *25*, 68–89. [CrossRef]
30. Qin, J.; Liu, X.; Sheng, X.; Wang, H.; Gao, S. Assisted reproductive technology and the risk of pregnancy-related complications and adverse pregnancy outcomes in singleton pregnancies: A meta-analysis of cohort studies. *Fertil. Steril.* **2016**, *105*, 73–85. [CrossRef]
31. Chen, Z.J.; Shi, Y.; Sun, Y.; Zhang, B.; Liang, X.; Cao, Y.; Yang, J.; Liu, J.; Wei, D.; Weng, N.; et al. Fresh versus Frozen Embryos for Infertility in the Polycystic Ovary Syndrome. *N. Engl. J. Med.* **2016**, *375*, 523–533. [CrossRef]
32. Shapiro, B.S.; Daneshmand, S.T.; Garner, F.C.; Aguirre, M.; Hudson, C.; Thomas, S. Evidence of impaired endometrial receptivity after ovarian stimulation for in vitro fertilization: A prospective rando—Mized trial comparing fresh and frozen-thawed embryo transfer in normal responders. *Fertil. Steril.* **2011**, *96*, 344–348. [CrossRef] [PubMed]
33. Lee, J.C.; Badell, M.L.; Kawwass, J.F. The impact of endometrial preparation for frozen embryo transfer on maternal and neonatal outcomes: A review. *Reprod. Biol. Endocrinol.* **2022**, *20*, 40. [CrossRef] [PubMed]
34. Kansal Kalra, S.; Ratcliffe, S.J.; Milman, L.; Gracia, C.R.; Coutifaris, C.; Barnhart, K.T. Perinatal morbidity after in vitro fertilization is lower with frozen embryo transfer. *Fertil. Steril.* **2011**, *95*, 548–553. [CrossRef] [PubMed]
35. Pinborg, A.; Henningsen, A.A.; Loft, A.; Malchau, S.S.; Forman, J.; Andersen, A.N. Large baby syndrome in singletons born after frozen embryo transfer (FET): Is it due to maternal factors or the cryotechnique? *Hum. Reprod.* **2014**, *29*, 618–627. [CrossRef]
36. Maheshwari, A.; Pandey, S.; Raja, E.A.; Shetty, A.; Hamilton, M.; Bhattacharya, S. Is frozen embryo transfer better for mothers and babies? Can cumulative meta-analysis provide a definitive answer? *Hum. Reprod. Update* **2018**, *24*, 35–58. [CrossRef] [PubMed]
37. Roque, M.; Haahr, T.; Geber, S.; Esteves, S.C.; Humaidan, P. Fresh versus elective frozen embryo transfer in IVF/ICSI cycles: A systematic review and meta-analysis of reproductive outcomes. *Hum. Reprod. Update* **2019**, *25*, 2–14. [CrossRef] [PubMed]
38. Ghobara, T.; Gelbaya, T.A.; Ayeleke, R.O. Cycle regimens for frozen-thawed embryo transfer. *Cochrane Database Syst. Rev.* **2017**, *7*, CD003414. [CrossRef]
39. Ginstrom Ernstad, E.; Wennerholm, U.B.; Khatibi, A.; Petzold, M.; Bergh, C. Neonatal and maternal outcome after frozen embryo transfer: Increased risks in programmed cycles. *Am. J. Obstet. Gynecol.* **2019**, *221*, 126.e1–126.e18. [CrossRef]
40. Conrad, K.P.; Baker, V.L. Corpus luteal contribution to maternal pregnancy physiology and outcomes in assisted reproductive technologies. *Am. J. Phys. Regul. Integr. Comp. Phys.* **2013**, *304*, R69–R72.

41. von Versen-Höynck, F.; Schaub, A.M.; Chi, Y.Y.; Chiu, K.H.; Liu, J.; Lingis, M.; Stan Williams, R.; Rhoton-Vlasak, A.; Nichols, W.W.; Fleischmann, R.R.; et al. Increased Preeclampsia Risk and Reduced Aortic Compliance With In Vitro Fertilization Cycles in the Absence of a Corpus Luteum. *Hypertension* **2019**, *73*, 640–649. [CrossRef]
42. Rienzi, L.; Gracia, C.; Maggiulli, R.; LaBarbera, A.R.; Kaser, D.J.; Ubaldi, F.M.; Vanderpoel, S.; Racowsky, C. Oocyte, embryo and blastocyst cryopreservation in ART: Systematic review and meta-analysis comparing slow-freezing versus vitrification to produce evidence for the development of global guidance. *Hum. Reprod. Update.* **2017**, *23*, 139–155. [CrossRef] [PubMed]
43. Gu, F.; Li, S.; Zheng, L.; Gu, J.; Li, T.; Du, H.; Gao, C.; Ding, C.; Quan, S.; Zhou, C.; et al. Perinatal outcomes of singletons following vitrification versus slow-freezing of embryos: A multicenter cohort study using propensity score analysis. *Hum. Reprod.* **2019**, *34*, 1788–1798. [CrossRef] [PubMed]
44. Brosens, I.; Pijnenborg, R.; Vercruysse, L.; Romero, R. The 'Great Obstetrical Syndromes' are associated with disorders of deep placentation. *Am. J. Obstet. Gynecol.* **2010**, *25*, 569–574. [CrossRef] [PubMed]
45. Rizzo, G.; Pietrolucci, M.E.; Mappa, I.; Bitsadze, V.; Khizroeva, J.; Makatsariya, A.; D'Antonio, F. Modeling Pulsatility Index nomograms from different maternal and fetal vessels by quantile regression at 24–40 weeks of gestation: A prospective cross-sectional study. *J. Matern. Fetal. Neonatal. Med.* **2022**, *35*, 1668–1676. [CrossRef] [PubMed]
46. Plasencia, W.; Maiz, N.; Bonino, S.; Kaihura, C.; Nicolaides, K. Uterine artery Doppler at 11+0 to 13+6 weeks in the prediction of pre-eclampsia. *Ultrasound Obstet. Gynecol.* **2007**, *30*, 742–749. [CrossRef]
47. Velauthar, L.; Plana, M.N.; Kalidindi, M.; Zamora, J.; Thilaganathan, B.; Illanes, S.E.; Khan, K.S.; Aquilina, J.; Thangaratinam, S. First-trimester uterine artery Doppler and adverse pregnancy outcome: A meta-analysis involving 55974 women. *Ultrasound Obstet. Gynecol.* **2014**, *43*, 500–507. [CrossRef] [PubMed]
48. Rizzo, G.; Capponi, A.; Cavicchioni, O.; Vendola, M.; Arduini, D. First trimester uterine Doppler and three-dimensional ultrasound placental volume calculation in predicting preeclampsia. *Eur. J. Obstet. Gynecol. Reprod. Biol.* **2008**, *138*, 147–151.
49. Carbone, I.F.; Cruz, J.J.; Sarquis, R.; Akolekar, R.; Nicolaides, K.H. Assisted conception and placental perfusion assessed by uterine artery Doppler at 11–13 weeks' gestation. *Hum. Reprod.* **2011**, *26*, 1659–1664.
50. Prefumo, F.; Fratelli, N.; Soares, S.C.; Thilaganathan, B. Uterine artery Doppler velocimetry at 11–14 weeks in singleton pregnancies conceived by assisted reproductive technology. *Ultrasound Obstet. Gynecol.* **2007**, *29*, 141–145. [CrossRef]
51. Rizzo, G.; Aiello, E.; Pietrolucci, M.E.; Arduini, D. Are There Differences in Placental Volume and Uterine Artery Doppler in Pregnancies Resulting From the Transfer of Fresh Versus Frozen-Thawed Embryos Through In Vitro Fertilization. *Reprod. Sci* **2016**, *23*, 1381–1386. [CrossRef]
52. Nelissen, E.C.; Dumoulin, J.C.; Busato, F.; Ponger, L.; Eijssen, L.M.; Evers, J.L.; Tost, J.; van Montfoort, A.P. Altered gene expression in human placentas after IVF/ICSI. *Hum. Reprod.* **2014**, *29*, 2821–2831. [CrossRef] [PubMed]
53. Gundogan, F.; Bianchi, D.W.; Scherjon, S.A.; Roberts, D.J. Placental pathology in egg donor pregnancies. *Fertil. Steril.* **2010**, *93*, 397–404. [CrossRef] [PubMed]
54. Cavoretto, P.I.; Farina, A.; Gaeta, G.; Sigismondi, C.; Spinillo, S.; Casiero, D.; Pozzoni, M.; Vigano, P.; Papaleo, E.; Candiani, M. Uterine artery Doppler in singleton pregnancies conceived after in-vitro fertilization or intracytoplasmic sperm injection with fresh vs. frozen blastocyst transfer: Longitudinal cohort study. *Ultrasound Obstet. Gynecol.* **2020**, *56*, 603–610. [CrossRef] [PubMed]
55. van Duijn, L.; Rousian, M.; Reijnders, I.F.; Willemsen, S.P.; Baart, E.B.; Laven, J.S.E.; Steegers-Theunissen, R.P.M. The influence of frozen-thawed and fresh embryo transfer on utero-placental (vascular) development: The Rotterdam Periconception cohort. *Hum. Reprod.* **2021**, *36*, 2091–2100. [CrossRef] [PubMed]
56. Perry, H.; Lehmann, H.; Mantovani, E.; Thilaganathan, B.; Khalil, A. Correlation between central and uterine hemodynamics in hypertensive disorders of pregnancy. *Ultrasound Obstet. Gynecol.* **2019**, *54*, 58–63. [CrossRef]
57. Arakaki, T.; Hasegawa, J.; Nakamura, M.; Hamada, S.; Muramoto, M.; Takita, H.; Ichizuka, K.; Sekizawa, A. Prediction of early- and late- onset pregnancy-induced hypertension using placental volume on three-dimensional ultrasound and uterine artery Doppler. *Ultrasound Obstet. Gyneco.* **2015**, *45*, 539–543. [CrossRef]
58. Schuchter, K.; Metzenbauer, M.; Hafner, E.; Philipp, K. Uterine artery Doppler and placental volume in the first trimester in the prediction of pregnancy complications. *Ultrasound Obstet. Gynecol.* **2001**, *18*, 590–592. [CrossRef]
59. Papastefanou, I.; Chrelias, C.; Siristatidis, C.; Kappou, D.; Eleftheriades, M.; Kassanos, D. Placental volume at 11 to 14 gestational weeks in pregnancies complicated with fetal growth restriction and preeclampsia. *Prenat. Diagn.* **2018**, *38*, 928–935. [CrossRef]
60. Rifouna, M.S.; Reus, A.D.; Koning, A.H.; van der Spek, P.J.; Exalto, N.; Steegers, E.A.; Laven, J.S. First trimester trophoblast and placental bed vascular volume measurements in IVF or IVF/ICSI pregnancies. *Hum. Reprod.* **2014**, *29*, 2644–2649. [CrossRef]
61. Rizzo, G.; Aiello, E.; Pietrolucci, M.E.; Arduini, D. Placental volume and uterine artery Doppler evaluation at 11 + 0 to 13 + 6 weeks' gestation in pregnancies conceived with in-vitro fertilization: Comparison between autologous and donor oocyte recipients. *Ultrasound Obstet. Gynecol.* **2016**, *47*, 726–731. [CrossRef]
62. Churchill, S.J.; Wang, E.T.; Akhlaghpour, M.; Goldstein, E.H.; Eschevarria, D.; Greene, N.; Macer, M.; Zore, T.; Williams, J., 3rd; Pisarska, M.D. Mode of conception does not appear to affect placental volume in the first trimester. *Fertil. Steril.* **2017**, *107*, 1341–1347.e1. [CrossRef] [PubMed]

63. Sundheimer, L.W.; Chan, J.L.; Buttle, R.; DiPentino, R.; Muramoto, O.; Castellano, K.; Wang, E.T.; Williams, J., 3rd; Pisarska, M.D. Mode of conception does not affect fetal or placental growth parameters or ratios in early gestation or at delivery. *J. Assist. Reprod. Genet.* **2018**, *35*, 1039–1046. [CrossRef] [PubMed]
64. Manna, C.; Lacconi, V.; Rizzo, G.; De Lorenzo, A.; Massimiani, M. Placental Dysfunction in Assisted Reproductive Pregnancies: Perinatal, Neonatal and Adult Life Outcomes. *Int. J. Mol. Sci.* **2022**, *23*, 659. [CrossRef] [PubMed]

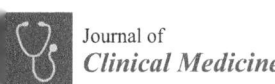

Systematic Review

Efficacy of Autologous Intrauterine Infusion of Platelet-Rich Plasma in Patients with Unexplained Repeated Implantation Failures in Embryo Transfer: A Systematic Review and Meta-Analysis

Muzi Li [1,2,3,4,5], Yan Kang [6], Qianfei Wang [1,2,3,4,5] and Lei Yan [1,2,3,4,5,*]

1. Center for Reproductive Medicine, Shandong University, Jinan 250100, China
2. Key Laboratory of Reproductive Endocrinology of Ministry of Education, Shandong University, Jinan 250100, China
3. Shandong Key Laboratory of Reproductive Medicine, Jinan 250012, China
4. Medical Integration and Practice Center, Shandong University, Jinan 250100, China
5. Gynecology Department, Reproductive Hospital Affiliated to Shandong University, Jinan 250001, China
6. Obstetrics Department, Shandong Provincial Maternal and Child Health Care Hospital, Jinan 250001, China
* Correspondence: yanlei@sdu.edu.cn

Abstract: (1) Background: Controversial conclusions have been made in previous studies regarding the influence of autologous platelet-rich plasma (PRP) in the reproductive outcomes of women with repeated implantation failures (RIF) who are undergoing embryo transfer (ET). (2) Methods: This study aimed to evaluate the effect of PRP intrauterine infusion in patients with unexplained RIF, who are undergoing in vitro fertilization (IVF) or intracytoplasmic injection (ICSI), by a systematic review and meta-analysis. (3) Results: A fixed-effects model was used, and 795 cases and 834 controls were included in these studies. The pooling of the results showed the beneficial effect of PRP which were compared with those of the control in terms of the clinical pregnancy rates (n = 10, risk ratio (RR) = 1.79, 95% confidence intervals (CI): 1.55, 2.06; $p < 0.01$, $I^2 = 40\%$), live birth rates (n = 4, RR = 2.92, 95% CI: 2.22, 3.85; $p < 0.01$, $I^2 = 83\%$), implantation rates (n = 3, RR = 1.74, 95% CI: 1.34, 2.26; $p < 0.01$, $I^2 = 0\%$), and positive serum β-HCG 14 days after the ET (n = 8, RR = 1.77, 95% CI: 1.54, 2.03; $p < 0.01$, $I^2 = 36\%$). However, we did not find that the miscarriage rates indicated a significant difference between the two groups (n = 6, RR = 1.04, 95% CI: 0.72, 1.51; $p = 0.83$, $I^2 = 0\%$). (4) Conclusions: The findings of this systemic review and meta-analysis suggest that PRP appears to improve the results of IVF/ICSI treatments in the cases of unexplained RIF.

Keywords: platelet-rich plasma; repeated implantation failures; embryo transfer; clinical pregnancy rates; intracytoplasmic injection; in vitro fertilization

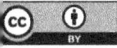

1. Introduction

A considerable proportion of couples worldwide suffer from infertility [1]. The common reasons for female infertility issues include ovulation disorders, fallopian-related disorders, uterine disorders, and unexplained infertility [2]. Although assisted reproductive technology (ART) has rapidly developed in recent years, the causes and treatments of repeated implantation failures (RIF, recurrent implantation failures) continue to plague reproductive specialists. There is no accepted formal definition for RIF due to the fact that RIF was initially considered to be a rather heterogeneous entity. Some studies have defined it as a failure of the implant after three or more embryo transfers (ETs) with high-quality embryos [3,4]. It was, however, also accepted that RIF was considered to be a disorder of infertility women who had undergone at least two ET failures [5,6]. Even so, quite a few specialists have suggested a more complete working definition, taking into account the maternal age, the number of embryos that were transferred, and the number of cycles that were completed [7,8]. The accumulative data have clarified that most of the etiology does not have the evidence base for a generalized application to be suggested by the relevant societies. The etiology of RIF was currently attributed to the dysfunction of the embryo and the endometrium, and Antonis Makrigiannakis et al., also divided it into several factors, namely anatomy, immunology, dysbiotic microbiota, and unexplained reasons, etc., in their review [2]. Moreover, this team has also described some of the main treatment protocols including endometrium injury, human chorionic gonadotropin, peripheral blood mononuclear cells, and platelet-rich plasma (PRP). RIF is a constant challenge in ART with it being a burden on health providers and infertile couples.

The extraction protocols of platelet rich-plasma also remain inconsistent, with there being no consensus around the world. It is generally defined as an autologous blood-derived concentrate of the platelets from the peripheral blood that has a platelet count that is 35 times higher than the baseline concentration with growth factors and other cytokines such as transforming growth factor beta (TGF-β) and interleukin-1β (IL-1β) [9–12]. Presently, PRP is widely used in knee osteoarthritis, erectile dysfunction, medical dermatology, periodontal regeneration, and facial rejuvenation [13–16].

In reproductive medicine, a poor ovarian reserve, premature ovarian failure, and a thin endometrium have been the main areas of the research of PRP by intraovarian injection or intrauterin infusion [17–19]. Studies found that PRP had high growth factor and cytokine concentrations, which are considered to be very important in cell proliferation, chemotaxis, cell differentiation, regeneration, and angiogenesis [20,21]. Fady I Sharara et al., reviewed the previous literature on the effects of autologous PRP in reproductive medicine, finding that PRP can increase the endometrial thickness in thin endometrium [22]. These reasons may explain why PRP could improve the implantation outcomes and be beneficial for embryo transfer.

There has been a surge in high-level studies investigating PRP for implantation failures. Therefore, in this systematic review and meta-analysis, we aimed at investigating the effect of the intrauterine infusion of autologous PRP in women with unexplained RIF who are undergoing IVF/ICSI cycles.

2. Methods

By complying with the guidelines of recommendations of the Cochrane Handbook for Systematic Reviews of Interventions and Preferred Reporting Items for Systematic Reviews and Meta-Analyses (PRISMA) to search for the relevant studies that had been published in the medical literature up to the time of this research, this systematic review and meta-analysis gathered statistics and evaluated the efficacy of autologous PRP intrauterine infusion on the pregnancy results for patients with RIF of unknown causes which were compared those who underwent no treatments or other treatments. Clinical pregnancy is the first outcome, and it is defined as the presence of a fetal heartbeat or the gestational sac in transvaginal ultrasonography 4–6 weeks after the embryo transfer. Live birth is defined as the delivery of a live-born child after 24 weeks of gestational age. Miscarriage is defined as s a fetal loss before 20 weeks of gestation.

2.1. Literature Search

We identified potential studies by searching Medline (PubMed), Embase, Cochrane Library, and Web of Science (WOS). Additionally, we identified eligible literature searches by using the references of published articles. The search terms included: ("RIF" OR "Repeated implantation failure" OR "Implantation failure" OR "Recurrent implantation failure" AND "Platelet-rich plasma" OR "PRP" OR "Autologous platelet-rich plasma" OR "Platelet-rich plasma gel" OR "Plasma, Platelet-Rich" OR "Platelet Rich Plasma"). Among these terms, platelet-rich plasma is a MESH, and the others are free terms. The terms were searched in the title and abstract parts of the studies. The database-specific indexing terminology is listed as ((((((Plasma, Platelet-Rich[Title/Abstract]) OR (Platelet Rich Plasma[Title/Abstract])) OR (PRP[Title/Abstract])) OR (Autologous Platelet-Rich Plasma[Title/Abstract])) OR (Platelet-

Rich Plasma Gel[Title/Abstract])) OR ("Platelet-Rich Plasm"[Mesh])) AND ((((Repeated implantation failure[Title/Abstract]) OR (implantation failure[Title/Abstract])) OR (recurrent implantation failure[Title/Abstract])) OR (RIF[Title/Abstract])).

2.2. Selection (Inclusion and Exclusion) Criteria

Two independent reviewers censored the titles and abstracts of the identified studies. Thereafter, the selected studies were thoroughly and completely read in order to made a decision about their inclusion or exclusion from this meta-analysis. Given that there is currently no consensus on the definition of RIF, we included medical records with a clear diagnosis in the studies. The randomized controlled trials and cohorts that underwent the PRP and RIF treatments were included in this review and they were required to meet all of the following six inclusion criteria. These inclusion criteria were: (1) interventions: the intrauterine infusion of PRP around the time of ET; (2) the controls: having undergone no treatment or other treatments; (3) the population were diagnosed as having had an RIF; (4) the pregnancy outcomes were confirmed; (5) only English language studies were accepted; (6) having an endometrial thickness of ≥ 7 mm. Other studies such as case reports, animal experiments, cell experiments, research that was irrelevant to PRP and RIF, bibliometric analyses, poor-quality literature, self-pro-post studies, reviews and abstracts were excluded. Clinical pregnancy rates were the primary outcome, and the secondary results were the live birth rates (LBR), positive serum β-HCG rates 14 days after the ET, the implantation rates, and the miscarriage rates. Clinical pregnancy was defined as a pregnancy that was diagnosed by ultrasonographic visualization of one or more gestational sacs or definitive clinical signs of pregnancy. In addition to an intra-uterine pregnancy, it includes a clinically documented ectopic pregnancy [23].

2.3. PRP Protocols

Peripheral venous blood was drawn using a syringe containing anticoagulant solution and centrifuged immediately to separate the red blood cells. The liquid supernatant was centrifuged again to separate the plasma and obtain the PRP with platelets. In addition, the peripheral blood was divided into three layers after the first centrifugation in the studies of Yangying Xu et al., and Mahvash Zargar et al., and the top layer was centrifuged again to obtain the PRP [3,6].

2.4. Statistical Analysis

We extracted the relative reproductive outcomes from the included studies. The RR and corresponding 95% CI for each study endpoint were calculated by the Mantel–Hansel method using the fixed-effects model between the intervention group and the control group according to the Review Manager 5.4. The heterogeneity of the studies was assessed graphically with forest plots and statistically by chi-square-based Q statistic and I^2 value. Heterogeneity, the statistical measure of homogeneity, was considered significant at a p-value of <0.05 in Q-test or $I^2 > 50\%$. According to the dosage of PRP (0.5–1 mL group and ≥ 1 mL group) and the study design (RCT and cohort), a subgroup analysis was used to identify the possible sources of heterogeneity for the effect of an intrauterine infusion of the PRP. A funnel plot was used to assess the reporting bias.

3. Results

3.1. Summary of Literature Research and Description of Studies

In total, 227 publications (38 from PubMed, 57 from Cochrane Library, 65 from Embase, and 67 from Web of Science) were searched using the terms above. All of the citations were imported into Endnote to eliminate 113 duplicates. Next, we scrutinized two case reports, eight animal or cell studies, thirty-one studies that were not part of the literature about PRP and RIF, one bibliometric analyses, twenty-one reviews, thirty-seven abstracts, one poor-quality study, and three self-pro-post control studies, and ten studies were finally analyzed. The flow diagram of the literature search and selection of studies is shown in

Figure 1. The details of the selected studies are showed in Table S1. Apart from the review, abstract, a bibliometric analysis, and the studies that were not related to PRP and RIF, we read the full texts to censor the studies. The exclusion reasons are presented in Table S2.

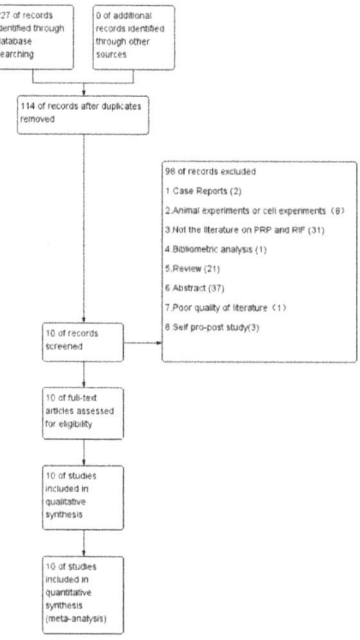

Figure 1. Flow diagram of the selection process.

3.2. Study Characteristics

Table S1 lists the characteristics of all of the selected studies. Eight studies were conducted in Iran [4–6,24–28], and another two studies were conducted, respectively, in China and India [3,29]. Six studies were RCTs, and four were cohorts. All of the control groups received no treatment, except one, which was compared with the granulocyte colony stimulating factor (GCSF) [26]. The population of one half of the studies was infused with a PRP of less than 1 mL; the other half received ≥1 mL. Only one study did not give an accurate time of intrauterine perfusion of the PRP; the others were conducted at 2–3 days before the ET [29].

3.3. Risk of Bias Assessment

The summary of the risks of the bias assessments are shown in Figure S1a,b. For a random sequence generation, five studies were judged to have low risks of bias, three were judged to have high risks, and two were judged to have unclear risks. Four of the trials were assessed as having high risks of bias, the others had unclear risks for the allocation concealment. Another bias, including the blinding of the participants and personnel, the blinding of outcome assessment, incomplete outcome data, selective reporting, and other bias were judged as low risks. All of the research selected the population from the same community sample and provided exacted diagnosis criteria for the interesting reproductive outcomes.

3.4. Clinical Pregnancy Rates

The summary results included 1629 participants (795 cases and 834 controls) from 10 studies. As shown in Figure 2, the comparison of the clinical pregnancy rates indicated that the intrauterine infusion of the PRP had a better effect on the clinical pregnancy outcomes when it was compared with that of the control group according to fixed-effects model analysis (n = 10, risk ratio (RR) = 1.79, 95% confidence intervals (CI): 1.55, 2.06; $p < 0.01$, $I^2 = 40\%$). In Figure S2, the funnel plot appears to be asymmetric, with some missingness at the lower left portion of the plot suggesting a possible publication bias, which means that some positive results from the small sample of studies with low precision were not published. The sensitivity analysis showed that the estimates of the summary RR ranged from 1.64 (95% CI: 1.39, 1.93) to 1.90 (95% CI: 1.63, 2.21), which meant that the pooled results were not overly influenced by a single study.

Study or Subgroup	EXPERIMENTAL Events	Total	CONTROL Events	Total	Weight	Risk Ratio M-H, Fixed, 95% CI
Ensieh S. Tehraninejad 2020	13	42	16	43	8.0%	0.83 [0.46, 1.51]
Leila Nazari 2019	26	49	13	48	6.7%	1.96 [1.15, 3.34]
Leila Nazari 2022	96	197	38	196	19.3%	2.51 [1.83, 3.46]
Leili Safdarian 2022	31	60	16	60	8.1%	1.94 [1.19, 3.15]
Mahvash Zargar 2021	4	38	1	39	0.5%	4.11 [0.48, 35.08]
Majiyd Abdul Noushin 2021	57	109	52	154	21.9%	1.55 [1.16, 2.06]
Marzieh Mehrafza 2019	27	67	12	56	6.6%	1.88 [1.05, 3.36]
Marzieh Zamaniyan 2020	29	55	10	43	5.7%	2.27 [1.25, 4.12]
Sara Ershadi 2022	13	40	11	45	5.2%	1.33 [0.67, 2.63]
Yangying Xu 2022	50	138	37	150	18.0%	1.47 [1.03, 2.10]
Total (95% CI)		795		834	100.0%	1.79 [1.55, 2.06]
Total events	346		206			

Heterogeneity: Chi² = 15.00, df = 9 (P = 0.09); I² = 40%
Test for overall effect: Z = 7.95 (P < 0.00001)

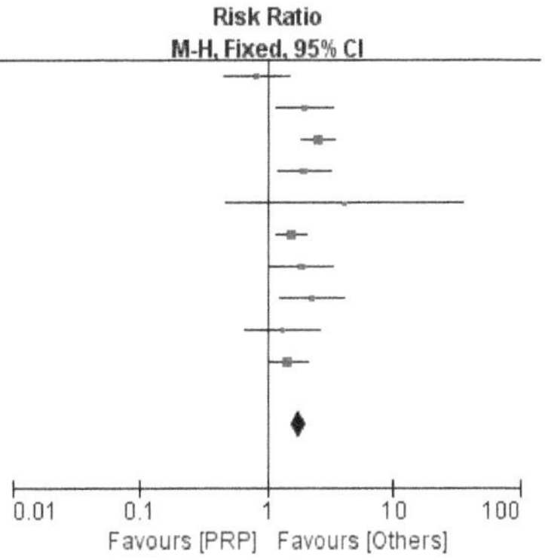

Favours [PRP]   Favours [Others]

Figure 2. Forest plot of RR, 95% CI, and heterogeneity in studies that evaluated the risk of clinical pregnancy in interventions versus controls [3–6,24–29].

Considering that we used *p*-values < 0.1 and there was an $I^2 = 0.45\%$ of heterogeneity testing in all of the cases and controls, a corresponding subgroup analysis was performed to recover what caused heterogeneity of the two groups. The PRP dosage and study design may be the sources of it, and so we analyzed the traits of the selected studies. When the women were treated at a 0.5–1 mL dose of PRP (n = 5, RR = 2.24, 95% CI: 1.80, 2.79; $p < 0.01$, $I^2 = 0\%$), the effect size was stronger than ≥1 mL (n = 5, RR = 1.48, 95% CI: 1.22, 1.80; $p < 0.01$, $I^2 = 23\%$), and more patients benefited in terms of the clinical pregnancy rates (Figure 3). Within the subgroups, there is only negligible heterogeneity. In Figure 4, the cohort studies (n = 4, OR = 1.79, 95% CI: 1.32, 2.43; $p < 0.01$, $I^2 = 36\%$) had a weaker effect when they were compared with the RCTs (n = 6, OR = 2.98, 95% CI: 2.29, 3.88; $p < 0.01$, $I^2 = 14\%$) in terms of the pregnancy outcomes, and the heterogeneity was not significant within the subgroups. With an asymmetric funnel plot of the risk ratios of the clinical pregnancy outcomes, we evaluated the reporting bias again, excluding the possible confounding factors, study design, and PRP dosage (Figures S3 and S4). In the study design subgroup, the funnel plot was symmetric, and the asymmetric reporting bias that is mentioned above could result from that.

3.5. Live Birth Rates

In Figure 5, four trials including 878 patients (433 cases and 445 controls) demonstrated that the live birth rates in patients that underwent an intrauterine infusion of PRP significantly increased when they were compared with the controls (n = 4, RR = 2.92, 95% CI: 2.22, 3.85; $p < 0.01$, $I^2 = 83\%$). We removed one study with high heterogeneity; the live birth rates remained statistically different between the two groups (n = 3, RR = 1.9, 95% CI: 1.39, 2.59; $p = 0.43$, $I^2 = 0$) (Figure S5) [4].

PRP OTHERS Risk Ratio Risk Ratio
Study or Subgroup Events Total Events Total Weight M-H, Fixed, 95% CI M-H, Fixed, 95% CI
1.2.1 Group(0.5-1ml)
Leila Nazari 2019 22 49 8 48 9.6% 2.69 [1.33, 5.45]
Leila Nazari 2022 96 197 38 196 45.5% 2.51 [1.83, 3.46]
Leili Safdarian 2022 31 60 16 60 19.1% 1.94 [1.19, 3.15]
Marzieh Zamaniyan 2020 29 55 10 43 13.4% 2.27 [1.25, 4.12]
Sara Ershadi 2022 13 40 11 45 12.4% 1.33 [0.67, 2.63]
Subtotal (95% CI) 401 392 100.0% 2.24 [1.80, 2.79]
Total events 191 83
Heterogeneity: Chi² = 3.36, df = 4 (P = 0.50); I² = 0%
Test for overall effect: Z = 7.27 (P < 0.00001)
1.2.2 Group2(≥1ml)
Ensieh S. Tehraninejad 2020 13 42 16 43 14.6% 0.83 [0.46, 1.51]
Mahvash Zargar 2021 4 38 1 39 0.9% 4.11 [0.48, 35.08]
Majiyd Abdul Noushin 2021 57 109 52 154 39.8% 1.55 [1.16, 2.06]
Marzieh Mehrafza 2019 27 67 12 56 12.1% 1.88 [1.05, 3.36]
Yangying Xu 2022 50 138 37 150 32.7% 1.47 [1.03, 2.10]
Subtotal (95% CI) 394 442 100.0% 1.48 [1.22, 1.80]
Total events 151 118
Heterogeneity: Chi² = 5.22, df = 4 (P = 0.27); I² = 23%
Test for overall effect: Z = 3.93 (P < 0.0001)
0.01 0.1 1 10 100
Favours [experimental] Favours [control]
Test for subgroup differences: Chi² = 7.69, df = 1 (P = 0.006), I² = 87.0%

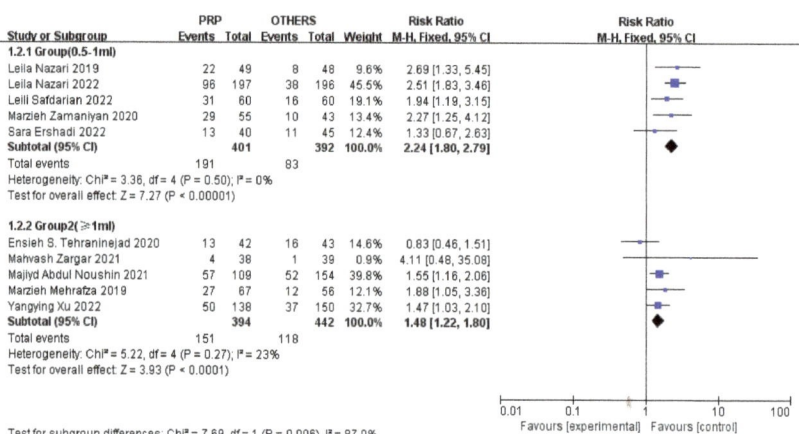

Figure 3. Forest plot of RR, 95% CI, and heterogeneity in studies that evaluated the risk of clinical pregnancy in interventions versus controls regarding doses of PRP [3–6,24–29].

Experimental Control Odds Ratio Odds Ratio
Study or Subgroup Events Total Events Total Weight M-H, Fixed, 95% CI M-H, Fixed, 95% CI
1.3.1 RCT
Leila Nazari 2019 22 49 8 48 6.9% 4.07 [1.58, 10.48]
Leila Nazari 2022 96 197 38 196 30.2% 3.95 [2.52, 6.20]
Leili Safdarian 2022 31 60 16 60 12.0% 2.94 [1.37, 6.31]
Mahvash Zargar 2021 57 109 52 154 31.8% 2.15 [1.30, 3.55]
Marzieh Zamaniyan 2020 29 55 10 43 8.2% 3.68 [1.52, 8.91]
Sara Ershadi 2022 13 40 11 45 10.8% 1.49 [0.58, 3.84]
Subtotal (95% CI) 510 546 100.0% 2.98 [2.29, 3.88]
Total events 248 135
Heterogeneity: Chi² = 5.82, df = 5 (P = 0.32); I² = 14%
Test for overall effect: Z = 8.09 (P < 0.00001)
1.3.2 Cohort
Ensieh S. Tehraninejad 2020 13 42 16 43 17.6% 0.76 [0.31, 1.86]
Majiyd Abdul Noushin 2021 57 109 52 154 33.2% 2.15 [1.30, 3.55]
Marzieh Mehrafza 2019 27 67 12 56 12.6% 2.48 [1.11, 5.53]
Yangying Xu 2022 50 138 37 150 36.5% 1.74 [1.04, 2.88]
Subtotal (95% CI) 356 403 100.0% 1.79 [1.32, 2.43]
Total events 147 117
Heterogeneity: Chi² = 4.67, df = 3 (P = 0.20); I² = 36%
Test for overall effect: Z = 3.76 (P = 0.0002)
0.01 0.1 1 10 100
Favours [experimental] Favours [control]
Test for subgroup differences: Chi² = 6.06, df = 1 (P = 0.01), I² = 83.5%

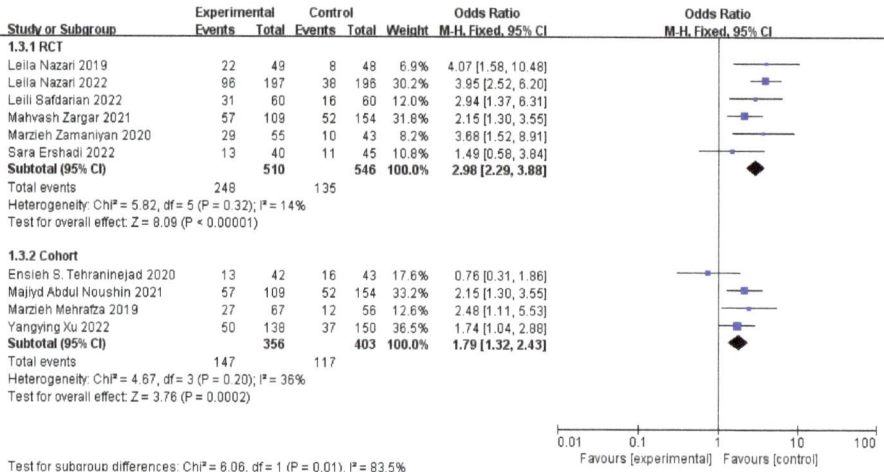

Figure 4. Forest plot of OR, 95% CI, and heterogeneity in studies that evaluated the risk of clinical pregnancy in interventions versus controls regarding study design [3–6,24–29].

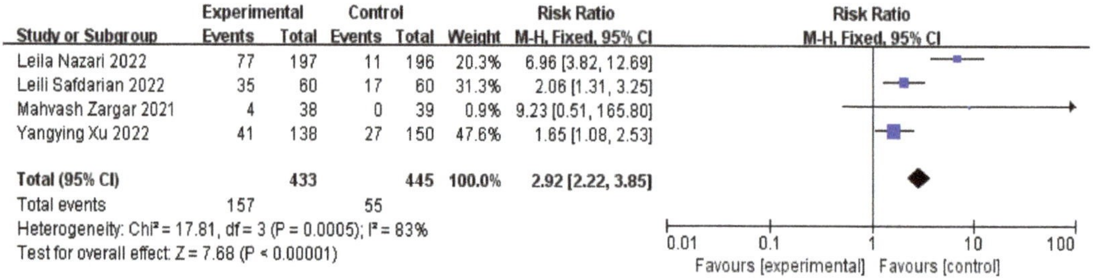

Experimental Control Risk Ratio Risk Ratio
Study or Subgroup Events Total Events Total Weight M-H, Fixed, 95% CI M-H, Fixed, 95% CI
Leila Nazari 2022 77 197 11 196 20.3% 6.96 [3.82, 12.69]
Leili Safdarian 2022 35 60 17 60 31.3% 2.06 [1.31, 3.25]
Mahvash Zargar 2021 4 38 0 39 0.9% 9.23 [0.51, 165.80]
Yangying Xu 2022 41 138 27 150 47.6% 1.65 [1.08, 2.53]
Total (95% CI) 433 445 100.0% 2.92 [2.22, 3.85]
Total events 157 55
Heterogeneity: Chi² = 17.81, df = 3 (P = 0.0005); I² = 83%
Test for overall effect: Z = 7.68 (P < 0.00001)
0.01 0.1 1 10 100
Favours [experimental] Favours [control]

Figure 5. Forest plot of RR, 95% CI, and heterogeneity in studies that evaluated the risk of live birth rates in interventions versus controls [3,4,6,27].

3.6. Positive Serum β-HCG Rates on 14 Days after ET and Implantation Rates

Six studies with 931 participants (440 cases and 491 controls) compared the serum β-HCG 14 days after the ET, and the positive rates of the experimental group were significantly higher than those of the control group (n = 8, RR = 1.77, 95% CI: 1.54, 2.03; $p < 0.01$, $I^2 = 36\%$) (Figure 6). One study was excluded owing to us not finding the test time of β-HCG [24]. The implantation rates were also evaluated by three studies involving 1061 women (549 cases and 512 controls), and it was shown that the intervention of PRP significantly increased the rates of the implantation when they were compared to those of the controls (n = 3, RR = 1.74, 95% CI: 1.34, 2.26; $p < 0.01$, $I^2 = 0$) (Figure 7). We excluded two studies because the data of one study could not be extracted, and the calculation formula of the other data was controversial [5,28]. Both the higher positive serum β-HCG rates 14 days after the ET and the implantation rates proved that the intrauterine infusion of PRP increased the possibility of implantation in comparison with that resulting from no treatment or other treatments for the women with RIF.

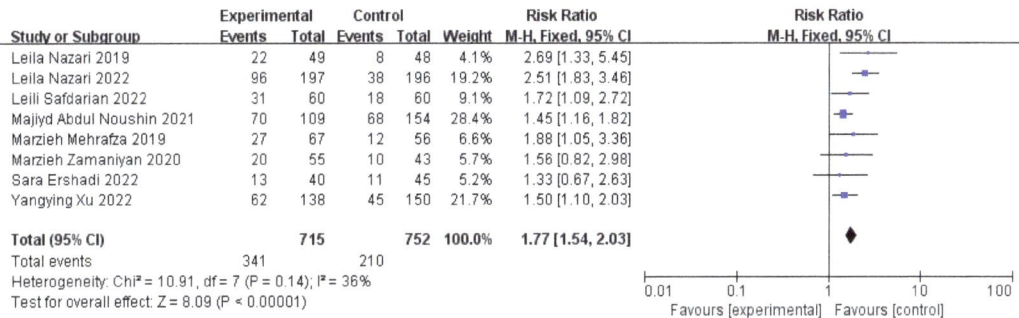

Figure 6. Forest plot of RR, 95% CI, and heterogeneity in studies that evaluated the risk of positive serum β-HCG rates 14 days after ET in interventions versus controls [3–5,25–29].

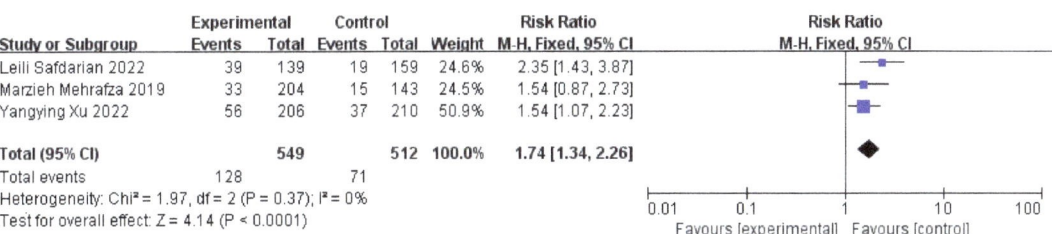

Figure 7. Forest plot of RR, 95% CI, and heterogeneity in studies that evaluated the risk of implantation rates after ET in interventions versus controls [3,26,27].

3.7. Miscarriage Rates

Next, we assessed the effect of PRP on the miscarriage rates for patients that experienced an RIF in six studies (440 cases and 491 controls). There was no significant difference between the intervention and the control group, and it seemed that no heterogeneity factor disturbed its analysis process (n = 6, RR = 1.04, 95% CI: 0.72, 1.51; $p = 0.83$, $I^2 = 0\%$) (Figure 8).

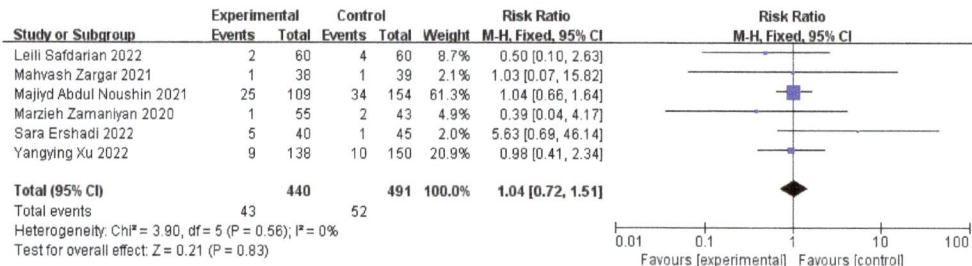

Figure 8. Forest plot of RR, 95% CI, and heterogeneity in studies that evaluated the risk of miscarriage rates after ET in interventions versus controls [3,5,6,27–29].

4. Discussion

In this study, 10 studies were included to assess the efficacy of the intrauterine perfusion of RPR for 1629 patients (795 cases and 834 controls) with unexplained repeated implantation failures, who were undergoing an embryo transfer. The endometrial thickness on the day of the HCG in our included population was no less than seven millimeters, and so the effect of a thin endometrium on the pregnancy outcomes was excluded.

In this meta-analysis, a fixed-effects model was used to assess the effect of the PRP in comparison with the control on the clinical pregnancy rates, live birth rates, implantation rates, and positive serum β-HCG 14 days after the ET and the miscarriage rates. RR and 95% CI showed that PRP group had better outcomes in terms of clinical pregnancy, live birth, implantation, and positive β-HCG 14 days after the embryo transfer. These results were consistent with PRP increasing the chance of pregnancy and delivery for females with RIF [4,25,27,28]. However, the PRP did not show significant advantages in improving the miscarriage rates, which was also proven in the findings of previous epidemiological studies [5,27,28]. Preferable embryo implantation, pregnancy, and live birth results suggest that the intrauterine infusion of PRP facilitates the embryo transfer in patients that have undergone an RIF. Unfortunately, not all of the included studies gave the research outcomes that we needed.

A subgroup analysis was carried out to disclose the reasons for the heterogeneity in the clinical pregnancy results between the two groups. The advantages of PRP were in improving the clinical pregnancy after the subgroup analysis regarding the PRP dosage (0.5–1 mL versus ≥1 mL) and the study design (cohort versus RCT). The effect size of 0.5–1 mL dose of PRP was stronger than a ≥1 mL one was, and more patients benefited in terms of the clinical pregnancy rates when they were treated with 0.5–1 mL dose of PRP. However, we did not think this result meant that a 0.5–1 mL dose of PRP was more suitable for patients with RIF because the required components were not reported in the included studies.

Autologous platelet-rich plasma is a platelet-rich whole blood extract without red or white blood cells. Because it is extracted from the patient's own peripheral blood, it is easy to obtain, inexpensive, and reduces the occurrence of an immune rejection. PRP is rich in growth factors, typically the platelet-derived growth factor (PDGF), the transforming growth factor (TGF), the vascular endothelial growth factor (VEGF), and the epidermal growth factor [30,31]. It induces regeneration and differentiation, accelerates endometrial damage repairment, and has anti-inflammatory properties [31–35]. Siwen Zhang et al., described in his study that PRP had a strong effect on endometrial regeneration, uterine damage restoration, and the increased proliferation of stromal cells, progenitor cells, and the vessel density of the endometrium [35]. These effects may explain why PRP improves the pregnancy outcomes in IVF/ICSI patients with RIF.

The heterogeneity analysis of the clinical pregnancy rates seemed high, although there were no significant differences. We designed a subgroup analysis regarding the PRP dosage, and the study design and reduced heterogeneity indicated that these two were confounding factors. The asymmetrical funnel plot indicated that there was a possible reporting bias. However, it changed to a symmetrical plot in the subgroup analysis of the study design, which suggested that the reason for the asymmetry may be attributed to the types of trials.

As there is no unified method to extract PRP from the peripheral blood, we have not yet obtained detailed key information such as the concentrations and activity of the platelets and growth factors to determine how PRP works. Thus, we cannot provide a reasonable explanation for the relationship between the PRP dosage and the IVF/ICSI outcomes in terms of RIF.

The design of the study and the outcomes that were measured affect the strength of the evidence according to evidence-based medicine (EBM) [36]. Randomized controlled trials are usually considered to be more convincing than cohort ones owing to the former's objectivity. Involving studies that included six RCTS and only four cohort studies also made this meta-analysis more objective and convincing.

It is the first that a meta-analysis and review was conducted to assess the intrauterine infusion of PRP to the influence reproductive outcomes of unexplained RIF patients undergoing an embryo transfer. In this review, we excluded the influence of endometrium thickness and childbearing age because some studies found that an endometrial thickness of ≤ 7 mm and a high reproductive age (all of the women included were below 40 years) may negatively impact the pregnancy results [37–40]. In addition, apart from one study that did not mention the exact time of the PRP infusion, all of the other populations used the PRP protocol two or three days before the ET [2]. This meta-analysis may provide a referable time point to initiate PRP.

It is undeniable that we did not give a strict definition of repeated implantation failures owing to a lack of consensus, and we included all of the patients who were diagnosed with a RIF by referring to the local criteria. Except for this, heterogeneity and a reporting bias existed in the process of the analysis, which had an impact on the credibility and objectivity of the article, but only based on the existing data, we may not completely rule out the occurrence of heterogeneity and bias. Meanwhile, the risk of bias graph and risk of bias summary also showed some risks in the selection bias. In addition, two studies involved some participants undergoing a fresh embryo transfer, however, we cannot extract them from the statistics to conduct a subgroup analysis. We cannot draw a conclusion as to which embryo transfer protocol benefits more from PRP. At the same time, our included studies did not report whether euploid tests were carried out or not. We suggest that the following studies can list more detailed data if they include more than one embryo transfer method.

Most suspiciously, most of the articles that we included did not control the variables. The other controls did not take any treatment besides one, which involved infusing GCSF [26]. However, during the intrauterine infusion PRP the insertion and removal of tubes is needed to finish the treatments. If the controls only took measures of no treatment, we were unable to assess the effect of the mechanical manipulation of the uterine cavity on the pregnancy outcomes [41,42].

A very limited number of studies were considered for an overly large number of confounding factors in this meta-analysis, and a further RCT should be conducted to prove these results.

5. Conclusions

This systematic review and meta-analysis proved that the intrauterine infusion of PRP has a positive effect on the pregnancy results for patients with unexplained repeated implantation failures, who are undergoing an embryo transfer.

Supplementary Materials: The following supporting information can be downloaded at: https://www.mdpi.com/article/10.3390/jcm11226753/s1, Figure S1: (a) Risk of bias graph and (b) risk of bias summary; Figure S2: Funnel plot of meta-analysis of 10 included studies; Figure S3: Funnel plot of meta-analysis of 10 included studies excluding PRP dosage; Figure S4: Funnel plot of meta-analysis of 10 included studies excluding study design; Figure S5: Forest plot of RR and 95% CI in studies that evaluated the risk of live birth rates in interventions versus controls; Table S1. Characteristics of the included studies; Table S2: Reasons for exclusion of studies.

Author Contributions: Conceptualization, M.L. and L.Y.; methodology, Y.K.; software, M.L. and Y.K.; validation, M.L., Q.W. and L.Y.; formal analysis, M.L.; investigation, Q.W.; resources, L.Y.; data curation, M.L. and Y.K.; writing—original draft preparation, M.L.; writing—review and editing, Y.K. and Q.W.; visualization, L.Y.; supervision, L.Y.; project administration, L.Y.; funding acquisition, L.Y. All authors have read and agreed to the published version of the manuscript.

Funding: This research was funded by BJHPA-2022-SHZHYXZHQNYJ-LCH-003 and 2020ZLYS02, Shandong Provincial Key Research and Development Program (2020ZLYS02), and the APC was funded by Shandong University.

Institutional Review Board Statement: Ethical approval (2020(63)) was waived by the Ethics Committee of the Reproductive Hospital Affiliated to Shandong University in view of this systematic review and meta-analysis, and all of the procedures that were performed were part of their routine care.

Informed Consent Statement: Not applicable.

Data Availability Statement: Not applicable.

Acknowledgments: Many people have offered me valuable help in my thesis writing, including my tutor and my classmates. Particularly, I would like to give my sincere gratitude to Lei Yan, my tutor who gave me great help by providing me with advice of great value and inspiration for new ideas. It was his suggestions that drew my attention to the number of deficiencies and made many things clearer. Without his strong support, this thesis could not take the present form. I also wish to sincerely thank my classmates. They graciously made considerable comments and sound suggestions for the outline of this paper. I would like to express my gratitude to all those who helped me during the writing of this thesis.

Conflicts of Interest: There is not any conflict of interest.

References

1. Pourakbari, R.; Ahmadi, H.; Yousefi, M.; Aghebati-Maleki, L. Cell Therapy in Female Infertility-Related Diseases: Emphasis on Recurrent Miscarriage and Repeated Implantation Failure. *Life Sci.* **2020**, *258*, 118181. [CrossRef] [PubMed]
2. Makrigiannakis, A.; Makrygiannakis, F.; Vrekoussis, T. Approaches to Improve Endometrial Receptivity in Case of Repeated Implantation Failures. *Front. Cell Dev. Biol.* **2021**, *9*, 613277. [CrossRef] [PubMed]
3. Xu, Y.; Hao, C.; Fang, J.; Liu, X.; Xue, P.; Miao, R. Intrauterine Perfusion of Autologous Platelet-Rich Plasma before Frozen-Thawed Embryo Transfer Improves the Clinical Pregnancy Rate of Women with Recurrent Implantation Failure. *Front. Med.* **2022**, *9*, 850002. [CrossRef] [PubMed]
4. Nazari, L.; Salehpour, S.; Hosseini, S.; Sheibani, S.; Hosseinirad, H. The Effects of Autologous Platelet-Rich Plasma on Pregnancy Outcomes in Repeated Implantation Failure Patients Undergoing Frozen Embryo Transfer: A Randomized Controlled Trial. *Reprod. Sci.* **2022**, *29*, 993–1000. [CrossRef] [PubMed]
5. Ershadi, S.; Noori, N.; Dashipoor, A.; Ghasemi, M.; Shamsa, N. Evaluation of the Effect of Intrauterine Injection of Platelet-Rich Plasma on the Pregnancy Rate of Patients with a History of Implantation Failure in the Fertilization Cycle. *J. Fam. Med. Prim. Care* **2022**, *11*, 2162–2166. [CrossRef]
6. Zargar, M.; Pazhouhanfar, R.; Najafian, M.; Choghakabodi, P.M. Effects of Intrauterine Autologous Platelet-Rich Plasma Infusions on Outcomes in Women with Repetitive in Vitro Fertilization Failures: A Prospective Randomized Study. *Clin. Exp. Obstetr. Gynecol.* **2021**, *48*, 180–185. [CrossRef]
7. Zhou, T.; Ni, T.; Li, Y.; Zhang, Q.; Yan, J.; Chen, Z.-J. Circfam120a Participates in Repeated Implantation Failure by Regulating Decidualization via the Mir-29/Abhd5 Axis. *FASEB J.* **2021**, *35*, e21872. [CrossRef]
8. Coughlan, C.; Ledger, W.; Wang, Q.; Liu, F.; Demirol, A.; Gurgan, T.; Cutting, R.; Ong, K.; Sallam, H.; Li, T.C. Recurrent Implantation Failure: Definition and Management. *Reprod. Biomed. Online* **2014**, *28*, 14–38. [CrossRef]
9. Yin, W.; Qi, X.; Zhang, Y.; Sheng, J.; Xu, Z.; Tao, S.; Xie, X.; Li, X.; Zhang, C. Advantages of Pure Platelet-Rich Plasma Compared with Leukocyte- and Platelet-Rich Plasma in Promoting Repair of Bone Defects. *J. Transl. Med.* **2016**, *14*, 73. [CrossRef]
10. Wang, D.; Rodeo, S.A. Platelet-Rich Plasma in Orthopaedic Surgery: A Critical Analysis Review. *JBJS Rev.* **2017**, *5*, e7. [CrossRef]

11. Scully, D.; Naseem, K.M.; Matsakas, A. Platelet Biology in Regenerative Medicine of Skeletal Muscle. *Acta Physiol.* **2018**, *223*, e13071. [CrossRef]
12. Wen, Y.H.; Lin, W.Y.; Lin, C.J.; Sun, Y.C.; Chang, P.Y.; Wang, H.Y.; Lu, J.J.; Yeh, W.L.; Chiueh, T.S. Sustained or Higher Levels of Growth Factors in Platelet-Rich Plasma During 7-Day Storage. *Clin. Chim. Acta* **2018**, *483*, 89–93. [CrossRef]
13. Mijiritsky, E.; Assaf, H.D.; Peleg, O.; Shacham, M.; Cerroni, L.; Mangani, L. Use of Prp, Prf and Cgf in Periodontal Regeneration and Facial Rejuvenation—A Narrative Review. *Biology* **2021**, *10*, 317. [CrossRef]
14. Raheem, O.A.; Natale, C.; Dick, B.; Reddy, A.G.; Yousif, A.; Khera, M.; Baum, N. Novel Treatments of Erectile Dysfunction: Review of the Current Literature. *Sex. Med. Rev.* **2021**, *9*, 123–132. [CrossRef]
15. Gilat, R.; Haunschild, E.D.; Knapik, D.M.; Evuarherhe, A.; Parvaresh, K.C.; Cole, B.J. Hyaluronic Acid and Platelet-Rich Plasma for the Management of Knee Osteoarthritis. *Int. Orthop.* **2021**, *45*, 345–354. [CrossRef]
16. Hesseler, M.J.; Shyam, N. Platelet-Rich Plasma and Its Utility in Medical Dermatology: A Systematic Review. *J. Am. Acad. Dermatol.* **2019**, *81*, 834–846. [CrossRef]
17. Chang, Y.; Li, J.; Wei, L.-N.; Pang, J.; Chen, J.; Liang, X. Autologous Platelet-Rich Plasma Infusion Improves Clinical Pregnancy Rate in Frozen Embryo Transfer Cycles for Women with Thin Endometrium. *Medicine* **2019**, *98*, e14062. [CrossRef]
18. Cakiroglu, Y.; Saltik, A.; Yuceturk, A.; Karaosmanoglu, O.; Kopuk, S.Y.; Scott, R.T.; Tiras, B.; Seli, E. Effects of Intraovarian Injection of Autologous Platelet Rich Plasma on Ovarian Reserve and Ivf Outcome Parameters in Women with Primary Ovarian Insufficiency. *Aging* **2020**, *12*, 10211–10222. [CrossRef]
19. Hsu, C.-C.; Hsu, L.; Hsu, I.; Chiu, Y.-J.; Dorjee, S. Live Birth in Woman with Premature Ovarian Insufficiency Receiving Ovarian Administration of Platelet-Rich Plasma (Prp) in Combination with Gonadotropin: A Case Report. *Front. Endocrinol.* **2020**, *11*, 50. [CrossRef]
20. Amable, P.R.; Carias, R.B.V.; Teixeira, M.V.T.; Pacheco, I.D.C.; Amaral, R.J.F.C.D.; Granjeiro, J.M.; Borojevic, R. Platelet-Rich Plasma Preparation for Regenerative Medicine: Optimization and Quantification of Cytokines and Growth Factors. *Stem Cell Res. Ther.* **2013**, *4*, 67. [CrossRef]
21. Sánchez-González, D.J.; Méndez-Bolaina, E.; Trejo-Bahena, N.I. Platelet-Rich Plasma Peptides: Key for Regeneration. *Int. J. Pept.* **2012**, *2012*, 532519. [CrossRef] [PubMed]
22. Sharara, F.I.; Lelea, L.L.; Rahman, S.; Klebanoff, J.S.; Moawad, G.N. A Narrative Review of Platelet-Rich Plasma (Prp) in Reproductive Medicine. Review. *J. Assist. Reprod. Genet.* **2021**, *38*, 1003–1012. [CrossRef] [PubMed]
23. Zegers-Hochschild, F.; Adamson, G.D.; Dyer, S.; Racowsky, C.; de Mouzon, J.; Sokol, R.; Rienzi, L.; Sunde, A.; Schmidt, L.; Cooke, I.D.; et al. The International Glossary on Infertility and Fertility Care, 2017. *Fertil. Steril.* **2017**, *108*, 393–406. [CrossRef] [PubMed]
24. Tehraninejad, E.S.; Kashani, N.G.; Hosseini, A.; Tarafdari, A. Autologous Platelet-Rich Plasma Infusion Does Not Improve Pregnancy Outcomes in Frozen Embryo Transfer Cycles in Women with History of Repeated Implantation Failure without Thin Endometrium. *J. Obstet. Gynaecol. Res.* **2021**, *47*, 147–151. [CrossRef] [PubMed]
25. Nazari, L.; Salehpour, S.; Hosseini, M.S.; Moghanjoughi, P.H. The Effects of Autologous Platelet-Rich Plasma in Repeated Implantation Failure: A Randomized Controlled Trial. *Hum. Fertil.* **2020**, *23*, 209–213. [CrossRef]
26. Mehrafza, M.; Kabodmehri, R.; Nikpouri, Z.; Pourseify, G.; Raoufi, A.; Eftekhari, A.; Samadnia, S.; Hosseini, A. Comparing the Impact of Autologous Platelet-Rich Plasma and Granulocyte Colony Stimulating Factor on Pregnancy Outcome in Patients with Repeated Implantation Failure. *J. Reprod. Infertil.* **2019**, *20*, 35–41.
27. Safdarian, L.; Aleyasin, A.; Aghahoseini, M.; Lak, P.; Mosa, S.H.; Sarvi, F.; Mahdavi, A. Efficacy of the Intrauterine Infusion of Platelet-Rich Plasma on Pregnancy Outcomes in Patients with Repeated Implantation Failure: A Randomized Control Trial. *Int. J. Women's Health Reprod. Sci.* **2022**, *10*, 38–44. [CrossRef]
28. Zamaniyan, M.; Peyvandi, S.; Gorji, H.H.; Moradi, S.; Jamal, J.; Aghmashhadi, F.Y.P.; Mohammadi, M.H. Effect of Platelet-Rich Plasma on Pregnancy Outcomes in Infertile Women with Recurrent Implantation Failure: A Randomized Controlled Trial. *Gynecol. Endocrinol.* **2021**, *37*, 141–145. [CrossRef]
29. Noushin, M.A.; Ashraf, M.; Thunga, C.; Singh, S.; Singh, S.; Basheer, R.; Ashraf, R.; Jayaprakasan, K. A Comparative Evaluation of Subendometrial and Intrauterine Platelet-Rich Plasma Treatment for Women with Recurrent Implantation Failure. *F & S Sci.* **2021**, *2*, 295–302. [CrossRef]
30. Arora, G.; Arora, S. Platelet-Rich Plasma-Where Do We Stand Today? A Critical Narrative Review and Analysis. *Dermatol. Ther.* **2021**, *34*, e14343. [CrossRef]
31. Baba, K.; Yamazaki, Y.; Sone, Y.; Sugimoto, Y.; Moriyama, K.; Sugimoto, T.; Kumazawa, K.; Shimakura, Y.; Takeda, A. An In vitro Long-Term Study of Cryopreserved Umbilical Cord Blood-Derived Platelet-Rich Plasma Containing Growth Factors-Pdgf-Bb, Tgf-B, and Vegf. *J. Cranio-Maxillo-Facial Surg.* **2019**, *47*, 668–675. [CrossRef]
32. Lee, M.J.; Yoon, K.S.; Oh, S.; Shin, S.; Jo, C.H. Allogenic Pure Platelet-Rich Plasma Therapy for Adhesive Capsulitis: A Bed-to-Bench Study with Propensity Score Matching Using a Corticosteroid Control Group. *Am. J. Sports Med.* **2021**, *49*, 2309–2320. [CrossRef]
33. Sun, Z.; Su, W.; Wang, L.; Cheng, Z.; Yang, F. Clinical Effect of Bushen Huoxue Method Combined with Platelet-Rich Plasma in the Treatment of Knee Osteoarthritis and Its Effect on Il-1, Il-6, Vegf, and Pge-2. *J. Healthc. Eng.* **2022**, *2022*, 9491439. [CrossRef]
34. Oneto, P.; Etulain, J. Prp in Wound Healing Applications. *Platelets* **2021**, *32*, 189–199. [CrossRef]
35. Zhang, S.; Li, P.; Yuan, Z.; Tan, J. Platelet-Rich Plasma Improves Therapeutic Effects of Menstrual Blood-Derived Stromal Cells in Rat Model of Intrauterine Adhesion. *Stem Cell Res. Ther.* **2019**, *10*, 61. [CrossRef]

36. Crumley, E.; Koufogiannakis, D. Developing Evidence-Based Librarianship: Practical Steps for Implementation. *Health Inf. Libr. J.* **2002**, *19*, 61–70. [CrossRef]
37. Liu, K.E.; Hartman, M.; Hartman, A.; Luo, Z.C.; Mahutte, N. The Impact of a Thin Endometrial Lining on Fresh and Frozen-Thaw Ivf Outcomes: An Analysis of over 40,000 Embryo Transfers. *Hum. Reprod.* **2018**, *33*, 1883–1888. [CrossRef]
38. Von Wolff, M.; Fäh, M.; Roumet, M.; Mitter, V.; Stute, P.; Griesinger, G.; Schwartz, A.K. Thin Endometrium Is Also Associated with Lower Clinical Pregnancy Rate in Unstimulated Menstrual Cycles: A Study Based on Natural Cycle Ivf. *Front. Endocrinol.* **2018**, *9*, 776. [CrossRef]
39. Correa-de-Araujo, R.; Yoon, S.S.S. Clinical Outcomes in High-Risk Pregnancies Due to Advanced Maternal Age. *J. Women's Health* **2021**, *30*, 160–167. [CrossRef]
40. Attali, E.; Yogev, Y. The Impact of Advanced Maternal Age on Pregnancy Outcome. *Best Pract. Res. Clin. Obstet. Gynaecol.* **2021**, *70*, 2–9. [CrossRef]
41. Panagiotopoulou, N.; Karavolos, S.; Choudhary, M. Endometrial Injury Prior to Assisted Reproductive Techniques for Recurrent Implantation Failure: A Systematic Literature Review. *Eur. J. Obstet. Gynecol. Reprod. Biol.* **2015**, *193*, 27–33. [CrossRef] [PubMed]
42. Sar-Shalom Nahshon, C.; Sagi-Dain, L.; Wiener-Megnazi, Z.; Dirnfeld, M. The Impact of Intentional Endometrial Injury on Reproductive Outcomes: A Systematic Review and Meta-Analysis. *Hum. Reprod. Update* **2019**, *25*, 95–113. [CrossRef] [PubMed]

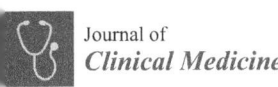

Article

Global Transcriptional Profiling of Granulosa Cells from Polycystic Ovary Syndrome Patients: Comparative Analyses of Patients with or without History of Ovarian Hyperstimulation Syndrome Reveals Distinct Biomarkers and Pathways

Maha H. Daghestani [1,*,†], Huda A. Alqahtani [1,†], AlBandary AlBakheet [2], Mashael Al Deery [3], Khalid A. Awartani [3], Mazin H. Daghestani [4], Namik Kaya [2], Arjumand Warsy [5], Serdar Coskun [6] and Dilek Colak [7,*]

1. Department of Zoology, College of Science, King Saud University, Riyadh 11495, Saudi Arabia
2. Department of Translational Genomics, Center for Genomic Medicine, King Faisal Specialist Hospital and Research Centre, Riyadh 11211, Saudi Arabia
3. Department of Obstetrics and Gynecology, King Faisal Specialist Hospital and Research Centre, Riyadh 11211, Saudi Arabia
4. Department of Obstetrics and Gynecology, Umm-Al-Qura University, Makkah 24382, Saudi Arabia
5. Central Laboratory, Center for Women Scientific and Medical Studies, King Saud University, Riyadh 11451, Saudi Arabia
6. Department of Pathology and Laboratory Medicine, King Faisal Specialist Hospital and Research Centre, Riyadh 11211, Saudi Arabia
7. Department of Molecular Oncology, King Faisal Specialist Hospital and Research Centre, Riyadh 11211, Saudi Arabia
* Correspondence: mdaghestani@ksu.edu.sa (M.H.D.); dkcolak@gmail.com (D.C.)
† These authors contributed equally to this work.

Abstract: Ovarian hyperstimulation syndrome (OHSS) is often a complication of polycystic ovarian syndrome (PCOS), the most frequent disorder of the endocrine system, which affects women in their reproductive years. The etiology of OHSS is multifactorial, though the factors involved are not apparent. In an attempt to unveil the molecular basis of OHSS, we conducted transcriptome analysis of total RNA extracted from granulosa cells from PCOS patients with a history of OHSS ($n = 6$) and compared them to those with no history of OHSS ($n = 18$). We identified 59 significantly dysregulated genes (48 down-regulated, 11 up-regulated) in the PCOS with OHSS group compared to the PCOS without OHSS group (p-value < 0.01, fold change >1.5). Functional, pathway and network analyses revealed genes involved in cellular development, inflammatory and immune response, cellular growth and proliferation (including *DCN, VIM, LIFR, GRN, IL33, INSR, KLF2, FOXO1, VEGF, RDX, PLCL1, PAPPA,* and *ZFP36*), and significant alterations in the PPAR, IL6, IL10, JAK/STAT and NF-κB signaling pathways. Array findings were validated using quantitative RT-PCR. To the best of our knowledge, this is the largest cohort of Saudi PCOS cases (with or without OHSS) to date that was analyzed using a transcriptomic approach. Our data demonstrate alterations in various gene networks and pathways that may be involved in the pathophysiology of OHSS. Further studies are warranted to confirm the findings.

Keywords: ovarian hyperstimulation syndrome (OHSS); polycystic ovarian syndrome (PCOS); genome-wide gene expression; functional pathway; gene ontology; transcriptome; network analyses; biomarker

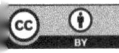

1. Introduction

Ovarian hyperstimulation syndrome (OHSS) is a rare, iatrogenic complication of ovarian hyperstimulation by assisted reproduction treatment and is potentially life-threatening [1–3]. Women with polycystic ovary syndrome (PCOS) are at a higher risk for developing OHSS due to having a large number of follicles on their ovaries and the tendency to over-respond to the hormones used for inducing fertility [2]. The causes of OHSS are generally unknown. Since complications can be severe and may even be life-threatening, it is critical to predict whether a woman going through gonadotropin therapy may develop OHSS.

Previous studies have reported several risk factors for the development of OHSS, such as young age, PCOS, low body mass index (BMI), and previous history of OHSS [4,5]. Granulosa cells (GC) are essential for ovarian folliculogenesis and are known to play a critical role in follicular development and oocyte maturation [6,7]. Several studies have indicated that GC dysfunction in women with PCOS may contribute to abnormal folliculogenesis [6,7]. Recent advances in omics technologies (genomics, transcriptomics, proteomics, and others) have enabled researchers to better understand the molecular characteristics of diseases and to identify disease biomarkers [7–11].

Genome-wide studies in various cells, including granulosa cells from women with PCOS and non-PCOS controls, have revealed several potential genes and pathways, such as the ERK/MAPK and VEGF signaling pathways [6,11]. However, OHSS (and PCOS) has a complex etiology and genetic basis and the disease pathogenesis and mechanism still largely remain unclear [5,6,12,13]. In this study, we aimed to identify the potentially essential genes and pathways in PCOS patients who would be prone to developing OHSS and to identify potential markers that may be linked to the OHSS and its pathobiology using a transcriptomic approach. To this purpose, we investigated if the PCOS patients who had developed OHSS have a distinct molecular profile in their granulosa cells as compared to those who did not in order to understand the biology of its development.

2. Materials and Methods

2.1. Patients

Twenty-four infertile women with PCOS undergoing IVF treatment were identified and examined by an IVF physician at Gynecology/IVF clinics at King Faisal Specialist Hospital and Research Center (KFSHRC). PCOS was defined according to the criteria established by the American Society of Reproductive Medicine and the European Society of Human Reproduction and Embryology (ASRM/ESHRE) [14]. The PCOS patients who are younger than 40 years, with FSH $\leq$ 12, body mass index (BMI) $\leq$ 35 kg/m^2 and not undergoing any immunosuppressive therapy, were asked to participate in the study. The study was approved by the institutional review board (IRB) of the King Faisal Specialist Hospital and Research Center (no.08-MED604-2; RAC#2100002; RAC#2110006) and it is performed in accordance with the current version of the Helsinki Declaration. Written informed consent was obtained from all patients before participation in the study.

The study included samples from 24 patients (n = 24) with PCOS. Pituitary down-regulation was performed by administering gonadotrophin-releasing hormone (GnRH) agonist long or short protocols as described earlier [10]. Six patients had a positive history of OHSS (four patients had a history of OHSS and two had it in the current cycle) (referred to as "OHSS" group; n = 6) and the control group was without any history of OHSS (referred to as PCOS; n = 18). All OHSS cases were severe or moderate. Granulosa cells (3 mL) were collected into 15 mL regular falcon conical tubes from participating subjects undergoing control ovarian stimulation as described previously [10] for microarray and quantitative RT-PCR (qRT-PCR) experiments.

2.2. RNA Isolation

The total RNA was isolated from granulosa cells using Trizol or Total RNA Isolation Kit™ (ThermoFisher Scientific, Waltham, MA, USA) according to manufacturer's instructions. The quality and quantity of RNA were determined by measuring absorbance spectra on a UV/Vis spectrophotometer, NanoDrop® ND-1000 (ThermoFisher Scientific, Waltham, MA, USA). Further quality check was carried out using the RNA 6000 Nano Assay and 2100 Bioanalyzer (Agilent Technologies, Santa Clara, CA, USA). The high-quality RNA was either immediately used in the experiments (for the real-time RT-PCR and microarray experiments) or stored at $-80\ °C$ for further use.

2.3. Genome-Wide Gene Expression Profiling

Whole-genome gene expression profiling of samples from the OHSS ($n = 6$) and unrelated PCOS ($n = 18$) was performed using Affymetrix's Human Genome U133 Plus 2.0 Array (ThermoFisher Scientific, Waltham, MA, USA). High-quality RNA was converted into labeled cRNA, fragmented, hybridized onto the chip surface according to the manufacturer's protocols as described previously [15]. Briefly, the total RNA was converted into double-stranded cDNA, and then the cDNA was used for cRNA synthesis during which biotinylated UTPs and CTPs were incorporated into the cRNA. Target-labeled cRNA was fractionated and then hybridized onto the chip's surface. The experimental procedures and quality control procedures at each critical step (before hybridization as well as post-hybridization) were strictly followed according to the manufacturer's guidelines. Washing, staining, and scanning were performed according to the manufacturer's instructions and guidelines.

Microarray data normalization was performed using GC Robust Multi-array Average (GC-RMA) algorithm [16,17]. We performed independent two-sample t-test to identify genes whose expression significantly varied between OHSS and PCOS groups. Differentially expressed genes (DEGs) were defined as those with p-value < 0.01 and fold change (FC) ≥ 1.5. Two-dimensional hierarchical clustering is performed using Pearson's correlation with average linkage clustering. Functional annotation and biological term enrichment analysis were performed using DAVID Bioinformatics Resources [18]. Statistical analyses were performed using SPSS version 20 (SPSS, Inc., Chicago, IL, USA) and PARTEK Genomics Suite (Partek Inc., Chesterfield, MO, USA). All statistical tests were two-sided and p-value < 0.05 was considered statistically significant.

2.4. Functional, Pathway and Network Analyses

The functional, pathway, gene ontology enrichment, and network analyses were performed using Ingenuity Pathways Analysis (IPA) (QIAGEN Inc., Venlo, Netherlands; https://www.qiagenbioinformatics.com/products/ingenuity-pathway-analysis (accessed on 18 September 2020). The DEGs were mapped to their corresponding gene object in the Ingenuity Pathways Knowledge Base and significant gene interaction networks are identified. Scores of ≥ 2 were considered significant after applying a 99% confidence level. A right-tailed Fisher's exact test was used to calculate a p-value determining the probability that the biological function (or pathway) assigned to that data set is explained by chance alone.

2.5. Quantitative RT-PCR (qRT-PCR)

To validate our microarray results, confirmatory qRT-PCR was performed using the ABI 7500 Sequence Detection System (ThermoFisher Scientific, Waltham, MA, USA). For this purpose, 50 ng total RNA procured from the same microarray study samples were transcribed into cDNA using Sensiscript Kit (QIAGEN Inc., Venlo, The Netherlands) under the following conditions: 25 °C for 10 min, 42 °C for 2 h, and 70 °C for 15 min in a total volume of 20 µL. Then, 2–5 µL of cDNA was amplified under the following conditions: Initial denaturation of 5 min at 95 °C followed by 34 cycles of "denaturation at 95 °C for 1 min, annealing at 60 °C for 1 min and extension at 72 °C for 1 min" and a final extension of 10 min at 72 °C.

Twenty-one genes (*FOXO1, FOXO3, FOXP1, GPC4, GPSM1, IL33, INSR, KLF2, MAN2B2, MYO10, NAGA, PAPPA, PCSK5, PHEX, PLD2, RABGAP1, SIN3A, SQSTM1, TCF7L2, USP9X,* and *ZFP36*) were randomly selected amongst the significantly expressed genes (p-value < 0.01) and primers were designed using Primer 3 web-toolsoftware (https://primer3.ut.ee accessed on 18 September 2022). The list of primer sequences used in this study is presented in Table S1. After primer optimization, the PCR assays were performed in 6 µL of the cDNA using the QIAGEN Quantitech SYBR Green Kit (QIAGEN Inc., Venlo, Netherlands), employing GAPDH as the endogenous control gene. All reactions were conducted in triplicates. The data were analyzed using the delta delta CT method [19,20].

3. Results

3.1. Clinical Characteristics of the Patients

The study included 24 women with PCOS with or without a history of OHSS. Granulosa cells were isolated from six PCOS patients with a history of OHSS (referred to as OHSS) and 18 without OHSS (referred to as the PCOS group). The clinical features were similar between the two groups of patients in terms of age, weight, BMI, FSH, LH, total testosterone, and androstenedione (Mann–Whitney U-test p-value > 0.05) (Table 1).

Table 1. Comparison of clinical parameters between OHSS group and PCOS group.

	PCOS (n = 18)	OHSS (n = 6)	p-Value *
	Mean (SD)	Mean (SD)	
Age (years)	29.0 (3.7)	30.2 (6.3)	0.71
BMI (kg/m^2)	24.8 (1.2)	24.2 (1.4)	0.43
FSH (IU/L)	6.9 (2.2)	6.3 (1.1)	0.47
LH (IU/L)	13.0 (9.9)	7.5 (4.9)	0.14
Testosterone	2.5 (1.3)	2.2 (0.9)	0.76
Androstenedione	12.3 (6.8)	15.5 (4.8)	0.13

* Mann–Whitney U-test. BMI, Body mass index; FSH, Follicle stimulating hormone; LH, Lutenising hormone. OHSS refers to PCOS patients with a history of OHSS and PCOS refers to patients without any history of OHSS.

3.2. Identification of Differentially Expressed Genes

We analyzed the genome-wide mRNA expression profiling of 24 samples from OHSS and PCOS groups using Affymetrix's GeneChip® Human Genome U133 Plus 2.0 Arrays, which includes over 47,000 transcripts and variants using more than 54,000 probe sets. The array technology is a well-established and reliable method to assess global gene expression profiling [15,21]. Comparison of transcriptomes of OHSS with those PCOS patients with no history of OHSS revealed significant dysregulation of 1520 probes, corresponding to 1188 genes (p-value < 0.01), of which 65 probes (corresponding to 59 genes) had a greater than 1.5-fold change (FC) between the two groups (Table 2). The unsupervised principal component analysis (PCA) and hierarchical clustering in both dimensions (samples and genes) were performed using Pearson's correlation with average linkage clustering, where both analyses revealed clear discrimination of samples as PCOS and OHSS as well as the pattern of genes deregulation defining two main transcriptome clusters (Figure 1A,B, respectively) that clearly demonstrated the significant differences in gene expression profiles of having a positive or negative history of OHSS among the PCOS patients.

Table 2. Significantly altered probes in PCOS patients with history of OHSS as compared to no history of OHSS (p-value < 0.01 and >1.5-fold change).

Gene	Gene Title	p-Value	FC
PAPPA	pregnancy-associated plasma protein A, pappalysin 1	0.000798	1.86
DCN	Decorin	0.0044	1.76
PTPLA	protein tyrosine phosphatase-like (proline instead of catalytic arginine), member	0.005688	1.71
FKBP1A	FK506 binding protein 1A, 12 kDa	0.002428	1.7
SHOX2	short stature homeobox 2	0.008934	1.64
ELOVL5	ELOVL family member 5, elongation of long-chain fatty acids (FEN1/Elo2, SUR4/Elo)	0.000683	1.55
IL33	interleukin 33	0.003649	1.55

Table 2. *Cont.*

Gene	Gene Title	p-Value	FC
EIF5	eukaryotic translation initiation factor 5	0.007926	1.52
TMX1	thioredoxin-related transmembrane protein 1	0.000272	1.52
LIFR	leukemia inhibitory factor receptor alpha	0.00038	1.51
RDX	Radixin	0.005259	1.51
OBSL1	obscurin-like 1	0.009828	−1.5
RNPEP	arginylaminopeptidase (aminopeptidase B)	0.000196	−1.5
BAT3	HLA-B associated transcript 3	0.001025	−1.51
DYNC1H1	dynein, cytoplasmic 1, heavy chain 1	0.004793	−1.51
FOXP1	forkhead box P1	0.001132	−1.51
MAP4K4	mitogen-activated protein kinase kinasekinasekinase 4	0.000309	−1.51
GRN	Granulin	0.008224	−1.52
MED14	mediator complex subunit 14	0.001012	−1.52
HS3ST1	heparan sulfate (glucosamine) 3-O-sulfotransferase 1	0.007768	−1.53
SEC14L1	SEC14-like 1 (S. cerevisiae)	0.005745	−1.53
SNRNP200	small nuclear ribonucleoprotein 200k Da (U5)	0.001182	−1.53
BBS1	Bardet–Biedl syndrome 1	0.000834	−1.54
MAN2B2	mannosidase, alpha, class 2B, member 2	0.00033	−1.54
MYLIP	myosin regulatory light chain interacting protein	0.006807	−1.55
KIAA0513	KIAA0513	0.004853	−1.56
KDM5A	lysine (K)-specific demethylase 5A	0.000431	−1.57
PCSK5	proproteinconvertasesubtilisin/kexintype 5	0.002482	−1.58
GAS2L1	growth arrest-specific 2 like 1	0.005994	−1.59
MGC21881	hypothetical locus MGC21881	0.009274	−1.59
PLCL1	phospholipase C-like 1	0.009504	−1.59
ZSWIM5	zinc finger, SWIM-type containing 5	0.005745	−1.59
VIM	Vimentin	0.001645	−1.6
CRISPLD2	cysteine-rich secretory protein LCCL domain containing 2	0.00095	−1.61
GPSM1	G-protein signaling modulator 1	0.002004	−1.61
CHST3	carbohydrate (chondroitin 6) sulfotransferase 3	0.001192	−1.63
SCAP	SREBF chaperone	0.008736	−1.63
LAMP1	lysosomal-associated membrane protein 1	0.008512	−1.64
SH3PXD2B	SH3 and PX domains 2B	0.004433	−1.64
SP110	SP110 nuclear body protein	0.00000735	−1.66
PHEX	phosphate regulating endopeptidase homolog, X-linked	0.004347	−1.67
FOXO1	forkhead box O1	0.001054	−1.68
TPP1	tripeptidyl peptidase I	0.009215	−1.69
LGALS3BP	lectin, galactoside-binding, soluble, 3 binding protein	0.007244	−1.71
ABCA8	ATP-binding cassette, sub-family A (ABC1), member 8	0.004646	−1.76
CADM1	cell adhesion molecule 1	0.003501	−1.77
CLSTN1	calsyntenin 1	0.002802	−1.77
FOS	FBJ murine osteosarcoma viral oncogene homolog	0.00617	−1.81
MYO10	myosin X	0.004334	−1.86
KLF2	Kruppel-like factor 2 (lung)	0.003583	−1.87
INSR	insulin receptor	0.008567	−1.88
IER2	immediate early response 2	0.006056	−1.91
CNKSR3	CNKSR family member 3	0.004281	−1.99
GPC4	glypican 4	0.003565	−2.08
MYADM	myeloid-associated differentiation marker	0.002895	−2.14
PXDN	peroxidasin homolog (Drosophila)	0.00015	−2.15
DAPK1	death-associated protein kinase 1	0.001645	−2.17
ZFP36	zinc finger protein 36, C3H type, homolog (mouse)	0.000679	−2.38

FC, fold change between patients with history of OHSS as compared to PCOS patients. Negative sign indicates down-regulation.

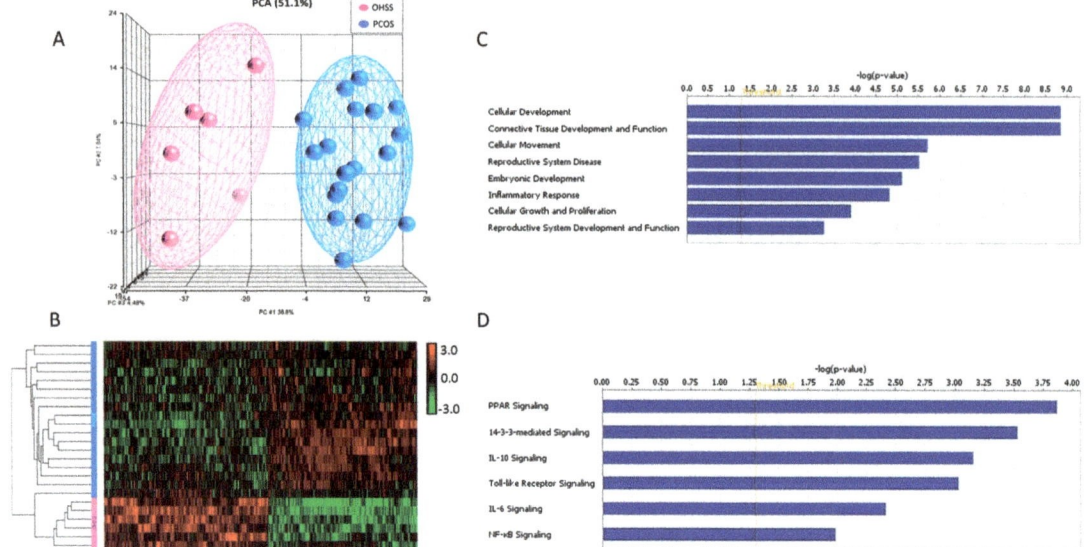

Figure 1. Global transcriptional changes associated with history of OHSS. (**A**) The unsupervised principal component analysis (PCA) and (**B**) two-dimensional hierarchical clustering analysis clearly distinguished individuals with PCOS with a positive history of OHSS from those without OHSS (**A**,**B**, respectively). The expression level of each gene across the samples is normalized to [−3, 3]. Hierarchical clustering was performed using Pearson's correlation with average linkage clustering. Pink spheres indicate OHSS, blue spheres indicate PCOS (without OHSS). Red and green in the heatmap denote highly and weakly expressed genes, respectively. (**C**) Over-represented biological functions and (**D**) significantly altered canonical pathways associated with DEG (up- or down-regulated) in OHSS patients. X-axis indicates the significance (−log p-value) of the functional/pathway association that is dependent on the number of genes in a class as well as biological relevance. The threshold line represents a p-value of 0.05.

3.3. Functional, Pathway and Gene Network Analysis of Dysregulated Genes

The gene ontology (GO) and functional analyses of differentially expressed genes in the OHSS group compared to PCOS were performed using IPA and DAVID Bioinformatics Resources [18,22]. The biological functions assigned to the data set were ranked according to the significance of the biological function to the dataset. As presented in Figure 1C, differentially expressed genes were enriched with functional categories including cellular development, connective tissue development and function, inflammatory and immune response, cellular growth and proliferation (including *DCN, FOXP1, GRN, IL33, INSR, KLF2, FOXO1, FOS, VIM, PAPPA,* and *ZFP36*). Significantly, altered canonical pathways in the OHSS included the PPAR, IL6, IL10, NF-κB and 14-3-3-mediated signaling pathways (Figure 1D).

To gain an in-depth insight into the interactions of the dysregulated genes involved in the different pathways, genes that were significantly dysregulated in the OHSS were mapped to the gene networks using the Ingenuity Pathway Analysis [22,23]. The network analysis revealed potentially important hub genes, including *DCN, IL33, VIM, VEGF, GPC4, KLF2, ELOVL5, KDM5A,* Immunoglobulin, *ZFP36*, and the NF-κB, FOXO, and JAK/STAT signaling pathways that may be relevant to the pathophysiology of OHSS (Figure 2).

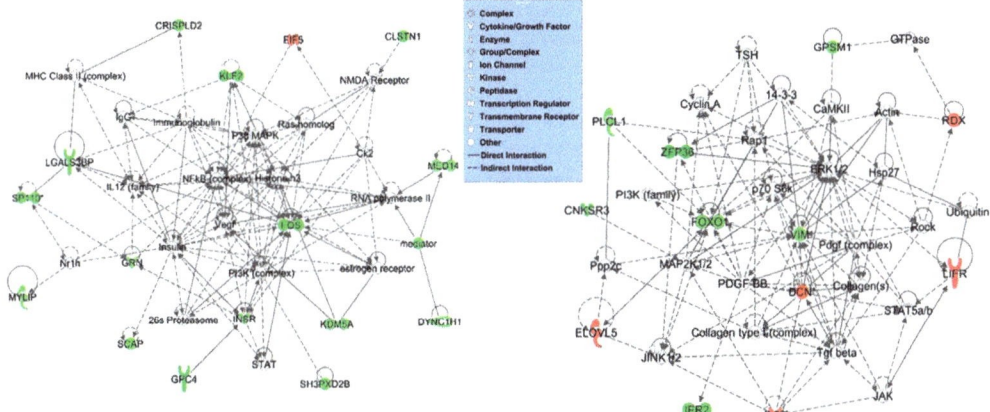

Figure 2. Gene interaction network analysis of significantly dysregulated genes in OHSS group. Top-scoring gene interaction networks with high relevancy scores are shown. Nodes represent genes and the edges indicate biological relationship between the nodes. Straight and dashed lines represent direct or indirect gene-to-gene interactions, respectively. The functional class of the gene product are represented with different shapes (see legend). Red/green indicated up- (down-) regulated in OHSS compared to PCOS group. The color intensity is correlated with fold change.

3.4. Confirmation of Gene Expression Using qRT-PCR

To validate the microarray results, confirmatory qRT-PCR was performed for randomly selected 21 significantly differentially expressed genes (p-value < 0.01), namely *FOXO1, FOXO3, FOXP1, GPC4, GPSM1, IL33, INSR, KLF2, MAN2B2, MYO10, NAGA, PAPPA, PCSK5, PHEX, PLD2, RABGAP1, SIN3A, SQSTM1, TCF7L2, USP9X*, and *ZFP36*, in OHSS compared to PCOS group (Figure S1). A strong correlation existed between the microarray and the qRT-PCR results (r = 0.9).

4. Discussion

In this study, we performed a transcriptomic comparison of PCOS patients with a history of OHSS to those patients with no history of OHSS using granulosa cells in order to identify potential markers for OHSS and to understand its biology. To the best of our knowledge, this is the largest cohort of Saudi PCOS cases (with or without OHSS) to date that was analyzed using a transcriptomic approach.

Our results revealed the potentially important roles of genes related to cellular development, connective tissue development and function, inflammatory and immune response, cellular growth and proliferation, and reproductive system development and function, including genes such as *FOXP1, FOXO1, DCN, IL33, INSR, KLF2, PAPPA, VIM*, and *ZFP36*, that have significant gene expression changes in the OHSS group compared to PCOS patients [24–26]. Forkhead box (FOX) transcription factor family members have critical aspects in modulating the genes that are important for various cellular processes such as cell growth, differentiation, and longevity and some of which have a crucial role in embryonic development [27], particularly in female reproduction [28]. Interestingly, Forkhead box P1 (*FOXP1*) is known to cause estrogen-dependent endometrial cancers through the KRAS pathway. Moreover, altered FOXP1 expression and Wnt-related β-catenin acetylation were observed in endometriotic stromal cells from endometriosis patients [29]. Knockdown experiments pointed out the dysregulation of genes involved in Wnt signaling and recapitulated the endometriotic cellular activities such as reducing collagen gel contraction and inhibiting cell proliferation [29]. Several studies have shown that the deletion of the *FOXO1* leads to embryonic cell death as a result of incomplete blood vessel development [30,31] and may have a critical role in placental morphogenesis in the developing embryo [32,33]. *FOXO1* was implicated in putatively regulating genes involved in lipid and sterol biosynthesis, suggesting that it may play a role in follicular steroidogenesis (Liu et al., 2009). Furthermore, the expression of *FOXO1* is shown to be associated with estrogen receptors alpha (ER-α) and beta (ER-β), which are produced primarily by the ovaries and the placenta during pregnancy. The follicle-stimulating hormone (FSH) stimulates the ovarian production of estrogens by the granulosa cells of the ovarian follicles and corpora lutea [34,35]. The pregnancy-associated plasma protein A (*PAPPA*) is significantly up-regulated in OHSS patients. *PAPPA* may have a role in female fertility by modulating ovarian function, preeclamptic placentae and steroidogenesis [24,36].

Zing finger protein (*ZFP36*), Kruppel-like factor 2 (*KLF2*), insulin receptor (*INSR*), elongation of very-long-chain fatty acid (*ELOVL5*) and Glypican-4 (*GPC4*) were found to be significantly altered in OHSS. *GPC4*, which is an adipokine that interacts with the INSR and influences insulin sensitivity [37], was down-regulated in OHSS, which may have a likely role in affecting the control of cell division, growth regulation, body fat distribution, insulin resistance, and arterial stiffness in OHSS [38]. Zing finger protein, *ZFP36*, was shown to be crucial for female fertility and early embryonic development [25] and influences ovulation and oocyte maturation [39,40]. Therefore, it was proposed as a promising candidate gene for obesity-associated metabolic complications [41]. Altered insulin functions have long been associated with abnormalities in female reproduction [42,43]. Conditions associated with insulin resistance, such as obesity and diabetes mellitus, are often accompanied by increased adiposity or hyperglycemia [44]. Obesity and diabetes are independently associated with an altered female reproductive function [13,45,46]. Interestingly, a recent study reported that *ELOVL5* is involved in embryonic development and lipid metabolism [47]. *KLF2* is expressed in endothelial cells and inhibited by the inflammatory cytokine interleukin-1, hence, implicated as a novel regulator response to proinflammatory stimuli [48]. KLF2's inhibition for endothelial cell migration and angiogenesis is partly attributed to its ability to inhibit the VEGF receptor (VEGFR) 2/kinase insert domain-containing receptor (KDR) expression [49]. Moreover, G-protein signaling modulator 1 (GPSM1) and Myosin X (MYO10) also displayed dysregulation in OHSS patients. *GPSM1* plays a critical role in regulating mitotic spindle orientation, cell polarity, and adenylyl cyclase activity [50] and *MYO10* has key functions in filopodia. Experiments with fibroblast-like cells have revealed that MYO10 localizes to the tips of filopodia and undergoes intrafilopodial motility [51].

The pathway and gene network analyses revealed significant alterations in the PPAR, IL6, IL10, FOXO, JAK/STAT and NF-κB signaling pathways and potentially critical roles of *IL33*, *VEGF*, *INSR*, *FOS*, *TGf-β*, *LIFR*, and immunoglobulin that may be relevant to the pathophysiology of OHSS [52–54]. Indeed, previous studies also reported the involvement of the immune system, cytokines, and growth factors in the pathogenesis of OHSS [52,53,55,56]. For example, *VEGF* was implicated as having a significant role in the development of OHSS [26,52,54,57]. *IL33* acts as both an extracellular cytokine and an intracellular nuclear factor with transcriptional regulatory properties [58]. IL33 was shown to have higher levels in PCOS patients compared to the controls [59]. Interestingly, dehydroepiandrosterone (DHEA)-induced PCOS in rats was shown to respond to omega-6 fatty acid (γ-linolenic acid (GLA)) treatment that led to a significant decrease in IL-33 levels in the rat's ovaries, hence, implicating GLA's potential use for likely human-related treatments for inflammatory responses in PCOS via the PPAR-γ pathway [60]. Previous studies have reported that the JAK/STAT pathway plays a critical role in the regulation of functions including immune regulation, growth, fertility, and embryogenesis [61–64].

A limitation of this study was that we had a relatively small sample size within the OHSS group. As the occurrence of OHSS is quite low (about 5% of treated women may encounter moderate and severe OHSS), we were able to recruit six patients with a history of OHSS ($n = 6$) (four patients had a history of OHSS and two had it in the current cycle) and 18 without any history of OHSS ($n = 18$) for our whole-genome expression analysis. This was, indeed, achieved after several years of sample collection. For whole-genome studies of such rare human diseases, including PCOS/OHSS, this number is considered a reasonable number to be able to identify differentially expressed genes (DEGs) for discovery-related investigations [6,54,65]. In addition, we used a stringent cutoff for selecting the DEGs; a p-value (of less than 0.01) as well as the fold change criteria. Furthermore, we performed an independent experimental method (qRT-PCR) to validate the microarray results and there was a strong correlation that existed between the microarray and qRT-PCR results ($r = 0.9$). Future studies may focus on investigating functional mechanisms and further validating the findings on a larger group of patient cohorts.

5. Conclusions

In conclusion, in this study, we identified markers and altered pathways that may have the potential to differentiate the patients who may be prone to developing OHSS and understanding the biology of its development, which opens new avenues for further research to confirm these findings.

Supplementary Materials: The following supporting information can be downloaded at: https://www.mdpi.com/article/10.3390/jcm11236941/s1. Figure S1: Confirmation of gene expression results by qRT-PCR for 21 genes (*FOXO1, FOXP1, GPC4, GPSM1, IL33, INSR, KLF2, MAN2B2, MYO10, PAPPA, PCSK5, PHEX, ZFP36*). A strong correlation existed between the microarray and qRT-PCR results ($r = 0.9$). Table S1: The sequences of 21 primers (forward and reverse) employing B-ACTIN as the endogenous control gene. Table S2: Microarray data for OHSS (PCOS patients with a positive history of OHSS; $n = 6$) and PCOS group (patients with PCOS and have no history of OHSS; $n = 18$) probed using Affymetrix's GeneChip® Human Genome U133 Plus 2.0 Arrays.

Author Contributions: N.K., D.C., M.H.D. (Maha H. Daghestani) and S.C. designed the study; K.A.A., M.A.D., M.H.D. (Mazin H. Daghestani) and S.C. enrolled the patients, collected clinical data, samples, and patient history; H.A.A. and A.A. performed the experiments; D.C. conducted the data analyses; M.H.D. (Maha H. Daghestani) received funding acquisition; N.K., D.C., M.H.D. (Maha H. Daghestani), and A.W. wrote the manuscript; all authors were involved in checking and finalization of the final manuscript. All authors have read and agreed to the published version of the manuscript.

Funding: This work was funded by the National Plan for Science, Technology, and Innovation (MAARIFAH), King Abdul-Aziz City for Science and Technology, Kingdom of Saudi Arabia, grant Number No 08-MED 604-2.

Institutional Review Board Statement: The study was approved by the institutional review board (IRB) of the King Faisal Specialist Hospital and Research Center (no.08-MED604-2; RAC#2100002; RAC#2110006) and was performed in accordance with the current version of the Helsinki Declaration.

Informed Consent Statement: Written informed consent was obtained from all patients before participation in the study.

Data Availability Statement: All data generated and analyzed in this study are included in this manuscript and its Supplementary Materials files.

Acknowledgments: We extend our appreciation to the National Plan for Science, Technology, and Innovation (MAARIFAH), King Abdul-Aziz City for Science and Technology, Kingdom of Saudi Arabia, for supporting this study through grant Number No 08-MED604-2. We are immensely grateful to the patients for their participation. Our sincere thanks and appreciation go to King Saud University and King Faisal Specialist Hospital and Research Center (KFSHRC), and Genetics Department, Microarray Core Facility for their kind and continuous support and help in allowing us to carry out this project.

Conflicts of Interest: The authors declare no conflict of interest. The funders had no role in the design of the study; in the collection, analyses, or interpretation of data; in the writing of the manuscript; or in the decision to publish the results.

References

1. Kumar, P.; Sait, S.F.; Sharma, A.; Kumar, M. Ovarian hyperstimulation syndrome. *J. Hum. Reprod. Sci.* **2011**, *4*, 70–75. [CrossRef] [PubMed]
2. Practice Committee of American Society for Reproductive Medicine. Ovarian hyperstimulation syndrome. *Fertil. Steril.* **2008**, *90*, S188–S193. [CrossRef] [PubMed]
3. Namavar Jahromi, B.M.; Parsanezhad, M.M.; Shomali, Z.M.; Bakhshai, P.M.; Alborzi, M.M.; Moin Vaziri, N.M.D.P.; Anvar, Z.P. Ovarian Hyperstimulation Syndrome: A Narrative Review of Its Pathophysiology, Risk Factors, Prevention, Classification, and Management. *Iran. J. Med. Sci.* **2018**, *43*, 248–260. [PubMed]
4. Sun, B.; Ma, Y.; Li, L.; Hu, L.; Wang, F.; Zhang, Y.; Dai, S.; Sun, Y. Factors Associated with Ovarian Hyperstimulation Syndrome (OHSS) Severity in Women With Polycystic Ovary Syndrome Undergoing IVF/ICSI. *Front. Endocrinol.* **2020**, *11*, 615957. [CrossRef]
5. Soave, I.; Marci, R. Ovarian stimulation in patients in risk of OHSS. *Minerva Ginecol.* **2014**, *66*, 165–178.
6. Lan, C.W.; Chen, M.J.; Tai, K.Y.; Yu, D.C.; Yang, Y.C.; Jan, P.S.; Yang, Y.S.; Chen, H.F.; Ho, H.N. Functional microarray analysis of differentially expressed genes in granulosa cells from women with polycystic ovary syndrome related to MAPK/ERK signaling. *Sci. Rep.* **2015**, *5*, 14994. [CrossRef]
7. Brinca, A.T.; Ramalhinho, A.C.; Sousa, A.; Oliani, A.H.; Breitenfeld, L.; Passarinha, L.A.; Gallardo, E. Follicular Fluid: A Powerful Tool for the Understanding and Diagnosis of Polycystic Ovary Syndrome. *Biomedicines* **2022**, *10*, 1254. [CrossRef]
8. Al-Harazi, O.; Kaya, I.H.; Al-Eid, M.; Alfantoukh, L.; Al Zahrani, A.S.; Al Sebayel, M.; Kaya, N.; Colak, D. Identification of Gene Signature as Diagnostic and Prognostic Blood Biomarker for Early Hepatocellular Carcinoma Using Integrated Cross-Species Transcriptomic and Network Analyses. *Front. Genet.* **2021**, *12*, 710049. [CrossRef]
9. Al-Harazi, O.; Kaya, I.H.; El Allali, A.; Colak, D. A Network-Based Methodology to Identify Subnetwork Markers for Diagnosis and Prognosis of Colorectal Cancer. *Front. Genet.* **2021**, *12*, 721949. [CrossRef]
10. Coskun, S.; Otu, H.H.; Awartani, K.A.; Al-Alwan, L.A.; Al-Hassan, S.; Al-Mayman, H.; Kaya, N.; Inan, M.S. Gene expression profiling of granulosa cells from PCOS patients following varying doses of human chorionic gonadotropin. *J. Assist. Reprod. Genet.* **2013**, *30*, 341–352. [CrossRef]
11. Scarfo, G.; Daniele, S.; Fusi, J.; Gesi, M.; Martini, C.; Franzoni, F.; Cela, V.; Artini, P.G. Metabolic and Molecular Mechanisms of Diet and Physical Exercise in the Management of Polycystic Ovarian Syndrome. *Biomedicines* **2022**, *10*, 1305. [CrossRef]
12. Wu, L.; Sun, Y.; Wan, J.; Luan, T.; Cheng, Q.; Tan, Y. A proteomic analysis identifies candidate early biomarkers to predict ovarian hyperstimulation syndrome in polycystic ovarian syndrome patients. *Mol. Med. Rep.* **2017**, *16*, 272–280. [CrossRef]
13. Morgante, G.; Darino, I.; Spano, A.; Luisi, S.; Luddi, A.; Piomboni, P.; Governini, L.; De Leo, V. PCOS Physiopathology and Vitamin D Deficiency: Biological Insights and Perspectives for Treatment. *J. Clin. Med.* **2022**, *11*, 4509. [CrossRef]
14. The Rotterdam ESHRE/ASRM-Sponsored PCOS Consensus Workshop Group. Revised 2003 consensus on diagnostic criteria and long-term health risks related to polycystic ovary syndrome. *Fertil. Steril.* **2004**, *81*, 19–25. [CrossRef]
15. Aldosary, M.; Al-Bakheet, A.; Al-Dhalaan, H.; Almass, R.; Alsagob, M.; Al-Younes, B.; AlQuait, L.; Mustafa, O.M.; Bulbul, M.; Rahbeeni, Z.; et al. Rett Syndrome, a Neurodevelopmental Disorder, Whole-Transcriptome, and Mitochondrial Genome Multiomics Analyses Identify Novel Variations and Disease Pathways. *OMICS* **2020**, *24*, 160–171. [CrossRef]
16. Wu, Z.; Irizarry, R.A. Preprocessing of oligonucleotide array data. *Nat. Biotechnol.* **2004**, *22*, 656–658. [CrossRef]
17. Wu, Z.; Irizarry, R.A. Stochastic models inspired by hybridization theory for short oligonucleotide arrays. *J. Comput. Biol.* **2005**, *12*, 882–893. [CrossRef]
18. Dennis, G., Jr.; Sherman, B.T.; Hosack, D.A.; Yang, J.; Gao, W.; Lane, H.C.; Lempicki, R.A. DAVID: Database for Annotation, Visualization, and Integrated Discovery. *Genome Biol.* **2003**, *4*, R60. [CrossRef]
19. Livak, K.J.; Schmittgen, T.D. Analysis of relative gene expression data using real-time quantitative PCR and the 2(-Delta Delta C(T)) Method. *Methods* **2001**, *25*, 402–408. [CrossRef]
20. Schmittgen, T.D. Real-time quantitative PCR. *Methods* **2001**, *25*, 383–385. [CrossRef]
21. Lee, N.H.; Saeed, A.I. Microarrays: An overview. *Methods Mol. Biol.* **2007**, *353*, 265–300. [CrossRef] [PubMed]
22. Al-Harazi, O.; El Allali, A.; Colak, D. Biomolecular Databases and Subnetwork Identification Approaches of Interest to Big Data Community: An Expert Review. *OMICS* **2019**, *23*, 138–151. [CrossRef] [PubMed]
23. Colak, D.; Al-Harazi, O.; Mustafa, O.M.; Meng, F.; Assiri, A.M.; Dhar, D.K.; Broering, D.C. RNA-Seq transcriptome profiling in three liver regeneration models in rats: Comparative analysis of partial hepatectomy, ALLPS, and PVL. *Sci. Rep.* **2020**, *10*, 5213. [CrossRef] [PubMed]
24. Nyegaard, M.; Overgaard, M.T.; Su, Y.Q.; Hamilton, A.E.; Kwintkiewicz, J.; Hsieh, M.; Nayak, N.R.; Conti, M.; Conover, C.A.; Giudice, L.C. Lack of functional pregnancy-associated plasma protein-A (PAPPA) compromises mouse ovarian steroidogenesis and female fertility. *Biol. Reprod.* **2010**, *82*, 1129–1138. [CrossRef]
25. Ramos, S.B.; Stumpo, D.J.; Kennington, E.A.; Phillips, R.S.; Bock, C.B.; Ribeiro-Neto, F.; Blackshear, P.J. The CCCH tandem zinc-finger protein Zfp36l2 is crucial for female fertility and early embryonic development. *Development* **2004**, *131*, 4883–4893. [CrossRef]
26. Rizk, B.; Aboulghar, M.; Smitz, J.; Ron-El, R. The role of vascular endothelial growth factor and interleukins in the pathogenesis of severe ovarian hyperstimulation syndrome. *Hum. Reprod. Update* **1997**, *3*, 255–266. [CrossRef]
27. Tuteja, G.; Kaestner, K.H. Forkhead transcription factors II. *Cell* **2007**, *131*, 192. [CrossRef]

28. Lu, J.; Wang, Z.; Cao, J.; Chen, Y.; Dong, Y. A novel and compact review on the role of oxidative stress in female reproduction. *Reprod. Biol. Endocrinol.* **2018**, *16*, 80. [CrossRef]
29. Shao, X.; Wei, X. FOXP1 enhances fibrosis via activating Wnt/beta-catenin signaling pathway in endometriosis. *Am. J. Transl. Res.* **2018**, *10*, 3610–3618.
30. van der Vos, K.E.; Coffer, P.J. FOXO-binding partners: It takes two to tango. *Oncogene* **2008**, *27*, 2289–2299. [CrossRef]
31. van der Vos, K.E.; Coffer, P.J. The extending network of FOXO transcriptional target genes. *Antioxid. Redox Signal.* **2011**, *14*, 579–592. [CrossRef]
32. Fan, H.Y.; O'Connor, A.; Shitanaka, M.; Shimada, M.; Liu, Z.; Richards, J.S. Beta-catenin (CTNNB1) promotes preovulatory follicular development but represses LH-mediated ovulation and luteinization. *Mol. Endocrinol.* **2010**, *24*, 1529–1542. [CrossRef]
33. Kohan-Ghadr, H.R.; Smith, L.C.; Arnold, D.R.; Murphy, B.D.; Lefebvre, R.C. Aberrant expression of E-cadherin and beta-catenin proteins in placenta of bovine embryos derived from somatic cell nuclear transfer. *Reprod. Fertil. Dev.* **2012**, *24*, 588–598. [CrossRef]
34. Regan, S.L.P.; Knight, P.G.; Yovich, J.L.; Leung, Y.; Arfuso, F.; Dharmarajan, A. Granulosa Cell Apoptosis in the Ovarian Follicle-A Changing View. *Front. Endocrinol.* **2018**, *9*, 61. [CrossRef]
35. Richards, J.S.; Ren, Y.A.; Candelaria, N.; Adams, J.E.; Rajkovic, A. Ovarian Follicular Theca Cell Recruitment, Differentiation, and Impact on Fertility: 2017 Update. *Endocr. Rev.* **2018**, *39*, 1–20. [CrossRef]
36. Wagner, P.K.; Otomo, A.; Christians, J.K. Regulation of pregnancy-associated plasma protein A2 (PAPPA2) in a human placental trophoblast cell line (BeWo). *Reprod. Biol. Endocrinol.* **2011**, *9*, 48. [CrossRef]
37. Ussar, S.; Bezy, O.; Bluher, M.; Kahn, C.R. Glypican-4 enhances insulin signaling via interaction with the insulin receptor and serves as a novel adipokine. *Diabetes* **2012**, *61*, 2289–2298. [CrossRef]
38. Yoo, H.J.; Hwang, S.Y.; Cho, G.J.; Hong, H.C.; Choi, H.Y.; Hwang, T.G.; Kim, S.M.; Bluher, M.; Youn, B.S.; Baik, S.H.; et al. Association of glypican-4 with body fat distribution, insulin resistance, and nonalcoholic fatty liver disease. *J. Clin. Endocrinol. Metab.* **2013**, *98*, 2897–2901. [CrossRef]
39. Ball, C.B.; Rodriguez, K.F.; Stumpo, D.J.; Ribeiro-Neto, F.; Korach, K.S.; Blackshear, P.J.; Birnbaumer, L.; Ramos, S.B. The RNA-binding protein, ZFP36L2, influences ovulation and oocyte maturation. *PLoS ONE* **2014**, *9*, e97324. [CrossRef]
40. Otsuka, H.; Fukao, A.; Funakami, Y.; Duncan, K.E.; Fujiwara, T. Emerging Evidence of Translational Control by AU-Rich Element-Binding Proteins. *Front. Genet.* **2019**, *10*, 332. [CrossRef]
41. Bouchard, L.; Tchernof, A.; Deshaies, Y.; Marceau, S.; Lescelleur, O.; Biron, S.; Vohl, M.C. ZFP36: A promising candidate gene for obesity-related metabolic complications identified by converging genomics. *Obes. Surg.* **2007**, *17*, 372–382. [CrossRef] [PubMed]
42. Diamanti-Kandarakis, E.; Dunaif, A. Insulin resistance and the polycystic ovary syndrome revisited: An update on mechanisms and implications. *Endocr. Rev.* **2012**, *33*, 981–1030. [CrossRef] [PubMed]
43. Diamanti-Kandarakis, E.; Kandarakis, H.A. Conservative management of gynecologic diseases: Insulin sensitizing agents in polycystic ovary syndrome. *Ann. N. Y. Acad. Sci.* **2003**, *997*, 322–329. [CrossRef] [PubMed]
44. Vega, G.L.; Adams-Huet, B.; Peshock, R.; Willett, D.; Shah, B.; Grundy, S.M. Influence of body fat content and distribution on variation in metabolic risk. *J. Clin. Endocrinol. Metab.* **2006**, *91*, 4459–4466. [CrossRef]
45. Eriksson, U.J. The pathogenesis of congenital malformations in diabetic pregnancy. *Diabetes Metab. Rev.* **1995**, *11*, 63–82. [CrossRef]
46. Kjaer, K.; Hagen, C.; Sando, S.H.; Eshoj, O. Epidemiology of menarche and menstrual disturbances in an unselected group of women with insulin-dependent diabetes mellitus compared to controls. *J. Clin. Endocrinol. Metab.* **1992**, *75*, 524–529. [CrossRef]
47. Lanzarini, F.; Pereira, F.A.; Camargo, J.; Oliveira, A.M.; Belaz, K.R.A.; Melendez-Perez, J.J.; Eberlin, M.N.; Brum, M.C.S.; Mesquita, F.S.; Sudano, M.J. ELOVL5 Participates in Embryonic Lipid Determination of Cellular Membranes and Cytoplasmic Droplets. *Int. J. Mol. Sci.* **2021**, *22*, 1311. [CrossRef]
48. SenBanerjee, S.; Lin, Z.; Atkins, G.B.; Greif, D.M.; Rao, R.M.; Kumar, A.; Feinberg, M.W.; Chen, Z.; Simon, D.I.; Luscinskas, F.W. KLF2 Is a novel transcriptional regulator of endothelial proinflammatory activation. *J. Exp. Med.* **2004**, *199*, 1305–1315. [CrossRef]
49. Guangqi, E.; Cao, Y.; Bhattacharya, S.; Dutta, S.; Wang, E.; Mukhopadhyay, D. Endogenous vascular endothelial growth factor-A (VEGF-A) maintains endothelial cell homeostasis by regulating VEGF receptor-2 transcription. *J. Biol. Chem.* **2012**, *287*, 3029–3041. [CrossRef]
50. Kwon, M.; Pavlov, T.S.; Nozu, K.; Rasmussen, S.A.; Ilatovskaya, D.V.; Lerch-Gaggl, A.; North, L.M.; Kim, H.; Qian, F.; Sweeney, W.E., Jr.; et al. G-protein signaling modulator 1 deficiency accelerates cystic disease in an orthologous mouse model of autosomal dominant polycystic kidney disease. *Proc. Natl. Acad. Sci. USA* **2012**, *109*, 21462–21467. [CrossRef]
51. Watanabe, T.M.; Tokuo, H.; Gonda, K.; Higuchi, H.; Ikebe, M. Myosin-X induces filopodia by multiple elongation mechanism. *J. Biol. Chem.* **2010**, *285*, 19605–19614. [CrossRef]
52. Chen, S.U.; Chou, C.H.; Lee, H.; Ho, C.H.; Lin, C.W.; Yang, Y.S. Lysophosphatidic acid up-regulates expression of interleukin-8 and -6 in granulosa-lutein cells through its receptors and nuclear factor-kappaB dependent pathways: Implications for angiogenesis of corpus luteum and ovarian hyperstimulation syndrome. *J. Clin. Endocrinol. Metab.* **2008**, *93*, 935–943. [CrossRef]
53. Wei, L.H.; Chou, C.H.; Chen, M.W.; Rose-John, S.; Kuo, M.L.; Chen, S.U.; Yang, Y.S. The role of IL-6 trans-signaling in vascular leakage: Implications for ovarian hyperstimulation syndrome in a murine model. *J. Clin. Endocrinol. Metab.* **2013**, *98*, E472–E484. [CrossRef]
54. Borgwardt, L.; Olsen, K.W.; Rossing, M.; Helweg-Larsen, R.B.; Toftager, M.; Pinborg, A.; Bogstad, J.; Lossl, K.; Zedeler, A.; Grondahl, M.L. Rare genetic variants suggest dysregulation of signalling pathways in low and high risk patients developing severe ovarian hyperstimulation syndrome. *J. Assist. Reprod. Genet.* **2020**, *37*, 2883–2892. [CrossRef]

55. Elchalal, U.; Schenker, J.G. The pathophysiology of ovarian hyperstimulation syndrome—Views and ideas. *Hum. Reprod.* **1997**, *12*, 1129–1137. [CrossRef]
56. Binder, H.; Dittrich, R.; Einhaus, F.; Krieg, J.; Muller, A.; Strauss, R.; Beckmann, M.W.; Cupisti, S. Update on ovarian hyperstimulation syndrome: Part 1—Incidence and pathogenesis. *Int. J. Fertil. Womens Med.* **2007**, *52*, 11–26.
57. Goldsman, M.P.; Pedram, A.; Dominguez, C.E.; Ciuffardi, I.; Levin, E.; Asch, R.H. Increased capillary permeability induced by human follicular fluid: A hypothesis for an ovarian origin of the hyperstimulation syndrome. *Fertil. Steril.* **1995**, *63*, 268–272. [CrossRef]
58. Carriere, V.; Roussel, L.; Ortega, N.; Lacorre, D.A.; Americh, L.; Aguilar, L.; Bouche, G.; Girard, J.P. IL-33, the IL-1-like cytokine ligand for ST2 receptor, is a chromatin-associated nuclear factor in vivo. *Proc. Natl. Acad. Sci. USA* **2007**, *104*, 282–287. [CrossRef]
59. Karakose, M.; Demircan, K.; Tutal, E.; Demirci, T.; Arslan, M.S.; Sahin, M.; Celik, H.T.; Kazanci, F.; Karakaya, J.; Cakal, E.; et al. Clinical significance of ADAMTS1, ADAMTS5, ADAMTS9 aggrecanases and IL-17A, IL-23, IL-33 cytokines in polycystic ovary syndrome. *J. Endocrinol. Investig.* **2016**, *39*, 1269–1275. [CrossRef]
60. Prabhu, Y.D.; Valsala Gopalakrishnan, A. gamma-Linolenic acid ameliorates DHEA induced pro-inflammatory response in polycystic ovary syndrome via PPAR-gamma signaling in rats. *Reprod. Biol.* **2020**, *20*, 348–356. [CrossRef]
61. Furqan, M.; Mukhi, N.; Lee, B.; Liu, D. Dysregulation of JAK-STAT pathway in hematological malignancies and JAK inhibitors for clinical application. *Biomark. Res.* **2013**, *1*, 5. [CrossRef] [PubMed]
62. Khatib, H.; Huang, W.; Mikheil, D.; Schutzkus, V.; Monson, R.L. Effects of signal transducer and activator of transcription (STAT) genes STAT1 and STAT3 genotypic combinations on fertilization and embryonic survival rates in Holstein cattle. *J. Dairy Sci.* **2009**, *92*, 6186–6191. [CrossRef] [PubMed]
63. Tsurumi, A.; Zhao, C.; Li, W.X. Canonical and non-canonical JAK/STAT transcriptional targets may be involved in distinct and overlapping cellular processes. *BMC Genom.* **2017**, *18*, 718. [CrossRef] [PubMed]
64. Baumer, D.; Trauner, J.; Hollfelder, D.; Cerny, A.; Schoppmeier, M. JAK-STAT signalling is required throughout telotrophic oogenesis and short-germ embryogenesis of the beetle Tribolium. *Dev. Biol.* **2011**, *350*, 169–182. [CrossRef]
65. Ferrero, H.; Diaz-Gimeno, P.; Sebastian-Leon, P.; Faus, A.; Gomez, R.; Pellicer, A. Dysregulated genes and their functional pathways in luteinized granulosa cells from PCOS patients after cabergoline treatment. *Reproduction* **2018**, *155*, 373–381. [CrossRef]

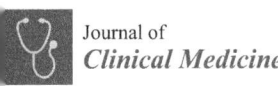

Review

The Impact of a Very Short Abstinence Period on Conventional Sperm Parameters and Sperm DNA Fragmentation: A Systematic Review and Meta-Analysis

Federica Barbagallo [1], Rossella Cannarella [1], Andrea Crafa [1], Claudio Manna [2,3], Sandro La Vignera [1], Rosita A. Condorelli [1,*] and Aldo E. Calogero [1]

1. Department of Clinical and Experimental Medicine, University of Catania, 95124 Catania, Italy
2. Biofertility IVF and Infertility Center, 00198 Rome, Italy
3. Department of Biomedicine and Prevention, University of Rome "Tor Vergata", 00133 Rome, Italy
* Correspondence: rosita.condorelli@unict.it

Abstract: Purpose: In recent years, a growing number of studies have supported the beneficial effects of a very short abstinence period on sperm parameters, especially in patients with oligoasthenozoospermia. However, the results are controversial and no consensus exists regarding whether to request a second semen collection in clinical practice. Therefore, this systematic review and meta-analysis aimed to evaluate the influence of a very short abstinence period (within 4 h) on conventional sperm parameters and sperm DNA fragmentation (SDF) rate. Materials and Methods: The literature search was performed using Scopus and PubMed databases. The meta-analysis was conducted according to the Preferred Reporting Items for Systematic Review and Meta-Analysis Protocol (PRISMA-P) guidelines. All eligible studies were selected according to the Population, Intervention, Comparison/Comparator, Outcomes, and Study design (PICOS) model. The quality of evidence of the included studies was analyzed through the Cambridge Quality Checklists. The standardized mean difference (SMD) was used to analyze the outcomes. Cochran-Q and I^2 statistics were used to evaluate statistical heterogeneity. Results: We assessed for eligibility 1334 abstracts, and 19 studies were finally included. All 19 articles evaluated the effects of a very short abstinence period on sperm parameters and, among these, 5 articles also evaluated the effects on SDF rate. The quantitative analysis showed a significant reduction in semen volume after a very short abstinence period in both normozoospermic men and patients with oligozoospermia, asthenozoospermia, and/or teratozoospermia (OAT) patients. We found a statistically significant increase in sperm concentration and total and progressive motility in the second ejaculation of patients with OAT. In contrast, the SDF rate decreased significantly in the second ejaculate of OAT patients. Conclusions: This is the first systematic review and meta-analysis investigating the impact of a very short abstinence period on sperm parameters and SDF rate. The results suggest that collecting a second consecutive ejaculation after a very short time from the first could represent a simple and useful strategy for obtaining better-quality spermatozoa, especially in patients with abnormal sperm parameters.

Keywords: ejaculatory abstinence; sexual abstinence period; consecutive ejaculation; sperm DNA fragmentation; couples infertility

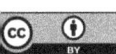

1. Introduction

The World Health Organization (WHO) defines infertility as the inability to conceive after at least 12 months of regular, unprotected sexual intercourse [1]. Infertility remains a global public health issue, affecting approximately 8–12% of couples of reproductive age [2]. The male factor is responsible for couples' infertility in about half of the cases [3]. Several causes contribute to the increasing prevalence of male infertility, which may be related to congenital, acquired, and idiopathic factors that impair spermatogenesis [3]. The causes of male infertility can be classified as factors acting at the pre-testicular, testicular, or post-testicular level. Nevertheless, despite several steps forward, male infertility remains a poorly understood area. In fact, to date, 50% of infertile patients have not received an etiological diagnosis and are defined as having idiopathic infertility [3]. Lifestyle and environmental factors, such as smoking [4], obesity [5], endocrine disruptors [6], exposure to heavy metals [7], or psychological stress [8], can play an important role in increasing the prevalence of male infertility.

Conventional sperm parameters (sperm concentration, motility, and morphology) are among the many predictors of male fertility and, to date, are still regarded as the cornerstone of fertility diagnosis despite the wide variability existing within and between men [9]. These variations may be attributed to several modifiable factors, including the latter and the length of sexual abstinence and the ejaculation frequency. Among these, sexual abstinence is often overlooked, although the length of sexual abstinence has been shown to influence sperm parameters. WHO laboratory manuals for the examination and processing human semen published since 1980 and the most recently released in 2021 [10] recommend that semen should be collected for semen analysis after a minimum of 2 days and a maximum of 7 days of sexual abstinence and this instruction has remained unchanged in all these years. However, the European Society of Human Reproduction and Embryology (ESHRE) recommends an abstinence period of only 3–4 days [11]. The basis for these recommendations is unclear and much evidence shows that a change in the current indications on the abstinence length is needed [12,13]. Many years ago, McLeod and Gold indicated that the period of abstinence should be based on the frequency of copulation [14]. They reported that a coital frequency of fewer than three times per week could result in delayed fertility due to a missing ovulatory window and/or impaired sperm parameters [14].

Several studies have investigated the influence of the length of sexual abstinence on sperm parameters, although the results are still controversial. Indeed, a longer abstinence period appears to improve semen fluid volume and sperm count whereas the effects on sperm motility, morphology, and DNA fragmentation (SDF) rate are still contradictory [15]. Furthermore, a growing number of studies have focused on the possibility to use a second ejaculation collected after a very short period of abstinence in infertile patients, especially in patients with oligoasthenozoospermia (OA). We previously reported that a second consecutive ejaculate (collected within 1 h from the first) resulted in better conventional sperm parameters (motility and morphology) and a lower percentage of spermatozoa with fragmented DNA in normozoospermic male partners of infertile couples and even more in patients with oligoasthenoteratozoospermia (OAT) [16]. Our findings were in line with the most recent literature [17–22]. However, no consensus exists on whether to request a second successive sample.

Therefore, this systematic review and meta-analysis aimed to evaluate the influence of a very short abstinence period on conventional sperm parameters and the SDF rate.

2. Materials and Methods

2.1. Sources

This study was performed by applying the Preferred Reporting Items for Systematic Review and Meta-Analysis Protocols (PRISMA-P) [23]. The PRISMA checklist is reported in Supplementary Table S1. The articles were selected through extensive searches in PubMed and Scopus databases from their establishment until June 2022. In detail, the following search string was used to search the Scopus database: TITLE-ABS-KEY (consecutive AND ejaculate) OR TITLE-ABS-KEY (consecutive AND ejaculation) OR TITLE-ABS-KEY (consecutive AND semen collection) OR TITLE-ABS-KEY (repeated AND ejaculate) OR TITLE-ABS-KEY (repeated AND ejaculation) OR TITLE-ABS-KEY (repeated AND semen collection) OR TITLE-ABS-KEY (second AND ejaculation) OR TITLE-ABS-KEY (second AND ejaculate). Additional manual searches were carried out using the reference lists of relevant studies. The search was limited to human studies and only English articles were selected. All abstracts and relevant full texts were evaluated. Two authors independently

(F.B. and A.C.) reviewed the abstracts and selected only the articles that were pertinent to the objective of this study. Any disagreement was resolved by discussion with a third investigator (R.C.). The reference lists of the identified articles were also used to find pertinent studies.

2.2. Study Selection

All the eligible studies were selected following the PICOS (Population, Intervention, Comparison/Comparator, Outcomes, Study design) model (Table 1). We considered for inclusion all studies that evaluated the effects of a very short abstinence period (within 4 h) on sperm parameters (volume, concentration, total and progressive motility, and morphology) and SDF rate. Case reports, comments, letters to the editor, systematic or narrative reviews, and studies that did not allow extracting the outcomes of interest were excluded from the analysis.

Table 1. Selection criteria in included studies (PICOS) (Population, Intervention, Comparison/Comparator, Outcomes, Study design) model of the current systematic review and meta-analysis.

	Inclusion	Exclusion
Population	Men of reproductive age	Azoospermia, age < 18 years
Intervention	Short-second ejaculation (within 4 h)	Second ejaculation > 4 h
Comparison	Ejaculation after an abstinence sexual period between 2–7 days	/
Outcome	Sperm conventional parameters (semen volume, sperm concentration, sperm progressive motility, sperm total motility, sperm morphology) and SDF	/
Study type	Observational, cohort, cross-sectional, and case–control	Case reports, comments, letters to the editor, systematic or narrative reviews, in vitro studies, studies on animals

Abbreviations: SDF, sperm DNA fragmentation.

2.3. Data Extraction

Data extraction was performed by one author (F.B.) and verified by a second one (A.C.). Disagreements were resolved by a third author (A.E.C.). The following data were collected: sperm conventional parameters (semen volume, sperm concentration, sperm progressive motility, sperm total motility, sperm morphology) and SDF of the first and second ejaculation, semen characteristics of patients enrolled (normozoospermic or OAT), abstinence period of first ejaculate, abstinence period of second ejaculate (within 4 h), and methods used for semen analysis and for the assessment of SDF.

2.4. Quality of Evidence

The quality assessment of the articles included in this systematic review and meta-analysis was performed using the "Cambridge Quality Checklists" [24]. This checklist comprises three domains designed to identify high-quality studies of correlates, risk factors, and causal risk factors. The checklist for correlates consists of five items that can be given a score of zero or one for a total of five. It evaluates the appropriateness of the sample size and the quality of the outcome measurements. The checklist for risk factors consists of three items; the selection of one of the three items excludes the other two, with a maximum score of 3 points. This checklist assigns high-quality scores only to those studies with appropriate time-ordered data. Finally, there is the checklist for causal risk factors that evaluates the type of study design, assigning the highest score to randomized clinical trials (RCTs) and the lowest score to cross-sectional studies without a control group. The maximum score is seven. To draw confident conclusions about correlates, the correlate score must be high. This means that the sample size must be large and the outcome assessment must be adequate and reproducible. To draw confident conclusions about risk factors, both the checklists for correlates and risk factor scores must be high. Thus, the studies that allow the most reliable conclusions to be drawn are prospective studies. To draw confident conclusions about causal risk factors, all three checklist scores must be high. Thus, in the absence of randomized clinical trials, confident conclusions can be drawn from studies with adequately controlled samples.

2.5. Statistic Analysis

The standard mean difference (SMD) with the 95% confidential interval (CI) was calculated for quantitative variables. The Cochran-Q and I^2 statistics were used to evaluate the statistical heterogeneity. Specifically, if I^2 resulted in being lower or equal to 50%, the variation in the studies was considered to be homogenous and the fixed effect model was adopted. If I^2 was higher than 50%, there was significant heterogeneity between studies, and the random effects model was used. All p-values lower than 0.05 were considered statistically significant. The analysis was performed using RevMan software v. 5.4 (Cochrane Collaboration, Oxford, UK) and Comprehensive Meta-Analysis Software (Version 2) (Englewood, NJ, USA).

We undertook the sensitivity analysis with the exclusion method one study at a time. Therefore, the pooled effect size and corresponding CI were calculated after exclusion of one study at a time. A study that resulted in the inference changing after its exclusion was labeled a "sensitive study".

We qualitatively analyzed the presence of publication bias from the asymmetry of the funnel plot, which suggested some missing studies on one side of the graph. Quantitative analysis of publication bias was performed using Egger's intercept test, which assessed statistical significance of publication bias. In case of publication bias, unbiased estimates were calculated using the "trim and fill" method [25].

3. Results

The aforementioned search strategy identified 1334 records. After the exclusion of 103 duplicates, the remaining 1231 articles were screened. Of these, 1202 were judged to be not pertinent for their topic after reading their titles and abstracts, 3 were excluded because they were reviews, and 4 were excluded because they were studies conducted on animals. One study was excluded because it was written in Chinese. Twenty-one studies were carefully read. Among these, two studies were excluded for their experimental design. Finally, 19 articles met our inclusion criteria and were, therefore, included in the analysis [16–22,26–37]. All 19 articles evaluated the effects of a very short abstinence period on sperm parameters and among these, 5 articles also evaluated the SDF rate [16,21,31,32,36] (Figure 1). All studies were judged to be of low quality after the assessment with the Cambridge Quality Checklists (Table 2). The main characteristics of the studies included in the systematic review and meta-analysis are reported in Table 3.

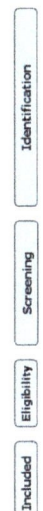
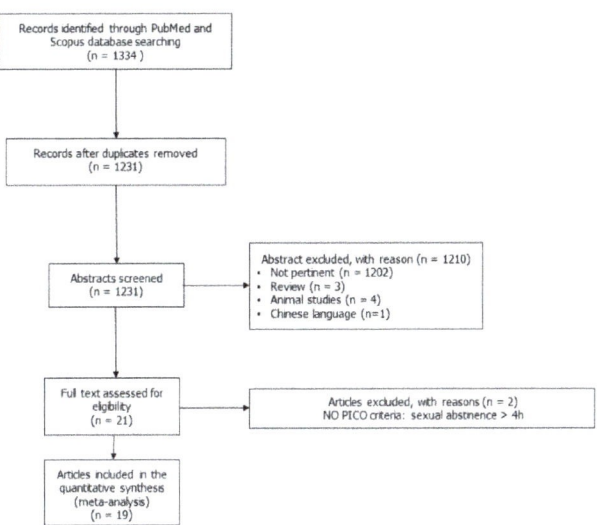

Figure 1. Flowchart of studies included.

Table 2. Evaluation of study quality using "The Cambridge Quality Checklists".

Authors and Year of Publication	Checklist for Correlates	Checklist for Risk Factors	Checklist for Casual Risk Factors	Total
Zverina et al., 1988 [26]	1	1	3	5/15
Tur-Kaspa et al., 1994 [27]	1	1	3	5/15
Barash et al., 1995 [28]	1	1	3	5/15
Bar-Hava et al., 2000 [29]	1	1	3	5/15
Sugiyam et al., 2008 [30]	1	1	3	5/15
Hussein et al., 2008 [31]	1	1	3	5/15
Bahadur et al., 2016 [17]	1	1	3	5/15
Ortiz et al., 2016 [18]	1	1	3	5/15
Mayorga-Torres et al., 2016 [32]	2	1	3	6/15
Alipour et al., 2017 [19]	2	1	3	6/15
Ragheb et al., 2018 [20]	1	1	3	5/15
Shen et al., 2019 [21]	2	1	3	6/15
Scarselli et al., 2019 [33]	2	1	3	6/15
Manna et al., 2020 [16]	2	1	3	6/15
Ciotti et al., 2021 [22]	1	1	3	5/15
Alipour et al., 2021 [34]	2	1	3	6/15
Barbagallo et al., 2021 [35]	2	1	3	6/15
Kulkarmi et al., 2022 [36]	1	1	3	6/15
Patel et al., 2022 [37]	1	1	3	5/15

Table 3. Effects of a very short abstinence period (within 4 h) on sperm conventional parameters and DNA fragmentation rate.

Authors and Years	Patients	Abstinence Period of First Ejaculate	Abstinence Period of Second Ejaculate	Method Used for Semen Analysis	Semen Parameters					Method of Evaluation of SDF	SDF
					Volume	Concentration	Total Motility	Progressive Motility	Normal Morphology		
Zverina et al., 1988 [26]	107 partners of infertile couples	3-6 days	60 min	NA	↓	-	↓	NA	-	NA	NA
Tur-Kaspa et al., 1994 [27]	27 Oligo	3 days	<4 h	NA	↓	-	-	NA	NA	NA	NA
	23 OAT	3 days	<4 h	NA	↓	↑	-	NA	NA	NA	NA
Baraish et al., 1995 [28]	36 OAT	3 days	2 h	NA	↓	-	↓	NA	-	NA	NA
Bar-Hava et al., 2000 [29]	109 severe OAT	NA	1 h	NA	↓	↓	↓	↑	NA	NA	NA
Sugiyam et al., 2008 [30]	32 OAT	3-5 days	30-60 min	NA	↓	-	↓	NA	NA	NA	NA
Hussein et al., 2008 [31]	20 Oligo or OAT	3 days	<1-3 h	WHO, 1999	↓	↓	NA	NA	NA	Comet assay	↓
	10 Normo	3 days			-	-	NA	NA	NA		↓
Bahadur et al., 2016 [17]	73 Oligo	2-7 days	40 min	WHO, 2010	↓	-	NA	NA	↑	NA	NA
Ortiz et al., 2016 [18]	32 OA	1-5 days	Less 1 h	WHO, 2010	↓	↓	↑	↑	NA	NA	NA
Mayorga-Torres et al., 2016 [32]	3 Normo	3-4 days	2 h	WHO, 2010	-	-	-	-	NA	SCSA	-
			4 h		-	-	-	-	NA		-
Alipour et al., 2017 [19]	43 Normo	At least 4 days	2 h	Sperm Class Analyzer CASA system	↓	↑	↑	NA	NA	NA	NA
Ragheb et al., 2018 [20]	157 OAT	3-7 days	1-3 h	WHO, 2010	↓	↑	↑	↑	↑	NA	NA
Shen et al., 2019 [21]	167 Normo	3-7 days	1-3 h	WHO, 2010	↓	↑	NA	NA	-	SCSA	-
	20 Normo	3-7 days	1-3 h	WHO, 2010	-	-	NA	NA	↑	SCSA	↓
Scarselli et al., 2019 [33]	22 OAT	2-5 days	1 h	WHO, 2010	↓	-	-	NA	-	NA	NA
Manna et al., 2020 [16]	30 Normo	2-7 days	1 h	WHO, 2010	↓	↑	-	-	-	SCD test (Halosperm kit)	↓
	36 OAT	2-7 days	1 h	WHO, 2010	↓	-	↑	↑	↑	SCD test (Halosperm kit)	↓
Ciotti et al., 2021 [22]	75 Severe OAT	2-3 days	2 h	NA	↓	-	↑	↑	↑	NA	NA
Alipour et al., 2021 [34]	31 Normo	4-7 days	2 h	WHO, 2010; Sperm Class Analyzer	↓	↑	-	↑	-	NA	NA
Barbagallo et al., 2021 [35]	90 Severe OA	2-7 days	1 h	WHO, 2010	NA	-	↑	↑	-	NA	NA
Kulkarmi et al., 2022 [36]	67 Oligo	2-7 days	1-3 h	WHO, 2010	↓	↑	-	↑	NA	SCD test (Qwik Check DFI test assay)	↓
Patel et al., 2022 [37]	41 Severe OAT	2-7 days	1 h	WHO, 2010	↓	NA	NA	-	-	NA	NA

Abbreviations: ↓ = reduction; ↑ = increase; - = no significant changes; NA = not available; SDF = sperm DNA fragmentation; CASA = computer-assisted sperm analysis; DFI = DNA fragmentation index; NA = not available; normo = normozoospermia; oligo = oligozoospermia; OA = oligoasthenozoospermia; OAT = oligoasthenoteratozoospermia; WHO = World Health Organization; SCD = sperm chromatin dispersion; SCSA = Sperm chromatin structure assay.

3.1. Effects of a Short Period of Abstinence on Semen Parameters

3.1.1. Semen Volume

Semen Volume: Qualitative Analysis

Eighteen studies evaluated the effect of a very short abstinence period on semen volume [16–22,26–34,36,37] (Table 3). Seventeen of them (94.4%) showed a lower semen volume after a very short sexual abstinence period [16–22,26–32,34,36,37]. Only one study did not find any significant change in semen volume in three healthy men after a very short abstinence period [32]. In detail, the authors evaluated the effects of four repeated ejaculations on the same day at two-hour intervals on semen parameters. Data of only the first two ejaculations (after 2 and 4 h, respectively) met our inclusion criteria and, therefore, they were included in our analysis. The authors showed a decreasing trend in semen volume in the second, third, and fourth collections after two hours of abstinence compared to the first one after 3–4 days of abstinence [32]. The very small sample size ($n = 3$) of this study may explain the lack of a statistically significant decrease in semen volume with shorter abstinence.

Semen Volume: Quantitative Analysis

The quantitative analysis of semen volume was performed in data extracted from 16 studies [16–20,22,27–34,36,37]. Although reported a reduction in semen volume, the study conducted by Shen et al. [21] was excluded from the quantitative analysis because no data regarding media, median, and standard deviation were reported in the article. The studies conducted by Tur-Kaspa et al. [27] and Alipour et al. [19,34] did not report data on median and standard deviation (SD) for semen volume, however, they were included in the quantitative analysis because they were calculated using the median, the minimum, and maximum values. Zverina et al. did not report if the men included in their study were normozoospermics or had OAT [26]. Furthermore, it was not possible to obtain these data from sperm parameters of the first semen collection because the authors did not report which WHO manual was used to perform semen analysis. For this reason, we decided to include the study conducted by Zverina et al. only in qualitative analysis but not in the quantitative one. The study by Hussein and colleagues [31] was considered twice since they evaluated the effects of a short period of abstinence on semen volume in a group of patients with oligo and/or asthenozoospermia and in a control group of fertile men. Mayorga-Torres and colleagues evaluated the effects of four repeated ejaculations on the same day at two-hour intervals (2, 4, 6, and 8 h) [32]. Therefore, Mayorga-Torres's study was considered twice because we included the data after 2 h and 4 h and we excluded data regarding the samples after 6 and 8 h [32]. Again, Manna's study [16] was also considered twice because it included a group of normozoospermic men and a group of patients with OAT. Furthermore, Tur-Kaspa and colleagues included two different groups: 27 patients with oligozoospermia and 23 OAT patients; therefore, this study was considered twice [27].

The statistical analysis showed a significant reduction in semen volume after a short period of abstinence in both normozoospermic men [SMD -1.16 (-1.44, -0.88); $p < 0.00001$] and oligozoospermic, asthenozoospermic, and/or teratozoospermic patients [SMD -1.49 (-2.25, -0.74); $p = 0.0001$] (Figure 2).

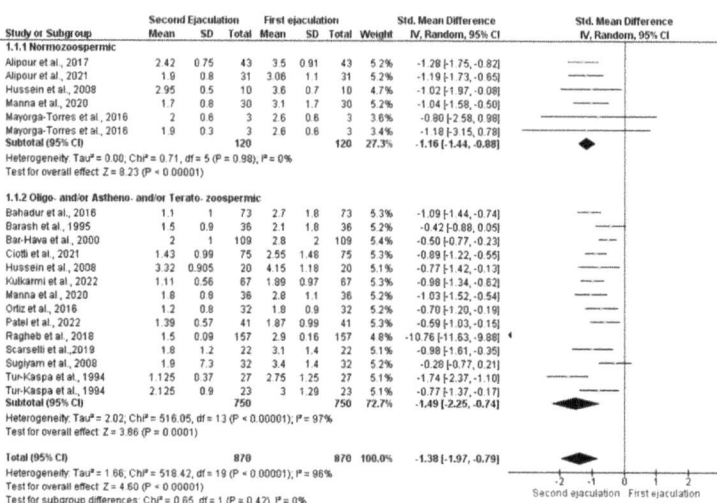

Figure 2. Forest plot of studies that evaluated the effects of a very short abstinence period on semen volume (expressed in mL). The following studies were included in the quantitative analysis (in order of appearance in the manuscript): Manna et al., 2020 [16], Bahadur et al., 2016 [17], Ortiz et al., 2016 [18], Alipour et al., 2017 [19], Ragheb et al., 2018 [20], Ciotti et al., 2021 [22], Tur-Kaspa et al., 1994 [27], Barash et al., 1995 [28], Bar-Hava et al., 2000 [29], Sugyam et al., 2008 [30], Hussein et al., 2008 [31], Mayorga-Torres et al., 2016 [32], Scarselli et al., 2019 [33], Alipour et al., 2021 [34], Kulkarmi et al., 2022 [36], and Patel et al., 2022 [37].

For the analysis of normozoospermic men, no inter-study heterogeneity was found, as demonstrated by the Q-test (Q-value = 0.71; p-value = 0.98) and I^2 = 0%. Egger's regression model and funnel plots reported no risk of bias (intercept = 0.096, 95% CI −0.96–1.16, p = 0.40) (Supplementary Figure S1A). At the sensitivity analysis, no study was sensitive enough to alter the above-reported results (Supplementary Figure S1B).

The analysis of patients with oligozoospermia, asthenozoospermia, and/or teratozoospermia showed the presence of inter-study heterogeneity (Q-value = 516.05; p-value = 0.000; I^2 = 97%) and, therefore, the random model was used. Egger's regression model and funnel plots reported risk of bias (intercept = −10.50, 95% CI −21.66–0.66, p = 0.03) (Supplementary Figure S2A). Three studies were the source of bias [20,27,29]. Once the data from these studies were excluded, heterogeneity decreased (Chi^2 = 21.91, I^2 = 30%) and the reduction in semen volume in the second sample remained significantly lower [SMD −0.79 (−0.96, −0.62); p < 0.00001]. However, at the sensitivity analysis, no study was sensitive enough to alter the above-reported results (Supplementary Figure S2B).

3.1.2. Sperm Concentration

Sperm Concentration: Qualitative Analysis

Eighteen studies evaluated the effects of a short abstinence period on sperm concentration (Table 3) [16–22,26–36]. Among these, six studies described an increase in sperm concentration in the second ejaculation after a very short abstinence period [18,20,21,27,29,36]. Five of the six studies which demonstrated an improvement in sperm concentration were conducted in patients with oligozoospermia, asthenozoospermia, and/or teratozoospermia, whereas one study was conducted on 167 couples who underwent their first round of IVF but information on semen parameters of the first ejaculate of male partners was not reported [21]. Among these six studies, Tur-Kaspa et al. [27] evaluated two different groups: 27 patients with oligozoospermia and 23 with OAT. The authors found a statistically significant increase in sperm concentration only in patients with OAT, whereas patients with oligozoospermia had higher but not significant sperm concentration in the second ejaculation. In contrast, four studies reported a reduction in sperm concentration in the second sample [16,19,31,34]. Interestingly, all these studies were conducted on normozoospermic patients. In particular, Hussein et al. [31] included 20 patients with altered sperm parameters and 10 normozoospermic men. They found a statistically significant reduction in sperm concentration only in the second group. Likewise, Manna et al. [16] reported a decrease in sperm concentration only in 30 normozoospermic men and not in patients with OAT. Alipour et al. found a statistically significant reduction in sperm concentration in the second ejaculate collected after 2 h of the first one in 31 normozoospermic men [34]. The remaining studies did not find statistically significant changes in sperm concentration after a short period of abstinence

Sperm Concentration: Quantitative Analysis

Data from 16 studies were included in the quantitative analysis for the evaluation of the impact of a short abstinence period on sperm concentration [16–20,22,27–36]. The study by Shen et al. [24] was excluded from the quantitative analysis because no data on mean, median, or standard deviation were reported. For the same reasons reported in the paragraph on semen volume, the studies conducted by Tur-Kaspa et al. [27], Hussein et al. [31], Mayorga-Torres et al. [32], and Manna et al. [16] were considered twice in the quantitative analysis. The studies conducted by Tur-Kaspa [27] and Alipour et al. in 2017 and 2021 [19,34] did not report data of mean and standard deviation for sperm concentration but they were included in the quantitative analysis because media ± SD were calculated using the median, the minimum, and maximum values. As reported for semen volume, the study conducted by Zverina et al. [26] was not included in the quantitative analysis because authors did not report if men included in their study were normozoospermic or OAT.

The statistical analysis showed a reduction in sperm concentration in the second ejaculation of normozoospermic men [SMD −0.73 (−1.13, −0.34); p = 00003]. In contrast, sperm concentration significantly increased in patients with abnormal sperm parameters [SMD 0.87 (0.22, 1.51); p = 0.009] (Figure 3).

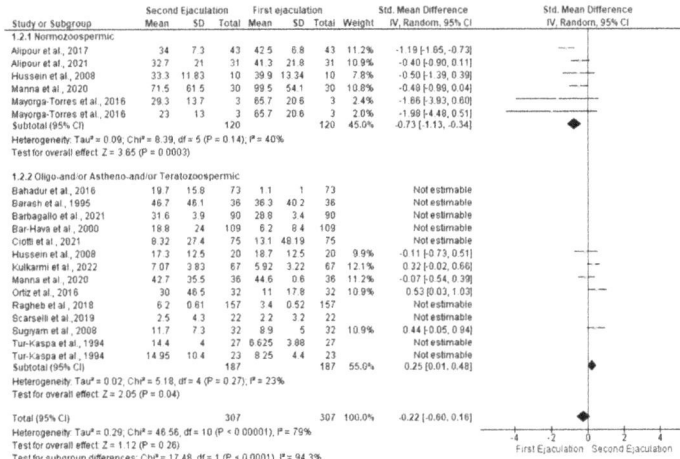

Figure 3. Forest plot of studies that evaluated the effects of a very short abstinence period on sperm concentration (expressed in mil/mL). The following studies were included in the quantitative analysis (in order of appearance in the manuscript): Manna et al., 2020 [16], Bahadur et al., 2016 [17], Ortiz et al., 2016 [18], Alipour et al., 2017 [19], Ragheb et al., 2018 [20], Ciotti et al., 2021 [22], Tur-Kaspa et al., 1994 [27], Barash et al., 1995 [28], Bar-Hava et al., 2000 [29], Sugyam et al., 2008 [30], Hussein et al., 2008 [31], Mayorga-Torres et al., 2016 [32], Scarselli et al., 2019 [33], Alipour et al., 2021 [34], Barbagallo et al.,2021 [35], and Kulkarmi et al., 2022 [36].

The I^2 (40%) revealed no inter-study heterogeneity in the studies conducted on normozoospermic men. However, this was not confirmed by the Q-test (Q-value = 11.141; p-value = 0.049). Egger's regression model and funnel plots reported no risk of bias (intercept = -1.38, 95% CI -5.03–2.27, $p = 0.18$) (Supplementary Figure S3A). At the sensitivity analysis, no study was sensitive enough to alter the above-reported results (Supplementary Figure S3B). The analysis of patients with abnormal sperm parameters revealed the presence of inter-study heterogeneity, as confirmed by the Q-test (Q-value = 440.766; p-value = 0.000) and $I^2 = 97\%$. The analysis of publication bias revealed no source of biases at Egger's regression model and funnel plots (intercept = 2.06, 95% CI -10.91–15.03, $p = 0.36$) (Supplementary Figure S4A). At the sensitivity analysis, no study was sensitive enough to alter the above-reported results (Supplementary Figure S4B).

3.1.3. Total Sperm Motility

Total Sperm Motility: Qualitative Analysis

Fifteen studies evaluated the impact of a very short abstinence period on total sperm motility [16,18–20,22,26–30,32–36] (Table 3). The study by Hussein et al. [31] was excluded because they did not report total sperm motility but only partial data regarding spermatozoa with rapid progressive (A), slow progressive (B), and non-progressive motility (C), and non-motile (D) spermatozoa. The authors described a significant increase in A and B and a significant decrease in C. The study by Bahadur et al. was excluded for the same reason [17]. They described a significant increase in A and a significant decrease in B, C, and D. Similarly, Shen et al. reported a significant improvement in motile sperm count in the second ejaculation compared to the first one [21]. Ten of the fifteen studies (66.6%) demonstrated a statistically significant increase in total sperm motility in the second ejaculate [16,18,20,22,28–30,35,36]. In particular, 10 out of 11 studies were conducted on patients with altered sperm parameters and only the study of Alipour et al. reported an increase in total sperm motility in 43 normozoospermic men [19]. Manna et al. [16] included 30 normozoospermic men and 36 OAT patients, although, in both groups, they found an increase in total sperm motility, the improvement reached statistical significance only in OAT patients. Four of the sixteen studies were unable to show significant alterations in sperm motility in the consecutive ejaculate collected within 4 h [27,32–34]. Only one study reported a statistically significant reduction in sperm motility [26]. However, this study was performed in 1988, and the WHO manual was not used to perform the semen analysis. The authors evaluated sperm motility and sperm velocity of the second ejaculation collected 1 h after the first one, in 107 men with an infertile marriage for at least one year. The different methodologies used could explain the different results from all the others.

Total Sperm Motility: Quantitative Analysis

The data on the effects of a short abstinence period on total sperm motility could be extracted from 14 studies [16,18–20,22,27–30,32–36]. The study conducted by Zverina et al. was not included in the quantitative analysis because the authors did not report if the men included in their study were normozoospermic or had OAT [26]. As for other sperm parameters, the studies conducted by Tur-Kaspa et al. [27], Mayorga-Torres et al. [32], Manna et al. [16] were considered twice in the quantitative analysis. For the studies conducted by Tur-Kaspa [27] et al. and Alipour et al. 2017 and 2022 [19,34], the mean of total sperm motility was calculated using the median, the minimum, and maximum values. The statistical analysis showed that a second ejaculation after a short period of abstinence improved total sperm motility only in patients with abnormal sperm parameters [SMD 7.59 (3.74, 11.44); $p = 0.0001$] without any significant changes in normozoospermic men [SMD 4.32 (-1.03, 9.66); $p = 0.11$] (Figure 4).

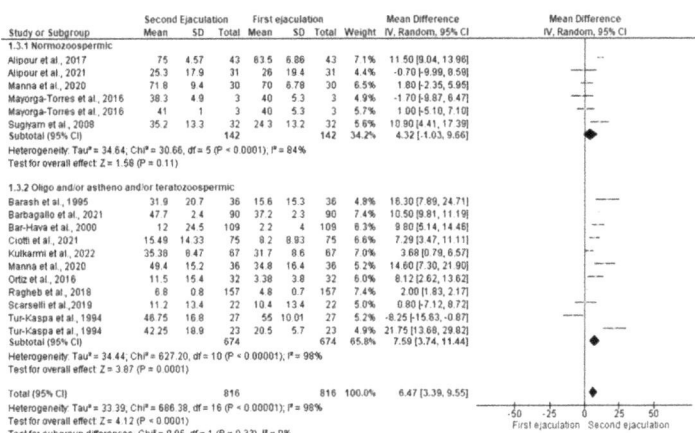

Figure 4. Forest plot of studies that evaluated the effects of a very short abstinence period on total sperm motility (expressed in percentage). The following studies were included in the quantitative analysis (in order of appearance in the manuscript): Manna et al., 2020 [16], Ortiz et al., 2016 [18], Alipour et al., 2017 [19], Ragheb et al., 2018 [20], Ciotti et al., 2021 [22], Tur-Kaspa et al., 1994 [27], Barash et al., 1995 [28], Bar-Hava et al., 2000 [29], Sugyam et al., 2008 [30], Mayorga-Torres et al., 2016 [32], Scarselli et al., 2019 [33], Alipour et al., 2021 [34], Barbagallo et al., 2021 [35], and Kulkarmi et al., 2022 [36].

In the analysis of normozoospermic men, inter-study heterogeneity was observed, as confirmed by the Q-test (Q-value = 37.389; p-value = 0.000) and the I^2 = 84%. Therefore, the random model was used. Egger's regression model and funnel plots reported no risk of bias (intercept = -1.207, 95% CI -10.03–7.61, $p = 0.36$) (Supplementary Figure S5A). At the sensitivity analysis, no study was sensitive enough to alter these results (Supplementary Figure S5B).

The analysis of subgroups with oligozoospermia, asthenozoospermia, and/or teratozoospermia (Chi^2 = 627.2, I^2 = 98%) found significant inter-study heterogeneity (Q-value = 340.336; p-value = 0.000; I^2 = 98%). At Egger's regression model and funnel plots, no risk of bias was found (intercept = 0.467, 95% CI -14.14–15.08, $p = 0.47$) (Supplementary Figure S6A). Furthermore, no study was sensitive enough to alter the above-mentioned results (Supplementary Figure S6B).

3.1.4. Progressive Sperm Motility

Progressive Sperm Motility: Qualitative Analysis

Ten studies evaluated the effects of a very short abstinence period on sperm progressive motility [16,18,20,22,29,32,34–37] (Table 3). The studies by Hussein et al. [31] and Bahadur et al. [17] were excluded because they did not report the value of progressive sperm motility (A + B) but only partial data regarding A, B, C, and D. However, Hussein et al. described a significant increase in A and B, whereas Bahadur et al. reported a significant increase in A and a significant decrease in B. Nine of the ten studies included described an increase in sperm progressive motility in the second ejaculate. Only two studies did not show any statistically significant change in the second ejaculate for progressive sperm motility [32,37]. In particular, the study conducted by Mayorga-Torres et al. [32] was conducted in three normozoospermic patients. Therefore, the small sample size of this study may explain the different results compared to other studies. Furthermore, most of the studies that showed an improvement of progressive sperm motility included patients with oligozoospermia, asthenozoospermia, and/or teratozoospermia. In particular, Manna et al., [16] included both normozoospermic and OAT patients, however, they found a statistically significant increase in progressive sperm motility only in the OAT group.

Progressive Sperm Motility: Quantitative Analysis

Data from ten studies were included in the quantitative analysis to evaluate the impact of a very short abstinence period on progressive sperm motility [16,18,20,22,29,32,34–37]. As for other parameters, the study by Shen et al. was not included in the quantitative analysis because no data on mean, median, or ST were reported [21]. The studies conducted by Mayorga-Torres et al. [32] and Manna et al. [16] were considered twice in the quantitative analysis for the same reasons reported previously.

As for total sperm motility, the statistical analysis showed that a second ejaculation after a very short abstinence period improved progressive sperm motility only in patients with abnormal sperm parameters [SMD 1.28 (0.58, 1.99); $p = 0.0004$] without any significant changes in normozoospermic men [SMD -1.55 (-6.96, 3.85); $p = 0.57$] (Figure 5).

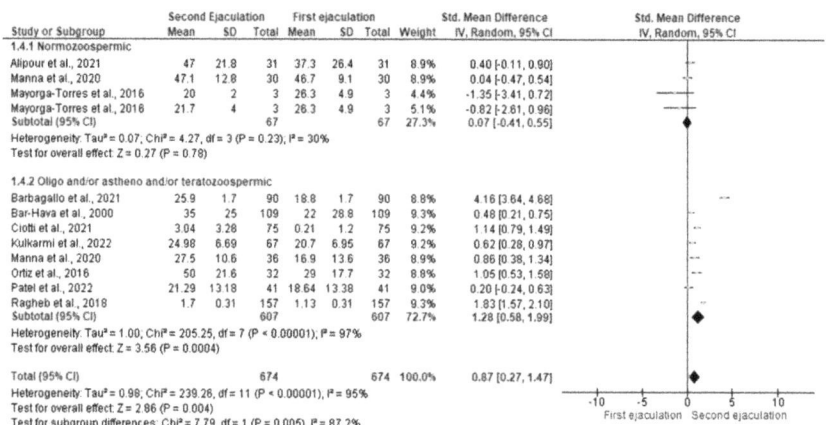

Figure 5. Forest plot of studies that evaluated the effects of a very short abstinence period on progressive sperm motility (expressed as a percentage). The following studies were included in the quantitative analysis (in order of appearance in the manuscript): Manna et al., 2020 [16], Ortiz et al., 2016 [18], Ragheb et al., 2018 [20], Ciotti et al., 2021 [22], Bar-Hava et al., 2000 [29], Mayorga-Torres et al., 2016 [32], Alipour et al., 2021 [34], Barbagallo et al., 2021 [35], Kulkarmi et al., 2022 [36], and Patel et al., 2022 [37].

The analysis of normozoospermic men found the presence of inter-study heterogeneity at the Q-test (Q-value = 6.645; p-value = 0.084), but not at the I^2 (30%). Egger's regression model and funnel plots showed the presence of risk of bias (intercept = -2.41, 95% CI -5.70–0.87, $p = 0.04$) (Supplementary Figure S7A). However, no study was sensitive enough to alter the above-mentioned results (Supplementary Figure S7B).

Furthermore, inter-study heterogeneity was found for the subgroups of oligozoospermic, asthenozoospermic, and/or teratozoospermic patients (Q-value = 207.899; p-value = 0.000; $I^2 = 97\%$). Egger's regression model and funnel plots reported no risk of bias (intercept = 4.364, 95% CI -14.98–23.71, $p = 0.30$) (Supplementary Figure S8A). At the sensitivity analysis, no study was sensitive enough to alter the above-reported results (Supplementary Figure S8B).

3.1.5. Sperm Morphology

Sperm Morphology: Qualitative Analysis

Ten studies investigated the impact of a very short abstinence period on sperm morphology [16,17,20–22,26,28,33,35,37] (Table 3). Five studies showed no statistically significant changes in sperm morphology in the second ejaculate [21,26,28,33,35]. The remaining five studies demonstrated that a very short abstinence period improved sperm morphology. In particular, Manna et al. [16] reported a statistically significant improvement of sperm morphology in the second ejaculation only in OAT patients and not in normozoospermic men. Almost all (four out of five) participants reported an improvement of sperm morphology after a very short abstinence period in a study conducted in patients with abnormal sperm parameters, whereas only one was conducted in normozoospermic men [21].

Sperm Morphology: Quantitative Analysis

Quantitative analysis on sperm morphology was evaluated on data from eight studies [16,17,20,22,28,33,35]. The study by Manna et al. [16] was considered twice because they included a group of normozoospermic men and a group of patients with OAT. The study by Shen et al. [21] was not included in the quantitative analysis because no data on mean, median, or standard deviation were reported. As for other sperm parameters, the study by Zverina et al. [26] was not included in the quantitative analysis because the authors did not report if the men included in their study were normozoospermics or OAT. In particular, the statistical analysis did not show a significant improvement in sperm morphology in patients with abnormal sperm parameters [SMD 0.35 (−0.03, 0.73); $p = 0.07$] (Figure 6).

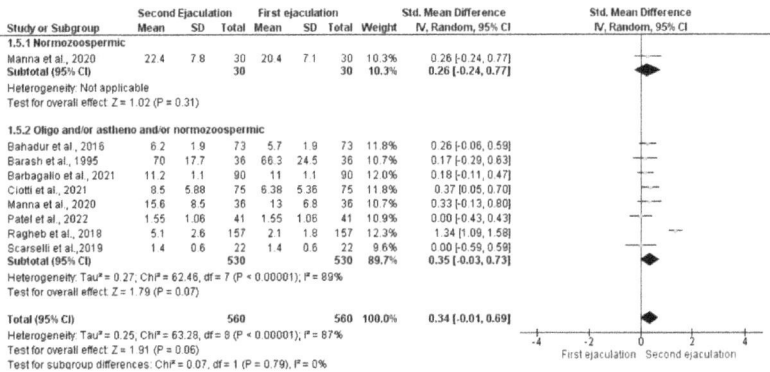

Figure 6. Forest plot of studies that evaluated the effects of a very short abstinence period on sperm morphology (expressed as a percentage). The following studies were included in the quantitative analysis (in order of appearance in the manuscript): Manna et al., 2020 [16], Bahadur et al., 2016 [17], Ragheb et al., 2018 [20], Ciotti et al., 2021 [22], Barash et al., 1995 [28], Sarselli et al., 2019 [33], Barbagallo et al., 2021 [35].

Only one study [25] included a subgroup of normozoospermic men. Therefore, analysis of publication bias and sensitivity analysis could not be performed in this sub-group. Inter-study heterogeneity was found for the subgroups of oligozoospermic, asthenozoospermic, and/or teratozoospermic patients (Q-value = 62.76; p-value = 0.000; I^2 = 89%). Egger's regression model and funnel plots reported the presence of risk of bias (intercept = −7.10, 95% CI −15.06–0.85, $p = 0.03$) (Supplementary Figure S9A). However, at the sensitivity analysis, no study was sensitive enough to alter the above-reported results (Supplementary Figure S9B).

3.1.6. Sperm DNA Fragmentation

Sperm DNA Fragmentation: Qualitative Analysis

Five studies investigated the effect of a very short abstinence period on the SDF rate [16,21,31,32,36] (Table 3). Four of the five studies reported a statistically significant reduction in the SDF rate after a very short abstinence period. In particular, Hussein et al. [31] found a statistically significant reduction in spermatozoa with severe DNA damage in the second ejaculation in both patients with abnormal sperm parameters and control men. In the study, SDF was evaluated using the Comet assay. Shen et al. reported a statistically significant reduction in SDF rate using the Sperm Chromatin Structure Assay (SCSA) in 167 patients; 61.1% of the patients enrolled in their study had normal sperm parameters [21]. According to Shen et al., Manna and colleagues reported a statistically significant reduction in SDF rate in both normozoospermic men and OAT patients using the Halosperm kit [16]. Furthermore, Kulkarmi et al. also showed lower SDF rates evaluated using the Qwik Check DFI test assay in conventional bright-field microscopy, in the second ejaculates compared to the first one of 67 oligozoospermic patients [36]. Only one study conducted by Torres et al. did not find any statistically significant change in the DNA fragmentation index evaluated using the SCSA kit. The small sample size (n = 3) could explain why this study did not find any change in the SDF rate. Indeed, the authors investigated SDF in only three healthy men at the second, third, and fourth evaluations after two hours of abstinence in comparison to the first evaluation after 2–4 days of abstinence [32].

Sperm DNA Fragmentation: Quantitative Analysis

Quantitative analysis of the SDF rate was evaluated in four studies [16,31,32,36]. The study by Shen et al. was not included in the quantitative analysis because no data on mean, median, or standard deviation was reported [21]. For the same reasons reported for other sperm parameters, the studies conducted by Torres et al. [32] and Manna et al. [16] were considered twice for quantitative analysis.

In particular, the statistical analysis showed that a second ejaculation after a very short abstinence period improved the SDF rate only in patients with abnormal sperm parameters [SMD −3.92 (−6.97, −0.87); p = 0.01] without any significant changes in normozoospermic men [SMD −2 (−4.72, 0.73); p = 0.15] (Figure 7).

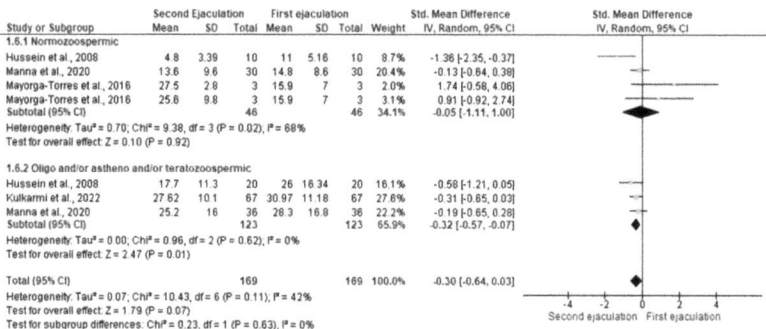

Figure 7. Forest plot of studies that evaluated the effects of a very short abstinence period on sperm DNA fragmentation (expressed as a percentage). The following studies were included in the quantitative analysis (in order of appearance in the manuscript): Manna et al., 2020 [16], Hussein et al., 2008 [31], Mayorga-Torres et al., 2016 [32], Kulkarmi et al., 2022 [36].

In the group of normozoospermic men, the analysis showed the presence of inter-study heterogeneity (Q-value = 13.648; p-value = 0.003; I^2 = 68%). No risk of bias was found at Egger's regression model and funnel plots (intercept = 1.610, 95% CI −8.507–11.727, p = 0.28) (Supplementary Figure S10A). No study was sensitive enough to alter the above-reported results (Supplementary Figure S10B).

In addition, no inter-study heterogeneity was found for the subgroups of oligozoospermic, asthenozoospermic, and/or teratozoospermic patients (Q-value = 1011; p-value = 0.603; I^2 = 0%). No risk of bias was found at Egger's regression model and funnel plots (intercept = −1.353, 95% CI −26.50–23.79, p = 0.309) (Supplementary Figure S11A). The study by Kulkarmi et al., 2022 [29] was sensitive enough to change these results. Indeed, its removal led to the loss of significance (Supplementary Figure S11B).

4. Discussion

The optimal period of sexual abstinence is still a matter of debate. Data on the effect of abstinence length on semen parameters are extremely heterogeneous and many publications from several decades ago are not yet conclusive. A systematic review conducted by

Hanson and colleagues including 28 studies investigated the impact of abstinence on semen parameters and fertility outcome. Analysis of publications showed that a longer abstinence was associated with increases in semen volume and sperm count. On the contrary, studies evaluating the effect of abstinence on motility, morphology, and SDF rate, although contradictory and not conclusive, showed a trend toward improvements with shorter abstinence period [15]. However, the authors did not establish any cut off to distinguish short and long abstinence period in their inclusion criteria.

Over time, many authors have supported the potential improvement of semen parameters in a second ejaculation collected after a very short period (within a few hours) from the first semen collection. However, data are still controversial. To our knowledge, this systematic review and meta-analysis, for the first time, pooled evidence for the influence of a very short abstinence period on sperm parameters and the SDF rate.

Our quantitative analysis showed a significant reduction in sperm volume after a very short abstinence period in both normozoospermic men and OAT patients. Sperm volume reflects the secretory activity of the accessory glands and the subsequent smooth muscle contractions that empty each gland in response to autonomous nerve stimulation elicited by sexual arousal [10]. Previous studies did not find consistent relationship between semen volume and fertility [14,38]. Of course, a minimal volume of semen is necessary for conception, and hypoposia should be investigated because it could reflect different pathological conditions (such as hypotestosteronemia, abnormalities of the neuroreceptor systems, retrograde ejaculation, and obstructive diseases) [9]. According to the last edition of the WHO manual for human sperm analysis, sperm volume should be equal to or more than 1.4 mL [10]. Sexual abstinence significantly influences sperm volume. Indeed, sperm volume was shown to increase by 11.9% per day in the first 4 days following ejaculation [39].

The present analysis also showed a decrease in sperm concentration in the second ejaculation of normozoospermic men and, conversely, a significant increase in patients with abnormal sperm parameters. Interestingly, also for total and progressive sperm motility, the improvement in the second ejaculation was statistically significant only in patients with OAT, without any changes in normozoospermic men. Furthermore, an improvement in sperm morphology was found in OAT patients but it did not reach statistical significance. Therefore, the results of the present meta-analysis support previous evidence on the beneficial effect of a very short abstinence period, especially in patients with abnormal sperm parameters.

The mechanism of sperm quality improvement in the second ejaculation collected after a short interval is unclear. Among the different reasons hypothesized, a different duration of the epididymal transit could play the main role. Human spermatozoa are produced in the seminiferous tubules and then stored in the epididymis. The length of spermatozoon epididymal transit time of spermatozoa ranges from 2 to 11 days [40] and its duration is possibly related to the rate of passage through the cauda which, in turn, can be influenced by the ejaculatory frequency [41]. During epididymal transit and storage, spermatozoa are exposed to high levels of reactive oxygen species (ROS). The hostile environment in the epididymis may be related to several causes, including dysfunctions or partial obstructions of the epididymis itself, stasis of seminal fluids, accumulation of senescent-degenerating spermatozoa, and packing of cells involved in the removal of aging spermatozoa [42,43]. Therefore, a short period of abstinence could decrease the time of exposure of spermatozoa to the harmful effects of ROS in the cauda epididymis and, in turn, may result in a "healthier" population of spermatozoa [13]. Previous studies have reported that prolonged exposure to ROS arising from dead spermatozoa and leukocytes may be one reason for the association between reduction in sperm quality and an increase in SDF rate with low ejaculation frequencies [44]. According to this hypothesis, Shen and colleagues found an increased total antioxidant capacity in ejaculates from short (1–3 h) compared with long (3–7 days) length of abstinence [21]. Moreover, Torres and colleagues found a decreasing trend of intracellular ROS production in four repeated ejaculations on the same day at two-hour intervals, and the difference became statistically significant at the fourth evaluation in comparison to the first one [32].

Interestingly, Johnson and Varner reported that the duration of epididymal transit was three times longer in patients with oligozoospermia than in men with normozoospermia [45]. Therefore, spermatozoa of patients with severe OA are stationed in the genital tract for a prolonged time and, in turn, are more damaged by oxidative stress. This might explain the greater improvement of sperm quality after a very short period of abstinence in patients with abnormal sperm parameters compared to normozoospermic men.

Furthermore, during the epididymal transit, several epigenetic modifications occur [46] and it is a fundamental step for spermatogenesis, sperm maturation, and the fertilization process [47]. In 2019, Shen and colleagues confirmed the potential molecular diversity of spermatozoa ejaculated after 1–3 h compared to 3–7 days by proteomic techniques [21]. Interestingly, the main differences were found in the expression of proteins highly involved in sperm motility and capacitation. The acrosome reaction capability of spermatozoa was markedly elevated after 1–3 h of abstinence [21]. To date, the role of these proteins in abstinence-related sperm function is still unclear. However, these findings suggest that a short abstinence period can alter the expression of sperm proteins, which may be one of the reasons why short sexual abstinence may improve sperm quality [48].

The investigation of biofunctional sperm parameters after a very short abstinence period could help us to understand the origin of this improvement. As reported in our results, a very short abstinence period is associated with a significant improvement in the SDF rate. This can be caused by extrinsic factors or intrinsic factors, including increased oxidative stress [49]. Therefore, the reduction in sperm SDF supports previous hypotheses that a short period of abstinence could decrease the time of exposure of spermatozoa to high levels of ROS. Few studies have investigated the effects of a very short sexual abstinence on other biofunctional sperm parameters. Shen and coworkers found a higher sperm mitochondrial membrane potential (MMP) in ejaculates from short (1–3 h) compared to long (3–7 days) length of abstinence [21]. MMP is a marker of sperm mitochondrial function that strictly correlates with sperm motility [50]. Mayorga-Torres and colleagues demonstrated that sperm MMP and plasma membrane integrity remained stable throughout four repeated ejaculations on the same day at two-hour intervals [32]. Scarselli et al. found an increase in the percentage of mature chromatin in ejaculates obtained after a very short abstinence time (1 h) [33]. Sperm chromatin structure could be important for the maintenance of the right epigenetic patterns during spermatogenesis. Epigenetic events in OAT patients directly influence embryogenesis. It is known that failure of ART treatment in couples with male partner infertility could be related to epigenetic alterations of blastocysts [47].

Furthermore, it was also speculated that the changes in seminal plasma composition after a very short period of abstinence might influence sperm quality. In particular, Alipour and colleagues compared the seminal plasma metabolomics profile of two consecutive ejaculates collected from normozoospermic men. The first sample was collected after an abstinence period of 4–7 days, whereas the second one was collected after a very short (2 h) abstinence period. The authors found a lower absolute amount of all metabolites in the second ejaculate [34]. This may be related to the insufficient time available for the secretion and accumulation of these metabolites by accessory sex glands, including the epididymis. However, the contemporary lower number of spermatozoa in the second ejaculate resulted in increased absolute amounts of pyruvate and taurine per spermatozoa, together with an improvement of sperm motility in these samples. Therefore, the authors speculated that changes in the seminal plasma composition might influence spermatozoa motility and kinematic parameters [34].

All the studies included in this systematic review and meta-analysis were judged as of fair quality at the quality analysis. Nevertheless, some limitations should be considered. The main limitation is that many of the included studies were observational. Furthermore, the analysis revealed a large heterogeneity in the studies included. This inter-study heterogeneity could be partly explained by the different methods to evaluate semen parameters and the SDF rate (Table 3). Many of the studies included have a relatively small sample size. The significance of data from smaller studies should not be ignored, although the larger studies included in our analysis had the statistical power to provide more convincing evidence. Another limitation is that the majority of publications included in the present meta-analysis evaluated different sperm parameters but not all studies evaluated the same parameters, making it difficult to draw a strong conclusion about some of these. Furthermore, cigarette smoking, caffeine intake, and lifestyle were not analyzed, although a significant relationship between the aforementioned factors with sperm quality was concluded by previous studies [4,51,52]. Further prospective randomized and larger studies are needed to evaluate the effects of a short abstinence period on sperm quality. Further studies should evaluate the effects of a very short abstinence period on biofunctional sperm parameters to better understand the reason for the improvement in sperm quality. Furthermore, future studies should evaluate the sperm parameters of the second ejaculation also based on the sexual abstinence length before the first collection.

5. Conclusions

This is the first systematic review and meta-analysis, which investigate the impact of a very short abstinence period on sperm parameters and the SDF rate. Our results suggest that a second ejaculation collected after a very short period from the first one contains spermatozoa of better quality, in terms of sperm concentration, total and progressive motility, and the SDF rate in patients with abnormal sperm parameters.

These results could have important implications in both natural and assisted reproductive technologies. For couples in reproductive age, these data suggest that more frequent intercourse with a very short sexual abstinence period could enhance conception.

Supplementary Materials: The following supporting information can be downloaded at: https://www.mdpi.com/article/10.3390/jcm11247303/s1, Table S1: PRISMA checklist; Figure S1: Funnel plot (A) and sensitivity analysis (B) of studies that evaluated the effects of a very short abstinence period on seminal fluid volume in normozoospermic men; Figure S2: Funnel plot (A) and sensitivity analysis (B) of studies that evaluated the effects of a very short abstinence period on seminal fluid volume in oligo- and/or astheno- and/or teratozoospermic men; Figure S3: Funnel plot (A) and sensitivity analysis (B) of studies that evaluated the effects of a very short abstinence period on sperm concentration in normozoospermic men; Figure S4: Funnel plot (A) and sensitivity analysis (B) of studies that evaluated the effects of a very short abstinence period on sperm concentration in oligo- and/or astheno- and/or teratozoospermic men; Figure S5: Funnel plot (A) and sensitivity analysis (B) of studies that evaluated the effects of a very short abstinence period on sperm total motility in normozoospermic men; Figure S6: Funnel plot (A) and sensitivity analysis (B) of studies that evaluated the effects of a very short abstinence period on sperm total motility in oligo- and/or astheno- and/or teratozoospermic men; Figure S7: Funnel plot (A) and sensitivity analysis (B) of studies that evaluated the effects of a very short abstinence period on sperm progressive motility in normozoospermic men; Figure S8: Funnel plot (A) and sensitivity analysis (B) of studies that evaluated the effects of a very short abstinence period on sperm progressive motility in oligo- and/or astheno- and/or teratozoospermic men; Figure S9: Funnel plot (A) and sensitivity analysis (B) of studies that evaluated the effects of a very short abstinence period on sperm morphology in oligo- and/or astheno- and/or teratozoospermic men; Figure S10: Funnel plot (A) and sensitivity analysis (B) of studies that evaluated the effects of a very short abstinence period on sperm DNA fragmentation in normozoospermic men; Figure S11: Funnel plot (A) and sensitivity analysis (B) of studies that evaluated the effects of a very short abstinence period on sperm DNA fragmentation in oligo- and/or astheno- and/or teratozoospermic men. Reference [53] is cited in Supplementary Materials.

Author Contributions: Conceptualization, F.B. and A.E.C.; methodology, F.B., A.C. and R.C.; software, R.C.; validation, S.L.V. and R.A.C.; formal analysis, F.B., A.C. and R.C.; investigation, F.B., A.C. and R.C.; data curation, F.B., A.C. and R.C.; writing—original draft preparation, F.B.; writing—review and editing, A.E.C.; visualization, C.M., R.A.C. and S.L.V.; supervision, R.C. and A.E.C.; project administration, F.B. and A.E.C. All authors have read and agreed to the published version of the manuscript.

Funding: This research received no external funding.

Institutional Review Board Statement: Not applicable.

Informed Consent Statement: Not applicable.

Data Availability Statement: The data are available upon request from the corresponding author.

Conflicts of Interest: The authors declare that there is no conflict of interest that could be perceived as prejudicing the impartiality of the research reported.

References

1. Zegers-Hochschild, F.; Adamson, G.D.; Dyer, S.; Racowsky, C.; de Mouzon, J.; Sokol, R.; Rienzi, L.; Sunde, A.; Schmidt, L.; Cooke, I.D.; et al. The International Glossary on Infertility and Fertility Care, 2017. *Fertil. Steril.* **2017**, *108*, 393–406. [CrossRef] [PubMed]
2. Vander Borght, M.; Wyns, C. Fertility and infertility: Definition and epidemiology. *Clin. Biochem.* **2018**, *62*, 2–10. [CrossRef] [PubMed]
3. Agarwal, A.; Baskaran, S.; Parekh, N.; Cho, C.L.; Henkel, R.; Vij, S.; Arafa, M.; Panner Selvam, M.K.; Shah, R. Male infertility. *Lancet* **2021**, *397*, 319–333. [CrossRef] [PubMed]
4. Condorelli, R.A.; La Vignera, S.; Giacone, F.; Iacoviello, L.; Vicari, E.; Mongioi', L.; Calogero, A.E. In vitro effects of nicotine on sperm motility and bio-functional flow cytometry sperm parameters. *Int. J. Immunopathol. Pharmacol.* **2013**, *26*, 739–746. [CrossRef]
5. Barbagallo, F.; Condorelli, R.A.; Mongioì, L.M.; Cannarella, R.; Cimino, L.; Magagnini, M.C.; Crafa, A.; La Vignera, S.; Calogero, A.E. Molecular Mechanisms Underlying the Relationship between Obesity and Male Infertility. *Metabolites* **2021**, *11*, 840. [CrossRef]
6. Barbagallo, F.; Condorelli, R.A.; Mongioì, L.M.; Cannarella, R.; Aversa, A.; Calogero, A.E.; La Vignera, S. Effects of Bisphenols on Testicular Steroidogenesis. *Front. Endocrinol.* **2020**, *30*, 373. [CrossRef]
7. Calogero, A.E.; Fiore, M.; Giacone, F.; Altomare, M.; Asero, P.; Ledda, C.; Romeo, G.; Mongioì, L.M.; Copat, C.; Giuffrida, M.; et al. Exposure to multiple metals/metalloids and human semen quality: A cross-sectional study. *Ecotoxicol. Environ. Saf.* **2021**, *215*, 112165. [CrossRef]
8. Leisegang, K.; Dutta, S. Do lifestyle practices impede male fertility? *Andrologia* **2021**, *53*, e13595. [CrossRef]
9. Crafa, A.; Cannarella, R.; LA Vignera, S.; Barbagallo, F.; Condorelli, R.A.; Calogero, A.E. Semen analysis: A workflow for an appropriate assessment of the male fertility status. *Minerva Endocrinol.* **2022**, *47*, 77–88. [CrossRef]
10. World Health Organization. *WHO Laboratory Manual for the Examination and Processing of Human Semen*, 6th ed.; WHO Press: Geneva, Switzerland, 2021. Available online: https://www.who.int/publications/i/item/9789240030787 (accessed on 26 July 2021).
11. Kvist, U.; Björndahl, L. Manual on Basic Semen Analysis 2002. ESHRE & Oxford University Press: Oxford, UK, 2002.
12. Henkel, R.R.; Schill, W.B. Sperm preparation for ART. *Reprod. Biol. Endocrinol.* **2003**, *1*, 108. [CrossRef]
13. Levitas, E.; Lunenfeld, E.; Weiss, N.; Friger, M.; Har-Vardi, I.; Koifman, A.; Potashnik, G. Relationship between the duration of sexual abstinence and semen quality: Analysis of 9489 semen samples. *Fertil. Steril* **2005**, *83*, 1680–1686. [CrossRef] [PubMed]
14. Mac Leod, J.; Gold, R.Z. The male factor in fertility and infertility. IV. Sperm morphology in fertile and infertile marriage. *Fertil. Steril* **1951**, *2*, 394–414. [CrossRef]
15. Hanson, B.M.; Aston, K.I.; Jenkins, T.G.; Carrell, D.T.; Hotaling, J.M. The impact of ejaculatory abstinence on semen analysis parameters: A systematic review. *J. Assist. Reprod. Genet.* **2018**, *35*, 213–220. [CrossRef] [PubMed]
16. Manna, C.; Barbagallo, F.; Manzo, R.; Rahman, A.; Francomano, D.; Calogero, A.E. Sperm Parameters before and after Swim-Up of a Second Ejaculate after a Short Period of Abstinence. *J. Clin. Med.* **2020**, *9*, 1029. [CrossRef] [PubMed]
17. Bahadur, G.; Almossawi, O.; Zeirideen Zaid, R.; Ilahibuccus, A.; Al-Habib, A.; Muneer, A.; Okolo, S. Semen characteristics in consecutive ejaculates with short abstinence in subfertile males. *Reprod. Biomed. Online* **2016**, *32*, 323–328. [CrossRef] [PubMed]
18. Ortiz, A.; Ortiz, R.; Soto, E.; Hartmann, J.; Manzur, A.; Marconi, M. Evidence for obtaining a second successive semen sample for intrauterine insemination in selected patients: Results from 32 consecutive cases. *Clin. Exp. Reprod. Med.* **2016**, *43*, 102–105. [CrossRef]
19. Alipour, H.; Van Der Horst, G.; Christiansen, O.B.; Dardmeh, F.; Jørgensen, N.; Nielsen, H.I.; Hnida, C. Improved sperm kinematics in semen samples collected after 2 h versus 4–7 days of ejaculation abstinence. *Hum. Reprod.* **2017**, *32*, 1364–1372. [CrossRef]
20. Ragheb, A.M.; Ibrahim, R.M.; Elbatanouny, A.M.; Moussa, A.S.; Abdelbary, A.M.; Sayed, O.M.; Eladawy, M.S.; Shaker, H.A.; Hamdi, S.O. Role of sequential semen samples in infertile men candidates for assisted reproduction: A prospective study, African. *J. Urol.* **2018**, *24*, 363–367. [CrossRef]
21. Shen, Z.Q.; Shi, B.; Wang, T.R.; Jiao, J.; Shang, X.J.; Wu, Q.J.; Zhou, Y.M.; Cao, T.F.; Du, Q.; Wang, X.X.; et al. Characterization of the Sperm Proteome and Reproductive Outcomes with in Vitro, Fertilization after a Reduction in Male Ejaculatory Abstinence Period. *Mol. Cell. Proteom.* **2019**, *18*, S109–S117. [CrossRef]

22. Ciotti, P.M.; Calza, N.; Zuffa, S.; Notarangelo, L.; Nardi, E.; Damiano, G.; Cipriani, L.; Porcu, E. Two subsequent seminal productions: A good strategy to treat very severe oligoasthenoteratozoospermic infertile couples. *Andrology* **2021**, *9*, 1185–1191. [CrossRef]
23. Shamseer, L.; Moher, D.; Clarke, M.; Ghersi, D.; Liberati, A.; Petticrew, M.; Shekelle, P.; Stewart, L.A.; PRISMA-P Group. Preferred reporting items for systematic review and meta-analysis protocols (PRISMA-P) 2015: Elaboration and explanation. *BMJ* **2015**, *350*, 7647. [CrossRef] [PubMed]
24. Murray, J.; Farrington, D.P.; Eisner, M.P. Drawing conclusions about causes from systematic reviews of risk factors: The Cambridge Quality Checklists. *J. Exp. Criminol.* **2009**, *5*, 1–23. [CrossRef]
25. Duval, S.; Tweedie, R. Trim and fill: A simple funnel-plot-based method of testing and adjusting for publication bias in meta-analysis. *Biometrics* **2000**, *56*, 455–463. [CrossRef]
26. Zvěrina, J.; Pondělíčková, J. Changes in seminal parameters of ejaculates after repeated ejaculation. *Andrologia* **1988**, *20*, 52–54. [CrossRef] [PubMed]
27. Tur-Kaspa, I.; Maor, Y.; Levran, D.; Yonish, M.; Mashiach, S.; Dor, J. How often should infertile men have intercourse to achieve conception? *Fertil. Steril.* **1994**, *62*, 370–375. [CrossRef] [PubMed]
28. Barash, A.; Lurie, S.; Weissman, A.; Insler, V. Comparison of sperm parameters, in vitro fertilization results, and subsequent pregnancy rates using sequential ejaculates, collected two hours apart, from oligoasthenozoospermic men. *Fertil. Steril.* **1995**, *64*, 1008–1011. [CrossRef]
29. Bar-Hava, I.; Perri, T.; Ashkenazi, J.; Shelef, M.; Ben-Rafael, Z.; Orvieto, R. The rationale for requesting a second consecutive sperm ejaculate for assisted reproductive technology. *Gynecol. Endocrinol.* **2000**, *14*, 433–436. [CrossRef]
30. Sugiyam, R.; Al-Salem, J.A.; Nishi, Y.; Sugiyama, R.; Shirai, M.; Inoue, M.; Irahara, M. Improvement of sperm motility by short-interval sequential ejaculation in oligoasthenozoospermic patients. *Arch. Med. Sci.* **2008**, *4*, 438–442.
31. Hussein, T.M.; Elariny, A.F.; Elabd, M.M.; Elgarem, Y.F.; Elsawy, M.M. Effect of repeated sequential ejaculation on sperm DNA integrity in subfertile males with asthenozoospermia. *Andrologia* **2008**, *40*, 312–317. [CrossRef]
32. Mayorga-Torres, J.M.; Agarwal, A.; Roychoudhury, S.; Cadavid, A.; Cardona-Maya, W.D. Can a Short Term of Repeated Ejaculations Affect Seminal Parameters? *J. Reprod. Infertil.* **2016**, *17*, 177–183.
33. Scarselli, F.; Cursio, E.; Muzzì, S.; Casciani, V.; Ruberti, A.; Gatti, S.; Greco, P.; Varricchio, M.T.; Minasi, M.G.; Greco, E. How 1 h of abstinence improves sperm quality and increases embryo euploidy rate after PGT-A: A study on 106 sibling biopsied blastocysts. *J. Assist. Reprod. Genet.* **2019**, *36*, 1591–1597. [CrossRef] [PubMed]
34. Alipour, H.; Duus, R.K.; Wimmer, R.; Dardmeh, F.; Du Plessis, S.S.; Jørgensen, N.; Christiansen, O.B.; Hnida, C.; Nielsen, H.I.; Van Der Horst, G. Seminal plasma metabolomics profiles following long (4–7 days) and short (2 h) sexual abstinence periods. *Eur. J. Obstet. Gynecol. Reprod. Biol.* **2021**, *264*, 178–183. [CrossRef]
35. Barbagallo, F.; Calogero, A.E.; Condorelli, R.A.; Farrag, A.; Jannini, E.A.; La Vignera, S.; Manna, C. Does a Very Short Length of Abstinence Improve Assisted Reproductive Technique Outcomes in Infertile Patients with Severe Oligo-Asthenozoospermia? *J. Clin. Med.* **2021**, *10*, 4399. [CrossRef] [PubMed]
36. Kulkarni, V.; Kaingade, P.; Kulkarni, N.; Bhalerao, T.; Nikam, A. Assessment of semen parameters in consecutive ejaculates with short abstinence period in oligospermic males. *JBRA Assist. Reprod.* **2022**, *26*, 310–314. [CrossRef] [PubMed]
37. Patel, D.V.; Patel, T.; Maheshwari, N.; Soni, S.; Patel, R.G. Retrospective Analysis of the First Collection versus the Second Collection in Severe Oligo-asthenoteratozoospermia Cases in Self-Intracytoplasmic Sperm Injection Patients. *J. Hum. Reprod. Sci.* **2022**, *15*, 138–142. [CrossRef]
38. Santomauro, A.G.; Sciarra, J.J.; Varma, A.O. A clinical investigation of the role of the semen analysis and postcoital test in the evaluation of male infertility. *Fertil. Steril.* **1972**, *23*, 245–251. [CrossRef]
39. Carlsen, E.; Petersen, J.H.; Andersson, A.M.; Skakkebaek, N.E. Effects of ejaculatory frequency and season on variations in semen quality. *Fertil. Steril.* **2004**, *82*, 358–366. [CrossRef]
40. Joseph, P.N.; Sharma, R.K.; Agarwal, A.; Sirot, L.K. Men Ejaculate Larger Volumes of Semen, More Motile Sperm, and More Quickly when Exposed to Images of Novel Women. *Evol. Psychol. Sci.* **2015**, *1*, 195–200. [CrossRef]
41. Turner, T.T. De Graaf's thread: The human epididymis. *J. Androl.* **2008**, *29*, 237–250. [CrossRef]
42. Wilton, L.J.; Temple-Smith, P.D.; Baker, H.W.; de Kretser, D.M. Human male infertility caused by degeneration and death of sperm in the epididymis. *Fertil. Steril.* **1988**, *49*, 1052–1058. [CrossRef]
43. de Kretser, D.M.; Huidobro, C.; Southwick, G.J.; Temple-Smith, P.D. The role of the epididymis in human infertility. *J. Reprod. Fertil. Suppl.* **1998**, *53*, 271–275. [PubMed]
44. Borges, E.J.; Zanetti, B.F.; Setti, A.S.; Braga, D.P.A.F.; Provenza, R.R.; Iaconelli, A.J. Sperm DNA fragmentation is correlated with poor embryo development, lower implantation rate, and higher miscarriage rate in reproductive cycles of non-male factor infertility. *Fertil. Steril.* **2019**, *112*, 483–490. [CrossRef] [PubMed]
45. Johnson, L.; Varner, D.D. Effect of daily spermatozoan production but not age on transit time of spermatozoa through the human epididymis. *Biol. Reprod.* **1988**, *39*, 812–817. [CrossRef] [PubMed]
46. Sharma, U.; Conine, C.C.; Shea, J.M.; Boskovic, A.; Derr, A.G.; Bing, X.Y.; Belleannee, C.; Kucukural, A.; Serra, R.W.; Sun, F.; et al. Biogenesis and function of tRNA fragments during sperm maturation and fertilization in mammals. *Science* **2016**, *351*, 391–396. [CrossRef]

47. Denomme, M.M.; McCallie, B.R.; Parks, J.C.; Booher, K.; Schoolcraft, W.B.; Katz-Jaffe, M.G. Inheritance of epigenetic dysregulation from male factor infertility has a direct impact on reproductive potential. *Fertil. Steril.* **2018**, *110*, 419–428. [CrossRef]
48. Li, J.; Shi, Q.; Li, X.; Guo, J.; Zhang, L.; Quan, Y.; Ma, M.; Yang, Y. The Effect of Male Sexual Abstinence Periods on the Clinical Outcomes of Fresh Embryo Transfer Cycles Following Assisted Reproductive Technology: A Meta-Analysis. *Am. J. Mens. Health* **2020**, *14*, 1–8. [CrossRef]
49. Agarwal, A.; Majzoub, A.; Baskaran, S.; Panner Selvam, M.K.; Cho, C.L.; Henkel, R.; Finelli, R.; Leisegang, K.; Sengupta, P.; Barbarosie, C.; et al. Sperm DNA Fragmentation: A New Guideline for Clinicians. *World J. Mens. Health* **2020**, *38*, 412–471. [CrossRef]
50. Barbagallo, F.; La Vignera, S.; Cannarella, R.; Aversa, A.; Calogero, A.E.; Condorelli, R.A. Evaluation of Sperm Mitochondrial Function: A Key Organelle for Sperm Motility. *J. Clin. Med.* **2020**, *9*, 363. [CrossRef]
51. Ricci, E.; Viganò, P.; Cipriani, S.; Somigliana, E.; Chiaffarino, F.; Bulfoni, A.; Parazzini, F. Coffee and caffeine intake and male infertility: A systematic review. *Nutr. J.* **2017**, *16*, 37. [CrossRef]
52. Shi, X.; Chan, C.P.S.; Waters, T.; Chi, L.; Chan, D.Y.L.; Li, T.C. Lifestyle and demographic factors associated with human semen quality and sperm function. *Syst. Biol. Reprod. Med.* **2018**, *64*, 358–367. [CrossRef]
53. Moher, D.; Liberati, A.; Tetzlaff, J.; Altman, D.G.; The PRISMA Group. Preferred Reporting Items for Systematic Reviews and Meta-Analyses: The PRISMA Statement. *PLoS Med.* **2009**, *6*, e1000097. [CrossRef] [PubMed]

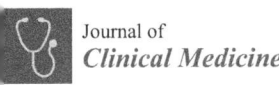

Article

Association of the Cumulative Live Birth Rate with the Factors in Assisted Reproductive Technology: A Retrospective Study of 16,583 Women

Qiumin Wang [1,2,3], Dan Qi [1,2,3], Lixia Zhang [1,4], Jingru Wang [1], Yanbo Du [1], Hong Lv [1,*] and Lei Yan [1,2,3,*]

1. Center for Reproductive Medicine, Shandong University, Jinan 250012, China
2. Key Laboratory of Reproductive Endocrinology of Ministry of Education, Shandong University, Jinan 250012, China
3. Shandong Key Laboratory of Reproductive Medicine, Jinan 250012, China
4. Maternal and Child Health and Family Planning Service Center of Yanggu County, Liaocheng 252300, China
* Correspondence: lvhong@sduivf.com (H.L.); yanlei@sdu.edu.cn (L.Y.)

Abstract: The cumulative live birth rate (CLBR) can better reflect the overall treatment effect by successive treatments, and continuous rather than categorical variables as exposure variables can increase the statistical power in detecting the potential correlation. Therefore, the dose–response relationships might find an optimal dose for the better CLBR, offering evidence-based references for clinicians. To determine the dose–response relationships of the factors and the optimal ranges of the factors in assisted reproductive technology (ART) associated with a higher CLBR, this study retrospectively analyzed 16,583 patients undergoing the first in vitro fertilization (IVF) or intracytoplasmic sperm injection (ICSI) from January 2017 to January 2019. Our study demonstrated the optimal ranges of age with a higher CLBR were under 32.10 years. We estimated the CLBR tends to increase with increased levels of AMH at AMH levels below 1.482 ng/mL, and the CLBR reaches a slightly high level at AMH levels in the range from 2.58–4.18 ng/mL. The optimal ranges of basal FSH with a higher CLBR were less than 9.13 IU. When the number of cryopreserved embryos was above 1.055 and the number of total transferred embryos was 2, the CLBR was significantly higher. In conclusion, there is a non-linear dose–response relationship between the CLBR with age, AMH, basal FSH, and the number of cryopreserved embryos and total transferred embryos. We proposed the optimal ranges of the five factors that were correlated with a higher CLBR in the first oocyte retrieval cycle, which may help consultation at IVF clinics.

Keywords: dose–response relationship; cumulative live birth; anti-Müllerian hormone; age; follicle-stimulating hormone; transferred embryos

1. Introduction

Currently, the incidence of infertility is gradually increasing, which is a global medical concern affecting between 8 and 30% of reproductive-age couples worldwide [1–4]; hence, the demand for infertility treatment is increasing [5]. Concomitant with the development of assisted reproductive technology (ART), an increasing number of infertility couples obtain a live birth through these technologies. Frozen embryo transfer (FET) is gaining popularity for its advantages of convenience, safety, and efficacy [6–8]. The cumulative live birth rate (CLBR) per oocyte retrieval (including fresh embryo transfer and subsequent FET) can better reflect the overall treatment effect by successive treatments [9]. Likewise, the CLBR is an important indicator of common concern for both clinicians and patients.

It has long been known that maternal age is the most significant factor affecting ART outcomes [10]. Previous research found that female obesity adversely affected the CLBR in their first in vitro fertilization (IVF) or intracytoplasmic sperm injection (ICSI) cycles [11]. Women with diminished ovarian reserves had substantially lower live birth rates [12], and

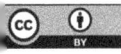

the anti-Müllerian hormone (AMH) levels, the basal follicle-stimulating hormone (FSH) levels, and AFC can be used as the indicators for ovarian reserve function [13–15]. There are also studies that found an additional predictor of the CLBR was the number of retrieved oocytes [16]. However, most of the previous research treated these factors as categorical variables, which hampered the establishment of clear dose–response relationships between these factors and the CLBR. Moreover, dose–response relationships might find an optimal dose for the better CLBR, offering evidence-based references for clinicians.

Therefore, we designed a retrospective study to determine the optimal ranges of the factors in ART associated with a higher CLBR in women undergoing the first IVF/ICSI.

2. Materials and Methods

2.1. Study Design and Population

This is a retrospective population-based study. Patients with a total of 30,530 retrieval cycles were collected in this study between January 2017 and January 2019 from the Center for Reproductive Medicine, Shandong University. The following cycles were excluded: all preimplantation genetic testing (PGT); IVF/ICSI with donor oocytes; gamete transfer; oocyte cryopreservation; not the first retrieval cycles; no AMH value or AMH > 1 year from oocyte retrieval; premature ovarian insufficiency (POI) or polycystic ovary syndrome (PCOS). The final sample size for analysis was 16,583. This study was approved by the institutional review board of the Center for Reproductive Medicine, Shandong University (2022–59).

2.2. IVF/ICSI Protocols

All patients received a controlled ovarian stimulation protocol, oocyte retrieval, fertilization, an embryo cultured and cryopreserved in vitro, and luteal phase support for fresh embryo transfer (ET), or endometrial preparation and luteal phase support for frozen embryo transfer, according to a routine method [17]. The protocols for controlled ovarian stimulation in our study included luteal phase gonadotropin-releasing hormone (GnRH) agonist long protocols (6536, 39.4%), GnRH agonist short protocols (4974, 30.0%), GnRH antagonist protocols (2842, 17.1%), follicular phase GnRH agonist long protocol (1375, 8.3%), mild stimulation protocol (258, 1.6%), natural cycle protocol (248, 1.5%), GnRH agonist ultrashort protocol (12, 0.1%), and other protocols (338, 2.0%). The IVF-ET protocols used in our center have been described in detail previously [7,18]. Ovarian response was monitored using ultrasonography and serum sex steroid levels. A dose from 4000 to 10,000 IU human chorionic gonadotropin (HCG) was administered when the size of at least two follicles reached 18 mm, and oocyte retrieval was performed from 34 to 36 h later. According to the male partner's sperm quality, oocytes were fertilized by conventional IVF/ICSI. All embryos were frozen, or up to two fresh embryos were transferred, at the cleavage or blastocyst stage after fertilization. Luteal phase support [18] was started after oocyte retrieval in women with fresh embryos transferred. Frozen blastocysts were thawed and transferred, and subsequently provided luteal phase support protocol according to the different endometrial preparation programs [19]. Pregnancy outcome follow-ups were carried out as previously described [20].

2.3. Outcome

Our primary outcome of interest was the CLBR in the first index retrieval cycle. The CLBR was defined as the percentage of live births per patient from the first index retrieval cycle, including all fresh or subsequent two years of frozen embryo transfer after the oocyte retrieval. Live birth (LB) was defined as the delivery of any viable infant at 28 weeks or more of gestation.

2.4. Statistical Analysis

All analyses and plotting were performed with IBM SPSS statistics 26.0, R 4.1.3, or GraphPad Prism 9. Continuous numeric variables were expressed as mean ± SD, and categorical variables were described as percentages. The Student's t-test was used for continuous numeric variables and the Chi-squared test was used for categorical variables. Multivariate logistic regression analyses were performed to identify the influencing factors of the CLBR. The candidate variables for multivariate logistic regression analyses were those with $p < 0.05$ after the univariate analyses. Multivariate logistic regression analyses (the backward logistic regression method) were conducted by fitting a logistic regression model. Logistic regression was expressed as an odds ratio (OR) with 95% confidence intervals (CI), and a forest plot was drawn by GraphPad Prism 9. The dose–response relationship between variables (age, AMH, basal FSH, the number of cryopreserved embryos, and total transferred embryos) and the odds ratio of the CLBR was evaluated by a restricted cubic spline (RSC) with covariates adjusted. Sensitivity analyses were performed to evaluate the stability of our findings by restricting the analytic samples to ovulatory women ($n = 16,474$) and women without endometriosis ($n = 15,605$), respectively. $p < 0.05$ was considered statistically significant.

3. Results

Of 30,530 retrieval cycles, 16,583 retrieval cycles/patients were included in the final analysis. The study population is presented in a flow chart (Figure 1).

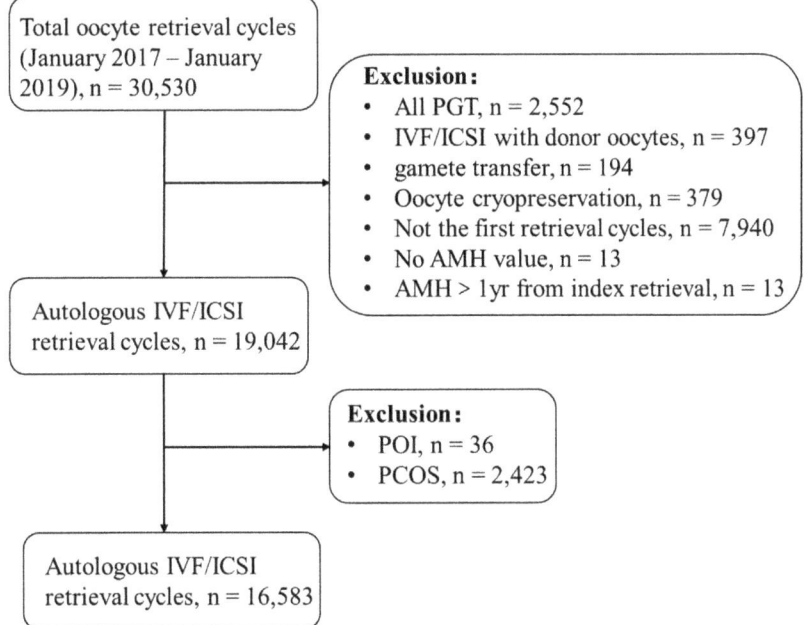

Figure 1. Flow chart of the study population. PGT: preimplantation genetic testing; IVF: in vitro fertilization; ICSI: intracytoplasmic sperm injection; AMH: anti-Müllerian hormone; POI: premature ovarian insufficiency; PCOS: polycystic ovary syndrome.

3.1. Characteristics of the Study Population

The characteristics of the 16,583 retrieval cycles/patients are shown in Table 1. A total of 7967 (48.04%) patients achieved a live birth. Compared to those who did not obtain a live birth, patients who obtained a live birth were younger (31.00 ± 4.15 vs. 34.221 ± 5.65, $p < 0.001$), had slightly lower BMI (23.67 ± 3.50 vs. 24.11 ± 3.47, $p < 0.001$), slightly shorter duration of infertility (3.62 ± 2.66 vs 3.84 ± 3.24, $p < 0.001$), and slightly lower FBG (5.24 ± 0.81 vs. 5.27 ± 0.79, $p = 0.028$). They had higher AMH levels (3.87 ± 2.75 vs. 2.74 ± 2.64, $p < 0.001$) and lower basal FSH (6.60 ± 1.93 vs. 7.54 ± 3.10, $p < 0.001$), and they were less likely to be parous women (51.30% vs. 62.50%, $p < 0.001$). There were differences in the incidence of uterine factor infertility (14.60% vs. 22.30%, $p < 0.001$), male factor infertility (17.30% vs. 12.60%, $p < 0.001$), and unexplained infertility (5.30% vs. 7.60%, $p < 0.001$) between patients who obtained a live birth or were not among infertility etiologies. Versus those who did not obtain a live birth, women who had a live birth had a lower total Gonadotropin dose (2000.39 ± 969.78 vs. 2211.21 ± 1207.59, $p < 0.001$), a slightly greater number of retrieved oocytes (11.19 ± 5.57 vs 7.69 ± 5.91, $p < 0.001$), more cryopreserved embryos (3.05 ± 2.51 vs. 1.35 ± 2.12, $p < 0.001$) and transferred embryos (1.83 ± 0.80 vs. 1.10 ± 1.14, $p < 0.001$), a higher proportion of cycles with oocytes retrieved (100.00% vs. 96.70%, $p < 0.001$), embryos cryopreserved (86.60% vs. 47.90%, $p < 0.001$), and total transferred embryos (100% vs. 59.30%, $p < 0.001$).

Table 1. Baseline and stimulation cycle characteristics.

Characteristic	Total (n = 16,583)	No Live Birth (n = 8616)	Live Birth (n = 7967)	p Value
Age	32.68 ± 5.24	34.22 ± 5.65	31.00 ± 4.15	<0.001
BMI	23.90 ± 3.49	24.11 ± 3.47	23.67 ± 3.50	<0.001
Duration of infertility	3.73 ± 2.98	3.84 ± 3.24	3.62 ± 2.66	<0.001
FBG	5.25 ± 0.80	5.27 ± 0.79	5.24 ± 0.81	0.028
AMH	3.28 ± 2.75	2.74 ± 2.64	3.87 ± 2.75	<0.001
Basal FSH	7.09 ± 2.64	7.54 ± 3.10	6.60 ± 1.93	<0.001
Gravidity ≥ 1 (%)	57.20	62.50	51.30	<0.001
Infertility etiology (%)				
Tubal factor	79.40	79.10	79.70	0.327
Uterine factor	18.60	22.30	14.60	<0.001
Male factor	14.80	12.60	17.30	<0.001
Unexplained	6.50	7.60	5.30	<0.001
Endometriosis	5.90	6.10	5.70	0.276
Ovulatory dysfunction	0.70	0.60	0.70	0.502
Total Gonadotropin dose (IU)	2109.92 ± 1104.77	2211.21 ± 1207.59	2000.39 ± 969.78	<0.001
No. of retrieved oocytes	9.37 ± 6.01	7.69 ± 5.91	11.19 ± 5.57	<0.001
Cycles with oocytes retrieved (%)	98.30	96.70	100.00	<0.001
No. of cryopreserved embryos	2.17 ± 2.47	1.35 ± 2.12	3.05 ± 2.51	<0.001
Cycles with embryos cryopreserved (%)	66.50	47.90	86.60	<0.001
No. of total transferred embryos	1.45 ± 1.06	1.10 ± 1.14	1.83 ± 0.80	<0.001
Cycles with transferred embryos (%)	78.80	59.30	100.00	<0.001

BMI: body mass index; FBG: fasting blood glucose; AMH: anti-Müllerian hormone; FSH: follicle-stimulating hormone.

3.2. Association of AMH and Other Factors with CLBR

A multivariate analysis was performed by logistic regression (the backward logistic regression method) to examine the association between the CLBR and those candidate variables with $p < 0.05$ after the univariate analyses. Those candidate variables included age, BMI, duration of infertility, FBG, AMH, basal FSH, infertility type, uterine factor infertility, male factor infertility, unexplained infertility, total Gonadotropin dose, the number of retrieved oocytes and cryopreserved embryos, and the number of total transferred embryos. In adjusted models, age (OR 0.910, 95%CI 0.903–0.917, $p < 0.001$), AMH (OR 1.021, 95%CI 1.006–1.037, $p = 0.005$), basal FSH (OR 0.967, 95%CI 0.951–0.983, $p < 0.001$), uterine infertility (OR 0.822, 95%CI 0.747–0.904, $p < 0.001$), male infertility (OR 1.185, 95%CI 1.072–1.309, $p = 0.001$), the number of cryopreserved embryos (OR 1.252, 95%CI 1. 231–1.274, $p < 0.001$), and the number of total transferred embryos (OR 2.033, 95%CI 1.954–2.115, $p < 0.001$) were significantly associated with the CLBR (Table 2 and Figure 2). That is, the CLBR increased with AMH, and the number of cryopreserved embryos and total transferred embryos decreased with age and basal FSH. These couples with male infertility more often had a CLBR, and those women with uterine infertility were significantly less likely to have a CLBR than women without uterine infertility. The other covariates (BMI, duration of infertility, FBG, infertility type, unexplained infertility, total Gonadotropin dose, and the number of retrieved oocytes) were unrelated to the CLBR and were not included in the multivariable-adjusted logistic regression model. In sensitivity analyses, the association of these factors with the CLBR was similar to the results in samples of women who were ovulatory ($n = 16{,}474$) or women without endometriosis ($n = 15{,}605$), respectively (Table 2).

Table 2. Multiple logistic regression analysis.

Parameter	Adjusted OR (95%CI)	p Value
Total population ($n = 16{,}583$)		
Age	0.910 (0.903–0.917)	<0.001
AMH	1.021 (1.006–1.037)	0.005
Basal FSH	0.967 (0.951–0.983)	<0.001
Uterine infertility	0.822 (0.747–0.904)	<0.001
Male infertility	1.185 (1.072–1.309)	0.001
No. of cryopreserved embryos	1.252 (1.231–1.274)	<0.001
No. of total transferred embryos	2.033 (1.954–2.115)	<0.001
Ovulatory Women ($n = 16{,}474$)		
Age	0.909 (0.902–0.917)	<0.001
AMH	1.023 (1.007–1.038)	0.003
Basal FSH	0.966 (0.950–0.982)	<0.001
Uterine infertility	0.824 (0.748–0.907)	<0.001
Male infertility	1.181 (1.069–1.306)	0.001
No. of cryopreserved embryos	1.252 (1.231–1.274)	<0.001
No. of total transferred embryos	2.035 (1.955–2.117)	<0.001
Women without endometriosis ($n = 15{,}605$)		
Age	0.910 (0.902–0.917)	<0.001
AMH	1.020 (1.004–1.036)	0.012
Basal FSH	0.968 (0.951–0.985)	<0.001
Uterine infertility	0.786 (0.711–0.869)	<0.001
Male infertility	1.175 (1.061–1.300)	0.002
Total Gonadotropin dose/100	0.997 (0.993–1.000)	0.090
No. of cryopreserved embryos	1.247 (1.225–1.269)	<0.001
No. of total transferred embryos	2.027 (1.946–2.112)	<0.001

AMH: anti-Müllerian hormone; FSH: follicle-stimulating hormone.

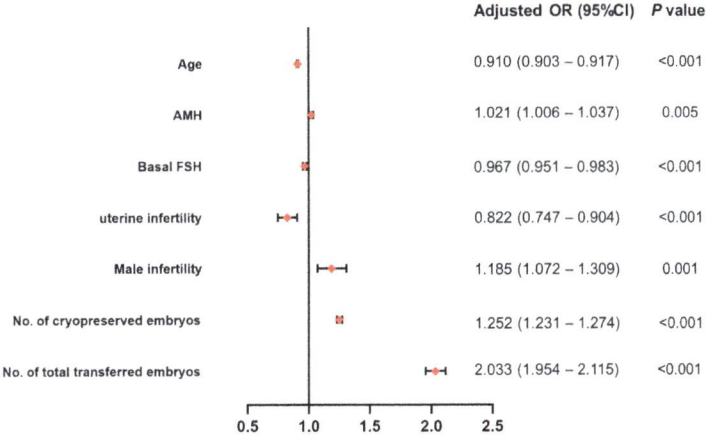

Figure 2. Forest plot of multivariable regression analyses. AMH: anti-Müllerian hormone; FSH: follicle-stimulating hormone. The red square is adjusted OR.

We further evaluated the dose–response relationship between the CLBR and AMH and other variables (age, basal FSH, and the number of cryopreserved embryos and transferred embryos) by a restricted cubic spline (RSC). The results of the RSC are presented in Figure 3. After adjusted AMH, basal FSH, and the number of cryopreserved embryos and transferred embryos, the CLBR decreased significantly with increasing age (non-linear, $p < 0.001$, Figure 3A). We found the CLBR with an inverse association above 32.10 years of age (OR 0.997, 95%CI 0.994–0.999). The association was more pronounced with increasing age, the OR of the CLBR was 0.016 (95%CI 0.010–0.025) when the age was 48 years. After adjusted age, basal FSH, and the number of cryopreserved embryos and transferred embryos, the CLBR increased significantly with increasing AMH levels (non-linear, $p < 0.001$, Figure 3B). We estimated the CLBR tends to increase with an increase in the levels of AMH at AMH levels below 1.482 ng/mL (OR 0.896, 95%CI 0.817–0.984) and the CLBR to reach a slightly high level at AMH levels in the range from 2.58–4.18 ng/mL (OR > 1.0, however, the 95%CI included 1.0). After adjusted age, AMH, and the number of cryopreserved embryos and transferred embryos, the CLBR was associated with basal FSH (non-linear, $p = 0.002$, Figure 3C). The CLBR was significantly decreased when basal FSH was more than 9.13 IU (OR 0.890, 95%CI 0.792–0.999). After adjusted age, basal FSH, AMH, and the number of total transferred embryos, the CLBR was positively correlated with the number of cryopreserved embryos (non-linear, $p < 0.001$, Figure 3D). When the number of cryopreserved embryos was above 1.055 (OR 1.038, 95%CI 1.035–1.041), the CLBR was significantly higher. After adjusted age, basal FSH, AMH, and the number of cryopreserved embryos, the CLBR was associated with the number of total transferred embryos (non-linear, $p < 0.001$, Figure 3E). The CLBR was significantly higher when the number of total transferred embryos was two (OR 1.252, 95%CI 1.151–1.361), and was decreased when the number of total transferred embryos was more than three (OR 0.595, 95%CI 0.535–0.662). When the number of total transferred embryos was eight, the OR of CLBR was only 0.077 (95%CI 0.047–0.127).

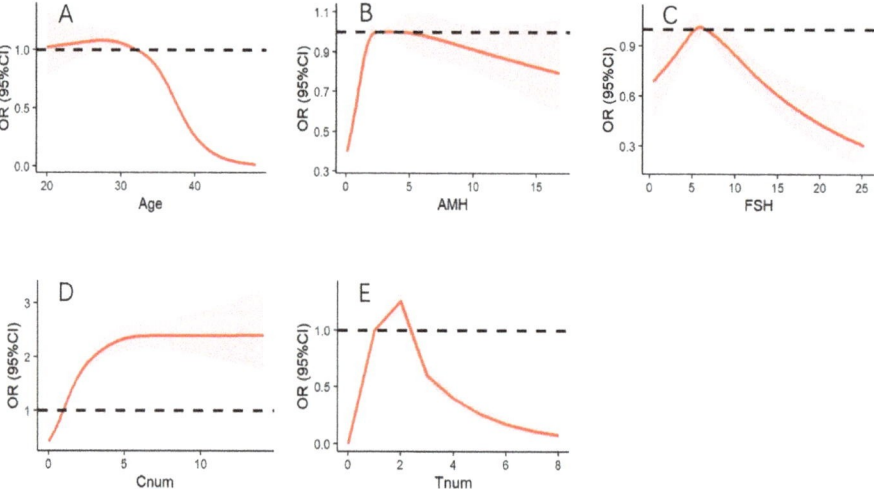

Figure 3. Association of the five factors with CLBR ((A). Association of age with CLBR; (B). Association of AMH with CLBR; (C). Association of FSH with CLBR; (D). Association of the number of cryopreserved embryos with CLBR; (E). Association of the number of total transferred embryos with CLBR). AMH: anti-Müllerian hormone; FSH: follicle-stimulating hormone; Cnum: number of cryopreserved embryos; Tnum: number of total transferred embryos.

In sensitivity analyses, the dose–response relationships between the CLBR and variables (age, AMH, basal FSH, the number of cryopreserved embryos, and the number of total transferred embryos) were similar to the above findings in ovulatory women or women without endometriosis (Figures S1 and S2).

4. Discussion

In this study, the CLBR was non-linearly associated with age, AMH, basal FSH, and the number of cryopreserved embryos and total transferred embryos. For the first time, we found the optimal ranges of the five factors that were correlated with a higher CLBR in the first oocyte retrieval cycle. The optimal ranges of age with a higher CLBR were under 32 years, the optimal ranges of AMH were from 2.58–4.18 ng/mL (but the differences were not significant), and the optimal ranges of basal FSH were less than 9.13 IU. When the number of cryopreserved embryos was above one and the number of total transferred embryos was two, the CLBR was significantly higher.

Considering the development of modern ART, the CLBR per oocyte retrieval cycle (including fresh embryos transferred and all frozen embryos transferred after oocyte retrieval) has become a more meaningful outcome for patients and clinicians [9]. Therefore, the CLBR served as the main outcome parameter in our study. Previous evidence has demonstrated that female age is a major factor influencing fertility [21] and that decreasing fecundity is associated with increasing age, due to a reduced ovarian reserve, poor quality of oocytes, and an increased incidence of embryonic aneuploidy [22,23]. Whether after assisted reproduction or not, the CLBR gradually decreased with an increase in the age of females [24]. The majority of studies [25–29] have reported that the CLBR decreases in females after the age of 35 compared with females under the age of 35; however, in our study, the age moved to 32 years. This result is consistent with the previous opinion [30]. The advanced upper limit of optimal reproductive age might be related to the increase in work stress, bad lifestyle, or environmental pollution today.

AMH is secreted by granulosa cells (GCs) of pre-antral and small antral follicles in the ovary [31]. AMH levels can reflect the number of pre-antral and small antral follicles [32]. Converging evidence revealed that AMH can be considered a reliable indicator of ovarian reserves [33,34] and for predicting the success rate of in vitro fertilization (IVF) [35–37]. Recently, a retrospective study with a large sample size pointed out that AMH highly correlates with the CLBR in women with diminished ovarian reserves (DOR) independent of age [14]. The similar result was found in a population of elderly women [38]. Low AMH levels have been reported to have a negative effect on live birth in women undergoing ART [29,39–41]. In our study, AMH levels below 1.482 n/mL were the risk factor of the CLBR, which indicated that a low AMH level is associated with poor ovarian reserves. The women with low AMH would yield fewer follicles, fewer transferable embryos, and, therefore, have fewer chances of transfer. AMH with specific ranges would provide better estimates of IVF outcomes [42]. At present, the optimal range of AMH levels has not been clarified. Previous research has found that serum levels of AMH above 3.5 ng/mL do not significantly increase the chance of a live birth [28], which is similar to our study findings in all subjects. Results of a recent study showed that the CLBR had a decreasing trend or was not significantly changed when the serum level of AMH was over 5 ng/mL in young women (under 35 years of age) or over 7 ng/mL in older women (above 35 years). Moreover, the optimal range of AMH levels was reported to be between 5 and 7 ng/mL in all women. [28]. However, the AMH range in that study was artificially set and this way is prone to anthropogenic impact. In the current analysis, RCS models allowed for departures from linearity, which can flexibly model the relationship of AMH and CLBR to determine the optimal range of AMH levels. Moreover, we used continuous rather than categorical variables, as exposure variables can increase the statistical power in detecting the potential correlation [43].

A previous study has concluded that high AMH levels might indicate more quantity of oocytes or embryos, rather than a higher quality of oocytes or embryos [44]. However, the specific mechanism of the high AMH levels affecting the quality of oocytes has not been clarified. There was no correlation between AMH levels with oocyte quality in women of advanced age [45]. Therefore, the CLBR is not significantly improved in the present study when the serum AMH level is above 4.18 ng/mL. It was speculated that a high AMH level might be associated with adverse perinatal outcomes. Recently, research found that high levels of serum AMH had a significantly higher risk of miscarriage in women with or without PCOS [46]. Similarly, an increased rate of miscarriage has been reported in women with high or low AMH levels [47]. High serum AMH levels were also associated with an increased risk of preterm delivery in women with PCOS [48]. The result was similar to those from another study, and another study proposed that closer monitoring during the third trimester in patients with serum levels of AMH over 9.3 ng/mL might be required [49]. In addition, we excluded the possible interference of the women with PCOS or POI to the results, and adjusted other potentially influencing factors such as age, basal FSH, or the number of cryopreserved embryos and total transferred embryos.

The basal FSH level is another clinical index to evaluate ovarian reserve, as basal FSH concentration increases when the ovarian reserve declines [50]. Compared with AMH, the ability of basal FSH to predict pregnancy outcomes was poor [35,51,52]. Our results showed that basal FSH was higher than 9.13 IU, and the CLBR was significantly decreased. Compared to previously published results, the cut-off of FSH in our study was a lower level, and a more accurate range could lead to more valuable information for the clinician. This could be useful for clinicians in clinical decision-making about ART for these patients. Over the past few decades, the number of FETs has continuously increased for the improvement of embryo culture conditions and the development of vitrification techniques [53]. FET is gaining popularity for its advantages of convenience, safety, and efficacy [6–8]. Our results were similar to those of the previous study [54–56], and the CLBR was positively correlated with the number of cryopreserved embryos. Fewer cryopreserved embryos reduces the chance to transfer; however, in our study, the CLBR no longer increased, as the number of cryopreserved embryos increased to a certain number. It might be that the top-quality embryos were given priority for transfer, so that transferring the surplus of poor embryos would not have significantly helped to increase the CLBR [57]. The same patients with several embryo transfers were unsuccessful, which may be associated with other factors, such as the patients with a thin endometrium. Further, we identified that the CLBR was significantly higher as the number of totals transferred was two. This result is different from the findings of previous research [58]. This could be due to high-quality embryos being preferentially selected for transfer, and women without obtained live birth needed to perform repeated embryo transfers. It is an important reminder for clinicians not to pursue the number of transfers, and prepared endometrium is an important factor affecting the success of ART when top-quality embryos are transferred [59].

There are strengths and weaknesses in the present study. First, the CLBR served as the main outcome parameter in our study. CLBR per oocyte retrieval can better reflect the overall treatment effect by successive treatments, and it has become a more meaningful outcome for patients and clinicians. Second, in this single-center and large-scale study, the embryos were cultured in the same laboratory conditions, which minimized potential bias to a large extent. Third, RCS models in the current analysis allowed for departures from linearity, which can flexibly model the relationship between these factors and the CLBR to determine the optimal ranges of these factors. We used continuous rather than categorical variables as exposure variables can increase the statistical power in detecting the potential correlation [43]. Dose–response relationships could find an optimal dose for the better CLBR, and we surmise that the results obtained in the present study are more precise and clinically more efficient than the previous research. In addition, we excluded the possible interference of the women with PCOS or POI from the results and adjusted other potentially influencing factors. However, the main limitation of our study was its retrospective nature; although, we attempted to mitigate these limitations by controlling for confounders and performing sensitivity analyses. Future prospective multicenter studies are required to verify our findings. Another limitation of our study was the lack of data on other risk factors, such as maternal lifestyle habits. Future studies should evaluate other potential confounders, such as work stress, lifestyle habits, or environmental pollution.

5. Conclusions

In conclusion, our study suggested that there is a non-linear dose–response relationship between the CLBR with age, AMH, basal FSH, and the number of cryopreserved embryos and total transferred embryos. We found the optimal ranges of the five factors that were correlated with a higher CLBR in the first oocyte retrieval cycle, which may provide a scientific basis for the clinical management and treatment of IVF. The results could guide clinicians to better manage the ART procedures and provide proper counseling services for infertile couples.

Supplementary Materials: The following supporting information can be downloaded at: https://www.mdpi.com/article/10.3390/jcm12020493/s1, Figure S1. Association of AMH and factors with CLBR in ovulatory women; Figure S2. Association of AMH and factors with CLBR in women without endometriosis. AMH, anti-Müllerian hormone; FSH, follicle-stimulating hormone; Cnum, No. of cryopreserved embryos; Tnum, No. of total transferred embryos.

Author Contributions: Q.W. contributed to statistical analysis and interpretation of data and drafting of the manuscript; D.Q., L.Z. and J.W. performed the statistical analysis and participated in the discussion; Y.D. and H.L. analyzed and interpreted the data; L.Y. and Q.W. participated in the discussion and critically revised the manuscript. All authors have read and agreed to the published version of the manuscript.

Funding: The study was funded by the National Natural Science Foundation of China (82071617), the Shandong Provincial Key Research and Development Program (2020ZLYS02), the Shandong Provincial Medical and Health Science and Technology Development Program (2019WS171), and the Shandong Provincial Natural Science Foundation (ZR2020MH072).

Institutional Review Board Statement: This study was approved by the institutional review board of the Center for Reproductive Medicine, Shandong University (2022-59).

Informed Consent Statement: Patient consent was waived due to the retrospective nature of this study.

Data Availability Statement: The data underlying this article will be shared upon reasonable request to the first or corresponding authors.

Acknowledgments: The authors thank the clinicians, nurses, and laboratory staff for their contribution. Moreover, the authors thank the infertile couples who participated in this study.

Conflicts of Interest: None of the authors declare any conflict of interest.

References

1. Sun, H.; Gong, T.T.; Jiang, Y.T.; Zhang, S.; Zhao, Y.H.; Wu, Q.J. Global, regional, and national prevalence and disability-adjusted life-years for infertility in 195 countries and territories, 1990–2017: Results from a global burden of disease study, 2017. *Aging* **2019**, *11*, 10952–10991. [CrossRef] [PubMed]
2. Zhou, Z.; Zheng, D.; Wu, H.; Li, R.; Xu, S.; Kang, Y.; Cao, Y.; Chen, X.; Zhu, Y.; Xu, S.; et al. Epidemiology of infertility in China: A population-based study. *BJOG* **2018**, *125*, 432–441. [CrossRef] [PubMed]
3. Vander Borght, M.; Wyns, C. Fertility and infertility: Definition and epidemiology. *Clin. Biochem.* **2018**, *62*, 2–10. [CrossRef]
4. Agarwal, A.; Baskaran, S.; Parekh, N.; Cho, C.L.; Henkel, R.; Vij, S.; Arafa, M.; Panner Selvam, M.K.; Shah, R. Male infertility. *Lancet* **2021**, *397*, 319–333. [CrossRef] [PubMed]
5. Sarac, M.; Koc, I. Prevalence and Risk Factors of Infertility in Turkey: Evidence from Demographic and Health Surveys, 1993–2013. *J. Biosoc. Sci.* **2018**, *50*, 472–490. [CrossRef] [PubMed]
6. Roque, M.; Haahr, T.; Geber, S.; Esteves, S.C.; Humaidan, P. Fresh versus elective frozen embryo transfer in IVF/ICSI cycles: A systematic review and meta-analysis of reproductive outcomes. *Hum. Reprod. Update* **2019**, *25*, 2–14. [CrossRef] [PubMed]
7. Shi, Y.; Sun, Y.; Hao, C.; Zhang, H.; Wei, D.; Zhang, Y.; Zhu, Y.; Deng, X.; Qi, X.; Li, H.; et al. Transfer of Fresh versus Frozen Embryos in Ovulatory Women. *N. Engl. J. Med.* **2018**, *378*, 126–136. [CrossRef]
8. Maheshwari, A.; Pandey, S.; Amalraj Raja, E.; Shetty, A.; Hamilton, M.; Bhattacharya, S. Is frozen embryo transfer better for mothers and babies? Can cumulative meta-analysis provide a definitive answer? *Hum. Reprod. Update* **2018**, *24*, 35–58. [CrossRef]

9. Maheshwari, A.; McLernon, D.; Bhattacharya, S. Cumulative live birth rate: Time for a consensus? *Hum. Reprod.* **2015**, *30*, 2703–2707. [CrossRef]
10. Zhou, Q.W.; Jing, S.; Xu, L.; Guo, H.; Lu, C.F.; Gong, F.; Lu, G.X.; Lin, G.; Gu, Y.F. Clinical and neonatal outcomes of patients of different ages following transfer of thawed cleavage embryos and blastocysts cultured from thawed cleavage-stage embryos. *PLoS ONE* **2018**, *13*, e0207340. [CrossRef]
11. Ding, W.; Zhang, F.L.; Liu, X.C.; Hu, L.L.; Dai, S.J.; Li, G.; Kong, H.J.; Guo, Y.H. Impact of Female Obesity on Cumulative Live Birth Rates in the First Complete Ovarian Stimulation Cycle. *Front. Endocrinol.* **2019**, *10*, 516. [CrossRef] [PubMed]
12. Stern, J.E.; Brown, M.B.; Wantman, E.; Kalra, S.K.; Luke, B. Live birth rates and birth outcomes by diagnosis using linked cycles from the SART CORS database. *J. Assist. Reprod. Genet.* **2013**, *30*, 1445–1450. [CrossRef] [PubMed]
13. Lew, R. Natural history of ovarian function including assessment of ovarian reserve and premature ovarian failure. *Best Pract. Res. Clin. Obstet. Gynaecol.* **2019**, *55*, 2–13. [CrossRef] [PubMed]
14. Tal, R.; Seifer, D.B.; Tal, R.; Granger, E.; Wantman, E.; Tal, O. AMH Highly Correlates with Cumulative Live Birth Rate in Women with Diminished Ovarian Reserve Independent of Age. *J. Clin. Endocrinol. Metab.* **2021**, *106*, 2754–2766. [CrossRef] [PubMed]
15. Ata, B.; Seyhan, A.; Seli, E. Diminished ovarian reserve versus ovarian aging: Overlaps and differences. *Curr. Opin. Obstet. Gynecol.* **2019**, *31*, 139–147. [CrossRef] [PubMed]
16. McLernon, D.J.; Raja, E.A.; Toner, J.P.; Baker, V.L.; Doody, K.J.; Seifer, D.B.; Sparks, A.E.; Wantman, E.; Lin, P.C.; Bhattacharya, S.; et al. Predicting personalized cumulative live birth following in vitro fertilization. *Fertil. Steril.* **2022**, *117*, 326–338. [CrossRef] [PubMed]
17. Pan, Y.; Hao, G.; Wang, Q.; Liu, H.; Wang, Z.; Jiang, Q.; Shi, Y.; Chen, Z.-J. Major Factors Affecting the Live Birth Rate after Frozen Embryo Transfer Among Young Women. *Front. Med.* **2020**, *7*, 94. [CrossRef] [PubMed]
18. Guo, Z.; Xu, X.; Zhang, L.; Zhang, L.; Yan, L.; Ma, J. Endometrial thickness is associated with incidence of small-for-gestational-age infants in fresh in vitro fertilization-intracytoplasmic sperm injection and embryo transfer cycles. *Fertil. Steril.* **2020**, *113*, 745–752. [CrossRef]
19. Zong, L.; Liu, P.; Zhou, L.; Wei, D.; Ding, L.; Qin, Y. Increased risk of maternal and neonatal complications in hormone replacement therapy cycles in frozen embryo transfer. *Reprod. Biol. Endocrinol.* **2020**, *18*, 36. [CrossRef]
20. Chen, Z.J.; Shi, Y.; Sun, Y.; Zhang, B.; Liang, X.; Cao, Y.; Yang, J.; Liu, J.; Wei, D.; Weng, N.; et al. Fresh versus Frozen Embryos for Infertility in the Polycystic Ovary Syndrome. *N. Engl. J. Med.* **2016**, *375*, 523–533. [CrossRef]
21. Xin, A.; Qu, R.; Chen, G.; Zhang, L.; Chen, J.; Tao, C.; Fu, J.; Tang, J.; Ru, Y.; Chen, Y.; et al. Disruption in ACTL7A causes acrosomal ultrastructural defects in human and mouse sperm as a novel male factor inducing early embryonic arrest. *Sci. Adv.* **2020**, *6*, eaaz4796. [CrossRef] [PubMed]
22. Sun, B.; Ma, Y.; Li, L.; Hu, L.; Wang, F.; Zhang, Y.; Dai, S.; Sun, Y. Factors Associated with Ovarian Hyperstimulation Syndrome (OHSS) Severity in Women with Polycystic Ovary Syndrome Undergoing IVF/ICSI. *Front. Endocrinol.* **2020**, *11*, 615957. [CrossRef] [PubMed]
23. Esteves, S.C.; Carvalho, J.F.; Martinhago, C.D.; Melo, A.A.; Bento, F.C.; Humaidan, P.; Alviggi, C. Estimation of age-dependent decrease in blastocyst euploidy by next generation sequencing: Development of a novel prediction model. *Panminerva Med.* **2019**, *61*, 3–10. [CrossRef] [PubMed]
24. Ng, E.H.; Ho, P.C. Ageing and ART: A waste of time and money? *Best Pract. Res. Clin. Obstet. Gynaecol.* **2007**, *21*, 5–20. [CrossRef] [PubMed]
25. Hogan, R.G.; Wang, A.Y.; Li, Z.; Hammarberg, K.; Johnson, L.; Mol, B.W.; Sullivan, E.A. Oocyte donor age has a significant impact on oocyte recipients' cumulative live-birth rate: A population-based cohort study. *Fertil. Steril.* **2019**, *112*, 724–730. [CrossRef] [PubMed]
26. Abuzeid, M.I.; Bolonduro, O.; La Chance, J.; Abozaid, T.; Urich, M.; Ullah, K.; Ali, T.; Ashraf, M.; Khan, I. Cumulative live birth rate and assisted reproduction: Impact of female age and transfer day. *Facts Views Vis. ObGyn* **2014**, *6*, 145–149. [PubMed]
27. Khalife, D.; Nassar, A.; Khalil, A.; Awwad, J.; Abu Musa, A.; Hannoun, A.; El Taha, L.; Khalifeh, F.; Abiad, M.; Ghazeeri, G. Cumulative Live-Birth Rates by Maternal Age after One or Multiple In Vitro Fertilization Cycles: An Institutional Experience. *Int. J. Fertil. Steril.* **2020**, *14*, 34–40.
28. Hu, K.L.; Liu, F.T.; Xu, H.; Li, R.; Qiao, J. Association of serum anti-Müllerian hormone and other factors with cumulative live birth rate following IVF. *Reprod. Biomed. Online* **2020**, *40*, 675–683. [CrossRef]
29. Zhang, B.; Meng, Y.; Jiang, X.; Liu, C.; Zhang, H.; Cui, L.; Chen, Z.J. IVF outcomes of women with discrepancies between age and serum anti-Müllerian hormone levels. *Reprod. Biol. Endocrinol.* **2019**, *17*, 58. [CrossRef]
30. American College of Obstetricians and Gynecologists Committee on Gynecologic Practice and Practice Committee. Female age-related fertility decline. Committee Opinion No. 589. *Fertil. Steril.* **2014**, *101*, 633–634. [CrossRef]
31. Sahmay, S.; Atakul, N.; Oncul, M.; Tuten, A.; Aydogan, B.; Seyisoglu, H. Serum anti-Müllerian hormone levels in the main phenotypes of polycystic ovary syndrome. *Eur. J. Obstet. Gynecol. Reprod. Biol.* **2013**, *170*, 157–161. [CrossRef] [PubMed]
32. Kotanidis, L.; Nikolettos, K.; Petousis, S.; Asimakopoulos, B.; Chatzimitrou, E.; Kolios, G.; Nikolettos, N. The use of serum anti-Mullerian hormone (AMH) levels and antral follicle count (AFC) to predict the number of oocytes collected and availability of embryos for cryopreservation in IVF. *J. Endocrinol. Investig.* **2016**, *39*, 1459–1464. [CrossRef] [PubMed]

33. Moolhuijsen, L.M.E.; Visser, J.A. Anti-Müllerian Hormone and Ovarian Reserve: Update on Assessing Ovarian Function. *J. Clin. Endocrinol. Metab.* **2020**, *105*, 3361–3373. [CrossRef]
34. Pankhurst, M.W. A putative role for anti-Müllerian hormone (AMH) in optimising ovarian reserve expenditure. *J. Endocrinol.* **2017**, *233*, R1–R13. [CrossRef] [PubMed]
35. Wang, S.; Zhang, Y.; Mensah, V.; Huber, W.J., 3rd; Huang, Y.T.; Alvero, R. Discordant anti-müllerian hormone (AMH) and follicle stimulating hormone (FSH) among women undergoing in vitro fertilization (IVF): Which one is the better predictor for live birth? *J. Ovarian Res.* **2018**, *11*, 60. [CrossRef] [PubMed]
36. Gomez, R.; Schorsch, M.; Hahn, T.; Henke, A.; Hoffmann, I.; Seufert, R.; Skala, C. The influence of AMH on IVF success. *Arch. Gynecol. Obstet.* **2016**, *293*, 667–673. [CrossRef]
37. Alson, S.S.E.; Bungum, L.J.; Giwercman, A.; Henic, E. Anti-müllerian hormone levels are associated with live birth rates in ART, but the predictive ability of anti-müllerian hormone is modest. *Eur. J. Obstet. Gynecol. Reprod. Biol.* **2018**, *225*, 199–204. [CrossRef]
38. Guan, Y.; Kong, P.; Xiao, Z.; Zhang, J.; He, J.; Geng, W.; Yan, J.; Sun, S.; Mu, M.; Du, X.; et al. Independent Variables for Determining the Cumulative Live Birth Rates of Aged Patients with Polycystic Ovary Syndrome or Tubal Factor Infertility: A Retrospective Cohort Study. *Front. Endocrinol.* **2021**, *12*, 728051. [CrossRef]
39. Lukaszuk, K.; Liss, J.; Kunicki, M.; Jakiel, G.; Wasniewski, T.; Woclawek-Potocka, I.; Pastuszek, E. Anti-Müllerian hormone (AMH) is a strong predictor of live birth in women undergoing assisted reproductive technology. *Reprod. Biol.* **2014**, *14*, 176–181. [CrossRef]
40. Peuranpää, P.; Hautamäki, H.; Halttunen-Nieminen, M.; Hydén-Granskog, C.; Tiitinen, A. Low anti-Müllerian hormone level is not a risk factor for early pregnancy loss in IVF/ICSI treatment. *Hum. Reprod.* **2020**, *35*, 504–515. [CrossRef]
41. Reijnders, I.F.; Nelen, W.L.; IntHout, J.; van Herwaarden, A.E.; Braat, D.D.; Fleischer, K. The value of Anti-Müllerian hormone in low and extremely low ovarian reserve in relation to live birth after in vitro fertilization. *Eur. J. Obstet. Gynecol. Reprod. Biol.* **2016**, *200*, 45–50. [CrossRef]
42. Keane, K.; Cruzat, V.F.; Wagle, S.; Chaudhary, N.; Newsholme, P.; Yovich, J. Specific ranges of anti-Mullerian hormone and antral follicle count correlate to provide a prognostic indicator for IVF outcome. *Reprod. Biol.* **2017**, *17*, 51–59. [CrossRef] [PubMed]
43. Altman, D.G.; Royston, P. The cost of dichotomising continuous variables. *BMJ* **2006**, *332*, 1080. [CrossRef]
44. Arce, J.C.; La Marca, A.; Mirner Klein, B.; Nyboe Andersen, A.; Fleming, R. Antimüllerian hormone in gonadotropin releasing-hormone antagonist cycles: Prediction of ovarian response and cumulative treatment outcome in good-prognosis patients. *Fertil. Steril.* **2013**, *99*, 1644–1653. [CrossRef] [PubMed]
45. Dai, X.; Wang, Y.; Yang, H.; Gao, T.; Yu, C.; Cao, F.; Xia, X.; Wu, J.; Zhou, X.; Chen, L. AMH has no role in predicting oocyte quality in women with advanced age undergoing IVF/ICSI cycles. *Sci. Rep.* **2020**, *10*, 19750. [CrossRef] [PubMed]
46. Liu, X.; Han, Y.; Wang, X.; Zhang, Y.; Du, A.; Yao, R.; Lv, J.; Luo, H. Serum anti-Müllerian hormone levels are associated with early miscarriage in the IVF/ICSI fresh cycle. *BMC Pregnancy Childbirth* **2022**, *22*, 279. [CrossRef]
47. Kostrzewa, M.; Żyła, M.; Garnysz, K.; Kaczmarek, B.; Szyłło, K.; Grzesiak, M. Anti-Müllerian hormone as a marker of abortion in the first trimester of spontaneous pregnancy. *Int. J. Gynaecol. Obstet.* **2020**, *149*, 66–70. [CrossRef]
48. Hu, K.L.; Liu, F.T.; Xu, H.; Li, R.; Qiao, J. High antimullerian hormone levels are associated with preterm delivery in patients with polycystic ovary syndrome. *Fertil. Steril.* **2020**, *113*, 444–452.e441. [CrossRef]
49. Kaing, A.; Jaswa, E.A.; Diamond, M.P.; Legro, R.S.; Cedars, M.I.; Huddleston, H.G. Highly elevated level of antimüllerian hormone associated with preterm delivery in polycystic ovary syndrome patients who underwent ovulation induction. *Fertil. Steril.* **2021**, *115*, 438–446. [CrossRef]
50. Valeri, C.; Pappalardo, S.; De Felici, M.; Manna, C. Correlation of oocyte morphometry parameters with woman's age. *J. Assist. Reprod. Genet.* **2011**, *28*, 545–552. [CrossRef]
51. Ligon, S.; Lustik, M.; Levy, G.; Pier, B. Low antimüllerian hormone (AMH) is associated with decreased live birth after in vitro fertilization when follicle-stimulating hormone and AMH are discordant. *Fertil. Steril.* **2019**, *112*, 73–81.e71. [CrossRef] [PubMed]
52. Nelson, S.M.; Yates, R.W.; Fleming, R. Serum anti-Müllerian hormone and FSH: Prediction of live birth and extremes of response in stimulated cycles—Implications for individualization of therapy. *Hum. Reprod.* **2007**, *22*, 2414–2421. [CrossRef] [PubMed]
53. du Boulet, B.; Ranisavljevic, N.; Mollevi, C.; Bringer-Deutsch, S.; Brouillet, S.; Anahory, T. Individualized luteal phase support based on serum progesterone levels in frozen-thawed embryo transfer cycles maximizes reproductive outcomes in a cohort undergoing preimplantation genetic testing. *Front. Endocrinol.* **2022**, *13*, 1051857. [CrossRef] [PubMed]
54. Aslan, K.; Kasapoglu, I.; Cakir, C.; Avci, B.; Uncu, G. Supernumerary embryos, do they show the cycle success in a fresh embryo transfer? A retrospective analysis. *Gynecol. Endocrinol. Off. J. Int. Soc. Gynecol. Endocrinol.* **2021**, *37*, 1107–1110. [CrossRef]
55. Hill, M.J.; Richter, K.S.; Heitmann, R.J.; Lewis, T.D.; DeCherney, A.H.; Graham, J.R.; Widra, E.; Levy, M.J. Number of supernumerary vitrified blastocysts is positively correlated with implantation and live birth in single-blastocyst embryo transfers. *Fertil. Steril.* **2013**, *99*, 1631–1636. [CrossRef]
56. Ibrahim, Y.; Stoddard, G.; Johnstone, E. A clinical counseling tool predicting supernumerary embryos after a fresh IVF cycle. *J. Assist. Reprod. Genet.* **2020**, *37*, 1137–1145. [CrossRef]
57. Kirillova, A.; Lysenkov, S.; Farmakovskaya, M.; Kiseleva, Y.; Martazanova, B.; Mishieva, N.; Abubakirov, A.; Sukhikh, G. Should we transfer poor quality embryos? *Fertil. Res. Pract.* **2020**, *6*, 2. [CrossRef]

58. Zhang, M.; Bu, T.; Tian, H.; Li, X.; Wang, D.; Wan, X.; Wang, Q.; Mao, X.; La, X. Use of Cumulative Live Birth Rate per Total Number of Embryos to Calculate the Success of IVF in Consecutive IVF Cycles in Women Aged ≥35 Years. *BioMed Res. Int.* **2019**, *2019*, 6159793. [CrossRef]
59. Vergaro, P.; Tiscornia, G.; Rodríguez, A.; Santaló, J.; Vassena, R. Transcriptomic analysis of the interaction of choriocarcinoma spheroids with receptive vs. non-receptive endometrial epithelium cell lines: An in vitro model for human implantation. *J. Assist. Reprod. Genet.* **2019**, *36*, 857–873. [CrossRef]

Disclaimer/Publisher's Note: The statements, opinions and data contained in all publications are solely those of the individual author(s) and contributor(s) and not of MDPI and/or the editor(s). MDPI and/or the editor(s) disclaim responsibility for any injury to people or property resulting from any ideas, methods, instructions or products referred to in the content.

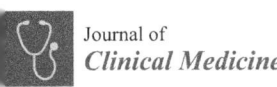

Article

Assisted Reproductive Technology without Embryo Discarding or Freezing in Women ≥40 Years: A 5-Year Retrospective Study at a Single Center in Italy

Claudio Manna [1,2,*], Federica Barbagallo [3], Francesca Sagnella [1], Ashraf Farrag [1] and Aldo E. Calogero [3]

1. Biofertility IVF and Infertility Center, 00128 Rome, Italy
2. Department of Biomedicine and Prevention, University of Rome "Tor Vergata", 00133 Rome, Italy
3. Department of Clinical and Experimental Medicine, University of Catania, 95123 Catania, Italy
* Correspondence: claudiomanna55@gmail.com

Abstract: The protocols commonly used in assisted reproductive technology (ART) consist of long-term embryo culture up to the blastocyst stage after the insemination of all mature oocytes, the freezing of all the embryos produced, and their subsequent transfer one by one. These practices, along with preimplantation genetic testing, although developed to improve the live birth rate (LBR) and reduce the risk of multiple pregnancies, are drawing attention to the possible increase in obstetric and perinatal risks, and adverse epigenetic consequences in offspring. Furthermore, ethical–legal concerns are growing regarding the increase in cryopreservation and storage of frozen embryos. In an attempt to reduce the risk associated with prolonged embryo culture and avoid embryo storage, we have chosen to inseminate a limited number of oocytes not exceeding the number of embryos to be transferred, after two days or less of culture. We retrospectively analyzed 245 ICSI cycles performed in 184 infertile couples with a female partner aged ≥40 from January 2016 to July 2021. The results showed a fertilization rate of 95.7%, a miscarriage rate of 48.9%, and a LBR of 10% with twin pregnancies of 16.7%. The cumulative LBR in our group of couples was 13%. No embryos were frozen. In conclusion, these results suggest that oocyte selection and embryo transfer at the cleaving stage constitute a practice that has a LBR comparable to that of the more commonly used protocols in older women who have reduced ovarian reserve.

Keywords: advanced maternal age; assisted reproductive technique; in-vitro fertilization; oocyte selection

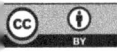

1. Introduction

Louise Brown was born in 1978 with the transfer into the uterus of a single embryo obtained after the laparoscopic retrieval of one oocyte without ovarian stimulation and in vitro fertilization (IVF) [1]. In the following decade, controlled ovarian stimulation (COS) made it possible to collect a higher number of oocytes with the simultaneous transfer into the uterus of more embryos, increasing the success rate of the assisted reproductive technique (ART). Subsequently, embryo freezing became a standard procedure in ART centers to avoid multiple pregnancies. With the development of the vitrification technique, oocyte freezing became possible, and the efficiency of embryo freezing improved.

Another relevant advance in ART is the extended embryo culture up to the blastocyst stage [2]. This procedure has shown a higher implantation potential and a better live birth rate (LBR) in fresh transfer compared to cleaving embryos [3]. However, other studies have shown similar results in cumulative LBR between the two stages of embryo culture [4,5].

Nowadays, a constant trend is to freeze all embryos produced in ART cycles and transfer them one by one—the so-called single embryo transfer (SET)—in a suitably prepared endometrium to reduce multiple pregnancies and maximize the cumulative LBR [6]. Indeed, several studies have shown that SET reduces multiple pregnancies at a rate similar to that of spontaneous pregnancies (3%); in the case of multiple embryo transfer, the rate of multiple pregnancy can be very high (20–50%) [7,8]. Multiple pregnancies are considered the main iatrogenic complication of ART, due to their association with adverse events in both mothers and children [9]. Furthermore, the costs of multiple pregnancies and deliveries are 2–7 times higher than those of singletons [10]. However, not all embryos reach the blastocyst stage (60% for the competence value of IVF laboratories, according to the ESHRE Vienna Consensus of 2017) [11] and in a significant number of cycles the transfer is canceled: 17% in the study of Sainte-Rose et al., especially in older women [12], and 18.8% in the study by De Croo et al. [13]. Furthermore, criticisms have been raised about the effects of the SET policy on the LBR, which does not leave couples the freedom to choose more blastocysts to transfer [14]. Finally, a longer in vitro culture time can be a stressful condition for embryos and can be a source of other possible concerns such as increased obstetric risk [15–19] and epigenetic risk [20–22]. Although the negative effects of a long culture on embryos is not fully proven, previous studies reported an increased risk of preterm birth (<37 weeks) [15], small-for-gestational age (SGA) [15] or large-for-gestational age (LGA) [15,19], placenta previa, and placental abruption [15] in pregnancies after blastocyst transfer as compared to pregnancies after cleavage-stage transfer. Furthermore, growing evidence suggests an association between ART and epigenetic modifications that can be transmitted to offspring [23]. Unphysiological conditions, including embryo culture, have the potential to contribute to epigenetic dysregulation [23].

The most challenging endeavor in the ART laboratory is the ability to identify the embryos with the best potential to produce a live birth. The morphological criteria are subjective. Even with "time-lapse" technology, it is not possible to identify with certainty embryos capable of successfully implanting [24]. Preimplantation genetic testing (PGT) is considered useful for discarding aneuploid (PGT-A) embryos to improve the implantation rate and reduce the miscarriage rate [25]. Many studies suggest that PGT-A can implement the use of elective SET (eSET), which selects first-quality embryos based on their morphology for transfer to patients undergoing ART [26], because the combination of the two approaches increases the live birth rate and reduces the multiple pregnancy rate [26]. There is also evidence that PGT-A in women between the ages of 35–40 can improve the clinical and live birth rates, and reduce the negative effects of maternal age on outcomes. However, the cumulative live birth rate does not appear to have improved [27,28]. Indeed, after more than 15 years, this technique still arouses some perplexity [29] because it is not possible to ascertain the ploidy of the whole embryo and, in particular, that of the inner cell mass with a sample of 5–7 cells taken from the trophectoderm. This uncertainty arises from several reasons: the high frequency of embryo mosaicism [30] due to chromosome instability [31], the ability of the embryo to recover from aneuploidy [32,33], and the birth of normal children after the transfer of aneuploid mosaic embryos [34]. Regarding mosaicism, a recent study conducted on 46 surplus cryopreserved preimplantation embryos demonstrated a low rate of cytogenetic concordance (48%) between the inner cell mass and trophectoderm. These results should suggest caution for the clinical application of PGT-A, considering that mosaicism was detected in 59% of embryos (n = 27/46) [35]. Accordingly, a recent meta-analysis showed no significant effect of PGT on the reduction of the miscarriage rate [36].

A particular concern in ART practice arises from embryo freezing, which leads to a growing number of embryos stored in cryobanks for an indefinite period of time. Indeed, there was a sharp increase in the United States (U.S.) from 2004 to 2013 of ART cycles in which all embryos have been frozen, and this resulted in a higher and increasing number of embryos stored [37], estimated to be 600,000 (or more) in the U.S. alone [38]. Concern about this topic can arise also in some countries where this practice is not allowed. In fact, in most countries, the mean age of women entering ART programs has seen an increasing trend (34.6% for the ART Italian registry and 20.4% for the U.S. Registry in 2019). Unfortunately, oocyte cryopreservation does not give acceptable results for a woman in the second half of her 30s and, particularly, for patients over 40 [39]. More recently, some authors describe a progression towards the industrialization of ART practices with possible negative consequences for couples such as a decline in ART birth rates [40], although personalized treatments should be a relevant aim for ART [41].

In this complex framework that shows possible limits and risks related to ART practices, we report the results of a personalized clinical practice used in a subgroup of women over 40 in our ART center. The protocol consisted of the selection of a limited number of oocytes to be injected, no more than the number of embryos to be transferred, and after a short time of embryo culture (two days or less). The primary aim of this retrospective study was to evaluate the success rate of this protocol in the light of some of the more widespread problems and emerging risks of ART practices.

2. Materials and Methods

2.1. Patient Selection

This clinical study included 245 ICSI cycles performed from January 2016 to July 2021 in 184 infertile couples with a female partner aged ≥40 years whose clinical charts were evaluated retrospectively. The mean age of the women was 42.4 ± 1.7 (range 40–47 years) and the mean of the previous failed ICSI attempts was 1.5 ± 1.9. The assessment of ovarian reserve was performed through antral follicular count (AFC) which was evaluated by the same experienced gynecologist (CM).

2.2. Controlled Ovarian Hyperstimulation

Controlled ovarian hyperstimulation protocols were performed using recombinant human follicle-stimulating hormone (rhFSH) (Gonal-F, Merck Serono, Geneva, Switzerland) according to ovarian reserve, and gonadotropin-releasing hormone (GnRH) antagonist (0.25 mg) from the day when a follicle reached 15 mm in diameter.

We also administered recombinant human luteinizing hormone (LH) at 75 IU (Luveris, Merck Serono, Geneva, Switzerland) every 12 h along with rhFSH increased by 75 IU during GnRH administration, according to data showing better outcomes in older female patients [42] and dramatic decrease in serum LH as a consequence of GnRH antagonist administration [43]. Follicular development monitoring was performed by real-time ultrasound scans from day 2 of the treatment cycle to the day of hCG administration based on the patient's response to stimulation. The response was monitored by ultrasound, and measurements of serum levels of 17ß-estradiol, progesterone, and FSH, including on weekends or holidays. When at least one ovarian follicle reached a diameter of 18–20 mm, ICSI was performed 36–38 h after administration of human chorionic gonadotropin (hCG, Gonasi, 10,000 IU) (IBSA, Lodi, Italy).

2.3. Oocyte Retrieval

Oocyte retrieval was scheduled on a 7-day basis and performed with local analgesia or under sedation 36–38 h after hCG administration based on response to ovarian stimulation.

2.4. Sperm Preparation

The first semen collection was obtained approximately 5–6 h before the microinjection of oocytes, which was scheduled approximately 40 h after the hCG administration to the female partner. All male partners had 2–7 days of abstinence, as suggested by the WHO 2010 criteria [44]. All semen samples were collected by ejaculation within the Fertility Center to minimize conditions that could alter sperm parameters/function. All semen analyses were performed by the same expert embryologist according to WHO 2010 criteria. The assessment of sperm motility was performed on a 10 µL drop on a slide with a 22×22 mm coverslip and a stage heated to 37 °C, with a reticule lens. The slides were examined with phase-contrast optics at a magnification of $400\times$. We evaluated 400 spermatozoa per replicate for an accurate assessment of motility. We asked male partners with severe oligoasthenozoospermia (OA) to provide a second consecutive ejaculation 1 h after the first, after explaining the possibility of having better sperm parameters in the second ejaculate [45,46].

2.5. Intracytoplasmic Sperm Injection Procedure

The ICSI procedure was performed with spermatozoa obtained by "swim-up" using the first or second ejaculate according to the sperm parameters of the male partner as described in Section 2.4. The "swim-up" technique was performed directly from the liquefied semen. For this purpose, several aliquots of semen were taken from each sample and placed in test tubes underneath an overlay of washing medium (Origio Italia Srl, Rome, Italy). Round-bottom tubes or four-well dishes were used to optimize the interface surface area between the semen layer and the culture medium. The samples were allowed to incubate at 37 °C in an incubator for 30–45 min. Spermatozoa with the best motility and ability to migrate were then collected.

Collected cumulus-enclosed oocytes were maintained in 500 µL of Continuous Single Culture™ Medium-Complete (CSCM-C) (Irvine Scientific, FujiFilm, Tilburg, the Netherlands) in 4-well multi-dishes (Nunclon Surface, Roskilde, Denmark) under oil (oil for embryo culture, Fuji Film, Europe), and maintained in the incubator for 2 h after their retrieval. Afterward, they were decumulated in hyaluronidase drops (Hyaluronidase Solution, Fuji Film, Europe). The ICSI procedure was performed according to the standard technique.

2.6. Selection of Oocytes and Transfer Policy

The choice of the oocyte to be inseminated was made after decumulation. The best oocytes to inseminate were those with the following characteristics: small perivitelline space and no granulation [47], intact first polar body (PB) [48,49], and a smooth surface [50]. We discarded oocytes with vacuolar cytoplasm or central granulation, ovoid-shaped formation [51], cytoplasmic inclusion [48], smooth endoplasmic reticulum (SER) aggregates [52], and refractive bodies [53]. Oocyte selection was also based on oolemma elasticity, a parameter that positively influences the outcome of ICSI. In particular, we have distinguished three different degrees based on the elasticity of the oolemma: grade A refers to oocytes that have penetrated the oolemma without the need for cytoplasmic aspiration (no elasticity); grade B refers to oocytes showing oolemma penetration requiring mild or moderate cytoplasmic aspiration (average elasticity); grade C refers to oocytes showing oolemma penetration requiring strong cytoplasmic aspiration (excessive elasticity). If no oocyte reached the highest grade, which is grade B, the closest grade was chosen based on the oolemma characteristics (grade C and, lastly, grade A).

Embryo culture was performed in a standard incubator at 37 °C under 6% CO_2 and 5% O_2 in CSCM-C (Irvine Scientific, FujiFilm, Tilburg, The Netherlands). Embryo transfer was usually performed after 2 days of culture. In some cases, the transfer was performed at the pronuclear stage. After 36–44 h of culture, all embryos were carefully examined with both a dissecting and an inverted microscope. The classification of the embryos was carried out according to the system proposed by Puissant [54]. The number and size of blastomeres as well as the presence or absence of anucleated fragments were carefully recorded so that embryos could be scored as follows: 4 = embryos with clear and regular blastomeres and no fragmentation or a maximum of five % of the embryo surface occupied with small anucleated fragments; 3 = embryos with few or no fragments but with unequal blastomeres (>1/3 difference in size); 2 = embryos with more fragments but less than 1/3 of the embryo surface; 1 = fragments on >1/3 of the embryo surface. Two points were added if the embryo had reached the 4-cell stage by 48 h after fertilization.

With regard to the maximum number of embryos to be transferred, we followed the guidelines of the Practice Committee of the American Society for Human Reproduction and Society for Assisted Reproductive Technology [9]. Therefore, in patients aged 40 years, three or four embryos could be transferred in the case of a particularly unfavorable prognosis; in patients aged 41–44 years, four embryos could be transferred, or even five when an unfavorable prognosis was present. A prognosis was considered unfavorable in the case of multiple previous ART cycle failures or no live births after an ART cycle. The informed consent was signed by the couples after an extensive discussion with the physicians on the maximum number of oocytes to be inseminated and, consequently, of embryos to be transferred. Eleven oocytes belonging to three couples were cryopreserved at their express request. In all cases, the selection of oocytes for the transfer of the resulting embryos was carried out according to the described criteria.

2.7. Ethical Approval

The study was conducted in the ART "Biofertility IVF Center" (Rome, Italy) on infertile couples undergoing ICSI treatment. It was reviewed and approved by the Institutional Review Board at the "Biofertility IVF Center", which indicated that ethical approval was not required for this study. Data collection followed the principles outlined in the Declaration of Helsinki. All patients provided their informed consent, agreeing to supply their anonymous information for this and future studies.

2.8. Statistical Analysis

Quantitative data were reported as mean $\pm$ SD throughout the study. The following rates were calculated: fertilization rate (FR = number of fertilized oocytes/number of oocytes inseminated), implantation rate (IR = number of gestational sacs/number of embryos transferred), clinical pregnancy rate (CPR = number of pregnancies with at least one fetal heartbeat/number of pick-up cycles with at least one oocyte retrieved), live birth delivery rate (LBR = number of deliveries with at least 1 live birth/number of pick-up with at least 1 oocyte retrieved), miscarriage rate (MR = number of spontaneous abortions/total number of pregnancies), and cumulative live birth rate (CLBR = number of deliveries with at least 1 live birth/total number of women with aspirated oocyte(s)) were calculated. Data were analyzed with SPSS 23.0 for Windows (SPSS Inc., Chicago, IL, USA).

3. Results

A total of 245 ICSI cycles performed in 184 couples with female partners aged $\geq$40 years were considered. Among the 184 couples enrolled, 39 couples underwent two ICSI cycles, 7 couples three attempts, and 2 couples four cycles.

Table 1 shows the clinical and demographic characteristics of the couples enrolled in this study and their previous failed ICSI attempts, which include both attempts performed in our and other ART centers. In six cycles, no oocytes were retrieved. Considering the repeated attempts for each couple, only two women had no transfer. Therefore, 182 women aged $\geq$40 years underwent 239 cycles with oocyte retrieval and embryo transfer. A total of 705 embryos were transferred with a mean number of 2.9 $\pm$ 1.4 embryos per transfer. In 35 cycles, the embryos were transferred at the pronuclear stage.

Twenty-four women have had at least one pregnancy. All pregnancies occurred in women between the ages of 40 and 44 years. As reported in the Materials and Methods section, according to the guidelines of the Practice Committee of the American Society for Human Reproduction and Society for Assisted Reproductive Technology [9], we transferred a maximum of five embryos when an unfavorable prognosis was present. In total, we transferred five embryos in 48 cycles of our cohort. Interestingly, all pregnancies occurred when at least three embryos were transferred, except in five cases where two embryos were transferred. In detail, if we consider the 24 cycles with pregnancy leading to delivery and live birth: in half of them (12 cycles), five embryos were transferred; in five cases, four embryos were transferred; in two cases, three and in five cases, two. Of the 24 pregnancies, four were twins; in three of those cases, five embryos were transferred, while in one case five embryos were transferred. No triplets occurred. In Table 3, we report the number and grade of embryos transferred and the related success rates. Four pregnancies with deliveries occurred among 35 cycles with embryo transfer at the pronuclear stage, with a LBR of 11.4% (4/35), and included the two cycles with women at 44 years ending with normal delivery. Table 4 presents the LBR based on the age of the women. The twenty-four women who achieved pregnancy had a previous mean failure of 1.9 $\pm$ 1.8. The causes of infertility of the couples enrolled are reported in Figure 1.

Table 1. Demographic and clinical characteristics of the female and male partners of the couples enrolled in this study.

Parameters	Results
Women	
Age (years, mean ± SD)	42.4 ± 1.7
Antral follicle count (mean ± SD)	8.4 ± 4.9
Total dosage of gonadotropin administered (IU) (mean ± SD)	3376.6 ± 1335.9
Men	
Age (years, mean ± SD)	43.9 ± 5.9
Sperm concentration (mil/mL, mean ± SD)	46.7 ± 40.6
Total sperm motility (%, mean ± SD)	47.4 ± 21.3
Progressive sperm motility (%, mean ± SD)	26.3 ± 16.8
Spermatozoa with normal morphology (%, mean ± SD)	15.2 ± 10.3
Couples	
Number of previous ART failures (mean ± SD)	1.5 ± 2

Legend: IU: international unit.

The outcomes of ICSI cycles are shown in Table 2.

Table 2. Intracytoplasmic sperm injection outcomes.

Fresh cycles	245
Number of oocytes retrieved (mean ± SD)	5.2 ± 4.1
Number of oocytes inseminated (mean ± SD)	3.1 ± 1.5
Number of oocytes fertilized (mean ± SD)	3.1 ± 1.5
Number of oocytes cryopreserved (mean ± SD)	0.06 ± 0.5
Peak of stimulated 17ß-estradiol (pg/mL)	1271.0 ± 744.5
Fertilization rate Number of fertilized oocytes/number of oocytes inseminated (%)	715/747 (95.7%)
Implantation rate Number of gestational sacs/number of embryos transferred (%)	47/705 (6.7%)
Clinical pregnancy rate Number of pregnancies with least 1 fetal heartbeat/number of pick-up cycles with at least 1 oocyte (%)	31/239 (13%)
Live birth delivery rate Number of deliveries with at least 1 live birth/number of pick-ups with at least 1 oocyte (%) • Singletons • Twins	24/239 (10%) 20 4 (16.7%)
Birth weight (g, mean ± SD)	3112.3 ± 698.9
Miscarriage rate Number of spontaneous abortion/total number of gestational sacs (%)	23/47 (48.9%)
Cumulative live birth rate Number of deliveries with at least 1 live birth/total number of women starting treatment (%)	24/184 (13%)

Table 3. Number and grade of embryos transferred and related success rates.

Number of Embryos Transferred	Total Number of Embryo-Transfers	Embryos Grade I	Embryos Grade II	Embryos Grade III–IV	PN	Live Births	Twin Birth	Multiple Births (≥ 3)
1	n = 42 (17.6%)	n = 23	n = 10	n = 4	n = 5	n = 0	n = 0	n = 0
2	n = 59 (24.7%)	n = 69	n = 32	n = 1	n = 16	n = 5	n = 0	n = 0
3	n = 55 (23.0%)	n = 97	n = 39	n = 5	n = 24	n = 2	n = 1	n = 0
4	n = 35 (14.6%)	n = 91	n = 27	n = 5	n = 17	n = 5	n = 0	n = 0
5	n = 48 (20.1%)	n = 156	n = 54	n = 14	n = 16	n = 12	n = 3	n = 0

Legend: grade I = blastomeres of equal size, without fragmentation or with <10% fragmentation; grade II = slight asymmetry between blastomeres and fragmentation of 10–25%; grade III–IV = asymmetric blastomeres and fragmentation of ≥ 35%. Abbreviations: PN = pronuclear stage.

Table 4. Live birth rates based on the woman's age and the number of cases (n).

Age of Women (Years)	Number of Live Births (%)
40 (n = 33)	7/24 (29.2%)
41 (n = 53)	6/24 (25%)
42 (n = 51)	5/24 (20.8%)
43 (n = 42)	4/24 (16.7%)
44 (n = 39)	2/24 (8.3%)
≥ 45 (n = 27)	0/24 (0%)

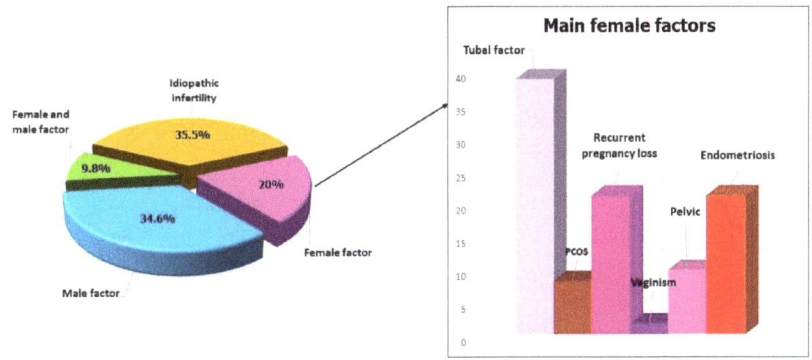

Figure 1. (**Left panel**): Main causes of infertility found in the 184 couples enrolled in this study. (**Right panel**): Detail of the main causes of female infertility.

4. Discussion

The results of the present study indicate that the selection of oocytes before ICSI to obtain a predetermined number of fresh cleaved embryos to be transferred is effective in terms of FR and LBR in a group of women ≥ 40 years. Our delivery rate (number of monitored deliveries/number of pick-ups or DR) was not lower than that of the Italian registry for the same age group (4.7% = 728/15,419) published in 2019 and not far from all age groups (11.2% = 5151/46,090) [55]. Furthermore, we reported a cumulative delivery rate (CLBR) for fresh cycle of 13%, whereas the Italian registry reported a CLBR of 5.9% for women aged between 40–42 years and 1.6% for women aged ≥ 43 years. With regard to

CLBR per pick up, the Italian registry listed 10.3% for women aged between 40–42 years and 3.2% for women aged ≥ 43 years, whereas the U.S. registry reported a cumulative transfer live birth delivery (LBD) rate per pick-up of 13% in 2019 [56]. It should be noted that the CLBR with frozen embryos rules out cycles unable to give enough embryos for freezing procedures.

With regard to the success rate of blastocyst transfer in aged women, Tannus and colleagues reported a higher LBR than ours (21.6%), although the mean AFC was 14, mean of previous failed cycles was 0.5, and oocytes collected was 11 [57]. Our patient group exhibited a less favorable AFC (8.4) and a higher number of previous failed ART cycles (1.5 ± 1.9) (Table 1). In another study conducted by De Croo and colleagues, in women with a mean age of 35 years, the comparison of LBRs with transfer at the blastocyst stage (1 or 2 embryos) versus cleaved embryos was 21.1% and 19.1%, respectively [13].

A specific and usual reason for long-term embryo culture up to the blastocyst stage is to perform PGT-A. Apart from the reduced rate of blastocyst formation in patients over 40 years of age, several concerns have been raised for the PGT-A technique, such as the high genetic mosaicism rate, which interferes with the precise evaluation of embryo chromosomal arrangement and the mismatch in the aneuploidy rate between the trophectoderm and the inner cell mass [29]. Furthermore, increased obstetric and perinatal risks are reported with PGT-A compared with non-PGT-A cycles, particularly the development of hypertension in pregnancy [58]. However, PGT-A has become the most widely utilized add-on procedure in ART practice [29] and is a reference for validating or at least comparing the results of many clinical trials in the U.S.

One of the possible advantages of reconsidering embryo transfer in the cleavage stage is the epigenetic risk after embryo exposure to a long culture environment in terms of fetal health. Many studies have shown that extended embryo culture significantly affects obstetric and perinatal outcomes [19,59–61]. Large-for-gestational age/macrosomia, hypertensive disorders, and perinatal mortality appear to increase with frozen embryo transfer [62]. Vroman and colleagues have demonstrated that embryo culture from the one-cell to blastocyst stage results in placental overgrowth, reduced fetal weight, and lower placental DNA methylation in rats [63]. Surprisingly, a recent study demonstrated that human genomic activation initiates at the one-cell stage [64].

There is evidence that the longer the in vitro cultures last (i.e., blastocyst transfer in comparison to the cleavage stage), the more epigenetic changes occur [65,66]. We know that only a percentage of fertilized oocytes arrive at the blastocyst stage in vitro and recent observations suggest that metabolic and epigenetic dysfunctions underlie the arrest of human ART embryos before their compaction [67].

From a biological point of view, we cannot rule out the existence of better "culture" conditions for embryos in uterus rather than in vitro (temperature, pH, osmolarity, and numerous unknown factors). Interestingly the LBR subsequent to transfer at the pronuclear stage (at 44 years, two of them delivered at term without obstetric or perinatal complications) does not seem negligible (11.4%), supporting the idea that an artificial incubator environment might be more stressful than that within the uterus for embryos in older women. Most of the studies on obstetric and perinatal risk in ART are linked to placental abnormalities that are increased when ART is the chosen treatment of infertility, particularly in more stressful conditions for embryos, such as long-term cultures and PGT-A [68].

Concerns about the possible consequences of ICSI for the health of the offspring have been reported since its first introduction into clinical practice [69]. Although ICSI use was associated with a significantly higher risk of congenital malformations [70], other studies did not report a significant difference in terms of congenital malformation between children conceived with IVF/ICSI compared to natural conception [71,72]. A recent systematic review and meta-analysis showed no differences in the epigenetic effects of offspring between couples treated with ICSI or traditional IVF [73]. In summary, after many decades of ICSI practice and according to most reports, children born after ICSI have perinatal outcomes comparable to those conceived after standard IVF.

With regard to the possible success rate of oocyte selection in ART practice, in 2004 and for many years, the Italian ART legislation limited the maximum number of oocytes to be fertilized during an ART cycle to three, and all resulting embryos had to be transferred at once due to the banning of embryo cryopreservation [74]. Ragni and colleagues, in a study including 1861 cycles performed in seven Italian fertility centers, showed that the pregnancy rate per oocyte retrieval and the rate of multiple pregnancies before and after the new law were 27 and 24.2% ($p = 0.18$), and 25.8 and 20.9% ($p = 0.11$), respectively [68]. It is worth noting that in countries such as Germany and Switzerland, it is impossible to cryopreserve embryos and selection is based on oocytes at the pronuclear stage.

Regarding the problem of twin pregnancy rate, our results (16.7%) appear acceptable, considering that the Italian registry showed a rate of 10.6% in 2019 and it was 16.9% in Europe [75]. Recent reports criticize the SET policy in favor of double embryo transfer at the blastocyst stage [6]. However, our transfers were performed at the cleavage stage, in which a higher number of embryos transferred is to be considered comparable with a lower number at the blastocyst stage. Considering the risk of twin or multiple-order pregnancies and their resultant cost, the results of our study should be taken with caution for general clinical practice. Indeed, as reported in Table 3, in a considerable number of cycles we decided to transfer three or more embryos because there was a poor prognosis. At present, insemination with the transfer of more than two embryos should not be a routinely offered practice, even though the latest U.S. guidelines allow the transfer of more than two embryos for older women, low-quality embryos, and repeated implantation failures. On the other hand, blastocyst transfer is associated with a higher risk of monozygotic twinning (MZT) [76] which has a more severe prognosis than dizygotic twinning for the risk of twin-to-twin transfusion due to their shared placenta. After 8435 frozen-thawed single blastocyst transfers with hormone replacement treatment, MZT was observed in 2.32% of cases [77], while the natural prevalence was 0.4% [78]. However, the transfer of a very limited number of embryos at their cleavage stage after insemination of selected oocytes may represent a practical option in cases of high risk for twin or multiple pregnancies.

Clinical trials with a mix of oocyte selection and embryo selection at the cleavage stage may be considered, even in couples with female partners under the age of 40. It could represent a kind of double selection in order to simultaneously reduce the obstetric/epigenetic risk and the risk of multiple pregnancies.

Regarding the efficiency of oocyte selection, we notice that our FR was higher (95.7%) compared with the usually reported data such as that of ESHRE/Alpha consensus ($\geq 65\%$ for competence value) [11], probably due to a selection of oocytes based on multiple morphologic elements studies [48,49,79].

We recognize that oocyte selection in ART is mostly still imperfect, mainly because it is subjective. However, with the introduction of artificial intelligence in ART, new tools may be available to promote more objective observations [80,81], as we have previously proved [82]. Nevertheless, we should not forget that even the current embryo selection is also a subjective laboratory procedure. The possible transition from embryo to oocyte selection, using more reliable methods, could provide us with valuable information on the relationship between oocyte quality and stimulation protocols and, consequently, embryo development.

In summary, our study showed the success rate and twin delivery rate in women over the age of 40 using a protocol with oocyte (rather than embryo) selection and transfer of embryos in the cleavage stage. Non-negligible LBR and moderate multiple pregnancy rates were recorded. No embryos were frozen.

The application in clinical practice of the results described in the present study can be relevant for geographical areas where embryo freezing is not possible for ethical reasons or law restrictions, or for couples with low prognosis with a female partner aged ≥ 40 who do not accept oocyte donation.

Furthermore, the financial implications and cost/benefits of this protocol, i.e., strong personalization and drug use, are to be considered. In this regard, milder stimulation for this group of patients based on their residual ovarian reserve could offer similar chances of success. The small size of this subgroup of patients undergoing ART and the lack of a control group are the main limitations of our study. However, we enrolled a particular group of couples with female partners aged ≥40 years, which made it difficult to establish a control group. Certainly, further prospective randomized controlled trials are needed to assess the relevance of our retrospective findings.

5. Conclusions

In conclusion, the possibility of oocyte selection and embryo transfer at the cleavage stage appears to be a reasonable strategy in older women who have reduced ovarian reserve and a high number of previous ART failures. As clinicians, we should consider current trends in reproductive medicine from a broad perspective, taking into account all possible consequences involving obstetricians, neonatologists, pediatricians and all other professionals interested in the long-term health consequences of ART laboratory practice. Although further studies are needed to confirm these findings, our preliminary results suggest that a return to more natural steps in reproductive medicine may be safer if the obstetric risks and epigenetic consequences on offspring linked to long-term culture protocols are confirmed in the future.

Author Contributions: Conceptualization, C.M.; methodology, A.F. and C.M.; formal analysis, F.B.; data curation, A.F. and F.S.; writing—original draft preparation, C.M.; writing—review and editing, F.B., A.E.C. and C.M.; supervision, A.E.C. and C.M. All authors have read and agreed to the published version of the manuscript.

Funding: This research received no external funding.

Informed Consent Statement: Informed consent was obtained from all subjects involved in the study.

Conflicts of Interest: The authors declare no conflict of interest.

References

1. Steptoe, P.C.; Edwards, R.G. Birth after the reimplantation of a human embryo. *Lancet* **1978**, *312*, 366. [CrossRef]
2. Gardner, D.K.; Lane, M. Culture and selection of viable blastocysts: A feasible proposition for human IVF? *Hum. Reprod. Updat.* **1997**, *3*, 367–382. [CrossRef] [PubMed]
3. Gardner, D.K.; Schoolcraft, W.B.; Wagley, L.; Schlenker, T.; Stevens, J.; Hesla, J. A prospective randomized trial of blastocyst culture and transfer in in- vitro fertilization. *Hum. Reprod.* **1998**, *13*, 3434–3440. [CrossRef]
4. Blake, D.A.; Farquhar, C.M.; Johnson, N.; Proctor, M. Cleavage stage versus blastocyst stage embryo transfer in assisted conception. *Cochrane Database Syst. Rev.* **2007**, *4*, CD002118. [CrossRef]
5. Glujovsky, D.; Retamar, A.M.Q.; Sedo, C.R.A.; Ciapponi, A.; Cornelisse, S.; Blake, D. Cleavage-stage versus blastocyst-stage embryo transfer in assisted reproductive technology. *Cochrane Database Syst. Rev.* **2022**, *2022*, 1465–1858. [CrossRef]
6. Vilska, S.; Tiitinen, A.; Hydén-Granskog, C.; Hovatta, O. Elective transfer of one embryo results in an acceptable pregnancy rate and eliminates the risk of multiple birth. *Hum. Reprod.* **1999**, *14*, 2392–2395. [CrossRef] [PubMed]
7. Kamath, M.S.; Mascarenhas, M.; Kirubakaran, R.; Bhattacharya, S. Number of embryos for transfer following in vitro fertili-sation or intra-cytoplasmic sperm injection. *Cochrane Database Syst. Rev.* **2020**, *8*, CD003416. [PubMed]
8. Monteleone, P.A.; Petersen, P.G.; Peregrino, P.F.; Miorin, J.; Gomes, A.P.; Fujii, M.G.; De Martin, H.; Bonetti, T.C.; Gonçalves, S.P. Should single embryo transfer be used in patients with any kind of infertility factor? Preliminary outcomes. *JBRA Assist. Reprod.* **2019**, *23*, 200–204. [CrossRef]
9. Practice Committee of the American Society for Reproductive Medicine; Practice Committee of the Society for Assisted Reproductive Technology. Guidance on the limits to the number of embryos to transfer: A committee opinion. *Fertil. Steril.* **2017**, *107*, 901–903. [CrossRef] [PubMed]
10. Chambers, G.M.; Ledger, W. The economic implications of multiple pregnancy following ART. *Semin. Fetal Neonatal Med.* **2014**, *19*, 254–261. [CrossRef]
11. ESHRE Special Interest Group of Embryology and Alpha Scientists in Reproductive Medicine. The Vienna consensus: Report of an expert meeting on the development of ART labor-atory performance indicators. *Reprod. Biomed. Online* **2017**, *35*, 494–510. [CrossRef] [PubMed]
12. Sainte-Rose, R.; Petit, C.; Dijols, L.; Frapsauce, C.; Guerif, F. Extended embryo culture is effective for patients of an advanced maternal age. *Sci. Rep.* **2021**, *11*, 13499. [CrossRef] [PubMed]
13. De Croo, I.; Colman, R.; De Sutter, P.; Tilleman, K. Blastocyst transfer for all? Higher cumulative live birth chance in a blas-tocyst-stage transfer policy compared to a cleavage-stage transfer policy. *Facts Views Vis. Obgyn.* **2019**, *11*, 169–176. [PubMed]

14. Gleicher, N.; Orvieto, R. Transferring more than one embryo simultaneously is justifiable in most patients. *Reprod. Biomed. Online* **2022**, *44*, 1–4. [CrossRef]
15. Ernstad, E.G.; Bergh, C.; Khatibi, A.; Källén, K.B.; Westlander, G.; Nilsson, S.; Wennerholm, U.-B. Neonatal and maternal outcome after blastocyst transfer: A population-based registry study. *Am. J. Obstet. Gynecol.* **2016**, *214*, 378.e1–378.e10. [CrossRef]
16. Makinen, S.; Soderstrom-Anttila, V.; Vainio, J.; Suikkari, A.-M.; Tuuri, T. Does long in vitro culture promote large for gestational age babies? *Hum. Reprod.* **2013**, *28*, 828–834. [CrossRef]
17. Ishihara, O.; Araki, R.; Kuwahara, A.; Itakura, A.; Saito, H.; Adamson, G.D. Impact of frozen-thawed single-blastocyst transfer on maternal and neonatal outcome: An analysis of 277,042 single-embryo transfer cycles from 2008 to 2010 in Japan. *Fertil. Steril.* **2014**, *101*, 128–133. [CrossRef]
18. Zhu, J.; Lin, S.; Li, M.; Chen, L.; Lian, Y.; Liu, P.; Qiao, J. Effect of in vitro culture period on birthweight of singleton newborns. *Hum. Reprod.* **2014**, *29*, 448–454. [CrossRef]
19. Huang, J.; Yang, X.; Wu, J.; Kuang, Y.; Wang, Y. Impact of Day 7 Blastocyst Transfer on Obstetric and Perinatal Outcome of Singletons Born After Vitrified-Warmed Embryo Transfer. *Front. Physiol.* **2020**, *11*, 74. [CrossRef]
20. Katari, S.; Turan, N.; Bibikova, M.; Erinle, O.; Chalian, R.; Foster, M.; Gaughan, J.P.; Coutifaris, C.; Sapienza, C. DNA methylation and gene expression differences in children conceived in vitro or in vivo. *Hum. Mol. Genet.* **2009**, *18*, 3769–3778. [CrossRef]
21. Nelissen, E.C.; van Montfoort, A.P.; Dumoulin, J.C.; Evers, J.L. Epigenetics and the placenta. *Hum. Reprod. Updat.* **2011**, *17*, 397–417. [CrossRef] [PubMed]
22. Novakovic, B.; Rakyan, V.; Ng, H.K.; Manuelpillai, U.; Dewi, C.; Wong, N.; Morley, R.; Down, T.; Beck, S.; Craig, J.M.; et al. Specific tumour-associated methylation in normal human term placenta and first-trimester cytotrophoblasts. *Mol. Hum. Reprod.* **2008**, *14*, 547–554. [CrossRef] [PubMed]
23. Sciorio, R.; Tramontano, L.; Rapalini, E.; Bellaminutti, S.; Bulletti, F.M.; D'Amato, A.; Manna, C.; Palagiano, A.; Bulletti, C.; Esteves, S.C. Risk of genetic and epigenetic alteration in children conceived following ART: Is it time to return to nature whenever possible? *Clin. Genet.* **2022**. [CrossRef]
24. ESHRE Working group on Time-lapse technology; Apter, S.; Ebner, T.; Freour, T.; Guns, Y.; Kovacic, B.; Le Clef, N.; Marques, M.; Meseguer, M.; Montjean, D.; et al. Good practice recommendations for the use of time-lapse technology. *Hum. Reprod. Open* **2020**, *2020*, hoaa008. [CrossRef] [PubMed]
25. Munné, S. Status of preimplantation genetic testing and embryo selection. *Reprod. Biomed. Online* **2018**, *37*, 393–396. [CrossRef]
26. Ubaldi, F.M.; Capalbo, A.; Colamaria, S.; Ferrero, S.; Maggiulli, R.; Vajta, G.; Sapienza, F.; Cimadomo, D.; Giuliani, M.; Gravotta, E.; et al. Reduction of multiple pregnancies in the advanced maternal age population after im-plementation of an elective single embryo transfer policy coupled with enhanced embryo selection: Pre-and post-intervention study. *Hum. Reprod.* **2015**, *30*, 2097–2106. [CrossRef]
27. Munné, S.; Kaplan, B.; Frattarelli, J.L.; Child, T.; Nakhuda, G.; Shamma, F.N.; Silverberg, K.; Kalista, T.; Handyside, A.H.; Katz-Jaffe, M.; et al. Preimplantation genetic testing for aneuploidy versus morphology as selection criteria for single frozen-thawed embryo transfer in good-prognosis patients: A multicenter randomized clinical trial. *Fertil. Steril.* **2019**, *112*, 1071–1079. [CrossRef]
28. Kang, H.J.; Melnick, A.P.; Stewart, J.D.; Xu, K.; Rosenwaks, Z. Preimplantation genetic screening: Who benefits? *Fertil. Steril.* **2016**, *106*, 597–602. [CrossRef]
29. Gleicher, N.; Patrizio, P.; Brivanlou, A. Preimplantation Genetic Testing for Aneuploidy—A Castle Built on Sand. *Trends Mol. Med.* **2021**, *27*, 731–742. [CrossRef]
30. Taylor, T.H.; Gitlin, S.A.; Patrick, J.L.; Crain, J.L.; Wilson, J.M.; Griffin, D.K. The origin, mechanisms, incidence and clinical consequences of chromosomal mosaicism in humans. *Hum. Reprod. Updat.* **2014**, *20*, 571–581. [CrossRef]
31. Vanneste, E.; Voet, T.; Le Caignec, C.; Ampe, M.; Konings, P.; Melotte, C.; Debrock, S.; Amyere, M.; Vikkula, M.; Schuit, F.; et al. Chromosome instability is common in human cleavage-stage embryos. *Nat. Med.* **2009**, *15*, 577–583. [CrossRef] [PubMed]
32. Bolton, H.; Graham, S.; Van Der Aa, N.; Kumar, P.; Theunis, K.; Gallardo, E.F.; Voet, T.; Zernicka-Goetz, M. Mouse model of chromosome mosaicism reveals lineage-specific depletion of aneuploid cells and normal developmental potential. *Nat. Commun.* **2016**, *7*, 11165. [CrossRef] [PubMed]
33. Orvieto, R.; Shimon, C.; Rienstein, S.; Jonish-Grossman, A.; Shani, H.; Aizer, A. Do human embryos have the ability of self-correction? *Reprod. Biol. Endocrinol.* **2020**, *18*, 98. [CrossRef] [PubMed]
34. Greco, E.; Minasi, M.G.; Fiorentino, F. Healthy Babies after Intrauterine Transfer of Mosaic Aneuploid Blastocysts. *N. Engl. J. Med.* **2015**, *373*, 2089–2090. [CrossRef] [PubMed]
35. Chavli, E.; van den Born, M.; Eleveld, C.; Boter, M.; van Marion, R.; Hoefsloot, L.; Laven, J.; Baart, E.; Van Opstal, D. Chromosomal mosaicism in human blastocysts: A cytogenetic comparison of trophectoderm and inner cell mass after next-generation sequencing. *Reprod. Biomed. Online* **2022**, *45*, 867–877. [CrossRef]
36. Simopoulou, M.; Sfakianoudis, K.; Maziotis, E.; Tsioulou, P.; Grigoriadis, S.; Rapani, A.; Giannelou, P.; Asimakopoulou, M.; Kokkali, G.; Pantou, A.; et al. PGT-A: Who and when? A systematic review and network meta-analysis of RCTs. *J. Assist. Reprod. Genet.* **2021**, *38*, 1939–1957. [CrossRef]
37. Christianson, M.S.; Stern, J.E.; Sun, F.; Zhang, H.; Styer, A.K.; Vitek, W.; Polotsky, A.J. Embryo cryopreservation and utilization in the United States from 2004–2013. *F&S Rep.* **2020**, *1*, 71–77. [CrossRef]
38. Hairston, J.C.; Kohlmeier, A.; Feinberg, E.C. Compassionate embryo transfer: Physician practices and perspectives. *Fertil. Steril.* **2020**, *114*, 552–557. [CrossRef]

39. Stoop, D. Social oocyte freezing. *Facts, Views Vis. ObGyn* **2010**, *2*, 31–34. [PubMed]
40. Gleicher, N.; Kushnir, V.A.; Barad, D.H. Worldwide decline of IVF birth rates and its probable causes. *Hum. Reprod. Open* **2019**, *2019*, hoz017. [CrossRef]
41. Simón, C. Personalized assisted reproductive technology. *Fertil. Steril.* **2013**, *100*, 922–923. [CrossRef]
42. Conforti, A.; Esteves, S.C.; Humaidan, P.; Longobardi, S.; D'Hooghe, T.; Orvieto, R.; Vaiarelli, A.; Cimadomo, D.; Rienzi, L.; Ubaldi, F.M.; et al. Recombinant human luteinizing hormone co-treatment in ovarian stimulation for assisted reproductive technology in women of advanced reproductive age: A systematic review and meta-analysis of randomized controlled trials. *Reprod. Biol. Endocrinol.* **2021**, *19*, 91. [CrossRef] [PubMed]
43. Westergaard, L.G.; Laursen, S.B.; Andersen, C.Y. Increased risk of early pregnancy loss by profound suppression of luteinizing hormone during ovarian stimulation in normogonadotrophic women undergoing assisted reproduction. *Hum. Reprod.* **2000**, *15*, 1003–1008. [CrossRef]
44. World Health Organization. *WHO Laboratory Manual for the Examination and Processing of Human Semen*, 5th ed.; World Health Organization: Geneva, Switzerland, 2010; ISBN 978-92-4-154778-9.
45. Manna, C.; Barbagallo, F.; Manzo, R.; Rahman, A.; Francomano, D.; Calogero, A.E. Sperm Parameters before and after Swim-Up of a Second Ejaculate after a Short Period of Abstinence. *J. Clin. Med.* **2020**, *9*, 1029. [CrossRef] [PubMed]
46. Barbagallo, F.; Calogero, A.E.; Condorelli, R.A.; Farrag, A.; Jannini, E.A.; La Vignera, S.; Manna, C. Does a Very Short Length of Abstinence Improve Assisted Reproductive Technique Outcomes in Infertile Patients with Severe Oligo-Asthenozoospermia? *J. Clin. Med.* **2021**, *10*, 4399. [CrossRef]
47. Ubaldi, F.; Rienzi, L. Morphological Selection of Gametes. *Placenta* **2008**, *29*, 115–120. [CrossRef]
48. Xia, P. Intracytoplasmic sperm injection: Correlation of oocyte grade based on polar body, perivitelline space and cytoplasmic inclusions with fertilization rate and embryo quality. *Hum. Reprod.* **1997**, *12*, 1750–1755. [CrossRef] [PubMed]
49. Ebner, T.; Yaman, C.; Moser, M.; Sommergruber, M.; Feichtinger, O.; Tews, G. Prognostic value of first polar body morphology on fertilization rate and embryo quality in intracytoplasmic sperm injection. *Hum. Reprod.* **2000**, *15*, 427–430. [CrossRef]
50. Ebner, T.; Moser, M.; Sommergruber, M.; Yaman, C.; Pfleger, U.; Tews, G. First polar body morphology and blastocyst formation rate in ICSI patients. *Hum. Reprod.* **2002**, *17*, 2415–2418. [CrossRef]
51. Ebner, T.; Moser, M.; Shebl, O.; Sommerguber, M.; Tews, G. Prognosis of oocytes showing aggregation of smooth endoplasmic reticulum. *Reprod. Biomed. Online* **2008**, *16*, 113–118. [CrossRef]
52. Setti, A.S.; Figueira, R.C.S.; de Almeida Ferreira Braga, D.P.; Azevedo, M.D.C.; Iaconelli, A.; Borges, E. Oocytes with smooth endoplasmic reticulum clusters originate blastocysts with impaired implantation potential. *Fertil. Steril.* **2016**, *106*, 1718–1724. [CrossRef]
53. Otsuki, J.; Nagai, Y.; Chiba, K. Lipofuscin bodies in human oocytes as an indicator of oocyte quality. *J. Assist. Reprod. Genet.* **2007**, *24*, 263–270. [CrossRef]
54. Puissant, F.; Van Rysselberge, M.; Barlow, P.; Deweze, J.; Leroy, F. Embryo scoring as a prognostic tool in IVF treatment. *Hum. Reprod.* **1987**, *2*, 705–708. [CrossRef] [PubMed]
55. *Assisted Reproductive Technology National Registry*; National Institute of Health: Rome, Italy, 2019.
56. *Assisted Reproductive Technology (ART) Fertility Clinic and National Summary Report 2019*; National Center for Chronic Disease Prevention and Health Promotion. US Dept of Health and Human Services 200: Washington, DC, USA, 2021.
57. Tannus, S.; Son, W.-Y.; Dahan, M. Elective single blastocyst transfer in advanced maternal age. *J. Assist. Reprod. Genet.* **2017**, *34*, 741–748. [CrossRef]
58. Makhijani, R.; Bartels, C.B.; Godiwala, P.; Bartolucci, A.; DiLuigi, A.; Nulsen, J.; Grow, D.; Benadiva, C.; Engmann, L. Impact of trophectoderm biopsy on obstetric and perinatal outcomes following frozen–thawed embryo transfer cycles. *Hum. Reprod.* **2021**, *36*, 340–348. [CrossRef] [PubMed]
59. Fernando, D.; Halliday, J.L.; Breheny, S.; Healy, D.L. Outcomes of singleton births after blastocyst versus non blastocyst transfer in assisted reproductive technology. *Fertil. Steril.* **2012**, *97*, 579–584. [CrossRef] [PubMed]
60. Martins, W.P.; Nastri, C.O.; Rienzi, L.; van der Poel, S.Z.; Gracia, C.; Racowsky, C. Blastocyst vs cleavage-stage embryo transfer: Systematic review and meta-analysis of reproductive outcomes. *Ultrasound Obstet. Gynecol.* **2016**, *49*, 583–591. [CrossRef]
61. Alviggi, C.; Conforti, A.; Carbone, I.F.; Borrelli, R.; De Placido, G.; Guerriero, S. Influence of cryopreservation on perinatal outcome after blastocyst- vs cleavage-stage embryo transfer: Systematic review and meta-analysis. *Ultrasound Obstet. Gynecol.* **2018**, *51*, 54–63. [CrossRef]
62. Orvieto, R.; Kirshenbaum, M.; Gleicher, N. Is Embryo Cryopreservation Causing Macrosomia—And What Else? *Front. Endocrinol.* **2020**, *11*, 19. [CrossRef]
63. Vrooman, L.A.; Rhon-Calderon, E.A.; Chao, O.Y.; Nguyen, D.K.; Narapareddy, L.; Dahiya, A.K.; Putt, M.E.; Schultz, R.M.; Bartolomei, M.S. Assisted reproductive technologies induce temporally specific placental defects and the preeclampsia risk marker sFLT1 in mouse. *Development* **2020**, *147*, dev186551. [CrossRef]
64. Asami, M.; Lam, B.Y.H.; Ma, M.K.; Rainbow, K.; Braun, S.; VerMilyea, M.D.; Yeo, G.S.H.; Perry, A.C.F. Human embryonic genome activation initiates at the one-cell stage. *Cell Stem. Cell* **2022**, *29*, 209–216.e4. [CrossRef] [PubMed]
65. Cagnone, G.; Sirard, M.-A. The embryonic stress response to in vitro culture: Insight from genomic analysis. *Reproduction* **2016**, *152*, R247–R261. [CrossRef]

66. Maheshwari, A.; Hamilton, M.; Bhattacharya, S. Should we be promoting embryo transfer at blastocyst stage? *Reprod. Biomed. Online* **2016**, *32*, 142–146. [CrossRef]
67. Yang, Y.; Shi, L.; Fu, X.; Ma, G.; Yang, Z.; Li, Y.; Zhou, Y.; Yuan, L.; Xia, Y.; Zhong, X.; et al. Metabolic and epigenetic dysfunctions underlie the arrest of in vitro fertilized human embryos in a senescent-like state. *PLoS Biol.* **2022**, *20*, e3001682. [CrossRef]
68. Ragni, G.; Allegra, A.; Anserini, P.; Causio, F.; Ferraretti, A.P.; Greco, E.; Palermo, R.; Somigliana, E. The 2004 Italian legislation regulating assisted reproduction technology: A multicentre survey on the results of IVF cycles. *Hum. Reprod.* **2005**, *20*, 2224–2228. [CrossRef] [PubMed]
69. Palermo, G.; Joris, H.; Devroey, P.; Van Steirteghem, A.C. Pregnancies after intracytoplasmic injection of single spermatozoon into an oocyte. *Lancet* **1992**, *340*, 17–18. [CrossRef]
70. Li, Z.; Wang, A.Y.; Bowman, M.; Hammarberg, K.; Farquhar, C.; Johnson, L.; Safi, N.; A Sullivan, E. ICSI does not increase the cumulative live birth rate in non-male factor infertility. *Hum. Reprod.* **2018**, *33*, 1322–1330. [CrossRef]
71. De Rycke, M.; Liebaers, I.; Van Steirteghem, A. Epigenetic risks related to assisted reproductive technologies: Risk analysis and epigenetic inheritance. *Hum. Reprod.* **2002**, *17*, 2487–2494. [CrossRef] [PubMed]
72. Ben Maamar, M.; Beck, D.; Nilsson, E.; McCarrey, J.R.; Skinner, M.K. Developmental alterations in DNA methylation during gametogenesis from primordial germ cells to sperm. *iScience* **2022**, *25*, 103786. [CrossRef]
73. Cannarella, R.; Crafa, A.; Mongioì, L.M.; Leggio, L.; Iraci, N.; La Vignera, S.; Condorelli, R.A.; Calogero, A.E. DNA Methylation in Offspring Conceived after Assisted Reproductive Techniques: A Systematic Review and Meta-Analysis. *J. Clin. Med.* **2022**, *11*, 5056. [CrossRef]
74. Manna, C.; Nardo, L.G. Italian law on assisted conception: Clinical and research implications. *Reprod. Biomed. Online* **2005**, *11*, 532–534. [CrossRef] [PubMed]
75. De Geyter, C.; Wyns, C.; Calhaz-Jorge, C.; de Mouzon, J.; Ferraretti, A.P.; Kupka, M.; Nyboe Andersen, A.; Nygren, K.G.; Goossens, V. 20 years of the European IVF-monitoring Consortium registry: What have we learned? A comparison with reg-istries from two other regions. *Hum. Reprod.* **2020**, *35*, 2832–2849. [CrossRef] [PubMed]
76. Ding, J.; Yin, T.; Zhang, Y.; Zhou, D.; Yang, J. The effect of blastocyst transfer on newborn sex ratio and monozygotic twinning rate: An updated systematic review and meta-analysis. *Reprod. Biomed. Online* **2018**, *37*, 292–303. [CrossRef] [PubMed]
77. Otsuki, J.; Iwasaki, T.; Katada, Y.; Sato, H.; Furuhashi, K.; Tsuji, Y.; Matsumoto, Y.; Shiotani, M. Grade and looseness of the inner cell mass may lead to the development of monochorionic diamniotic twins. *Fertil. Steril.* **2016**, *106*, 640–644. [CrossRef]
78. Bulmer, M.G. *The Biology of Twinning in Man*; Clarendon Press: Oxford, UK, 1970; ISBN1 10: 0198573472. ISBN2 13: 9780198573470.
79. Wilding, M.; Di Matteo, L.; D'Andretti, S.; Montanaro, N.; Capobianco, C.; Dale, B. An oocyte score for use in assisted reproduction. *J. Assist. Reprod. Genet.* **2007**, *24*, 350–358. [CrossRef]
80. Zaninovic, N.; Rosenwaks, Z. Artificial intelligence in human in vitro fertilization and embryology. *Fertil. Steril.* **2020**, *114*, 914–920. [CrossRef]
81. Manna, C.; Patrizi, G.; Rahman, A.; Sallam, H. Experimental results on the recognition of embryos in human assisted reproduction. *Reprod. Biomed. Online* **2004**, *8*, 460–469. [CrossRef]
82. Manna, C.; Nanni, L.; Lumini, A.; Pappalardo, S. Artificial intelligence techniques for embryo and oocyte classification. *Reprod. Biomed. Online* **2013**, *26*, 42–49. [CrossRef]

Disclaimer/Publisher's Note: The statements, opinions and data contained in all publications are solely those of the individual author(s) and contributor(s) and not of MDPI and/or the editor(s). MDPI and/or the editor(s) disclaim responsibility for any injury to people or property resulting from any ideas, methods, instructions or products referred to in the content.

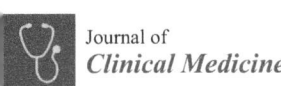

Article

Advanced Paternal Age Does Not Affect Medically-Relevant Obstetrical and Perinatal Outcomes following IVF or ICSI in Humans with Donated Oocytes

Ana Navarro-Gomezlechon [1,*,†], María Gil Juliá [1,†], Irene Hervás [1,2], Laura Mossetti [1,2], Rocío Rivera-Egea [3,‡] and Nicolás Garrido [1,‡]

1. IVI Foundation—Instituto de Investigación Sanitaria La Fe (IIS La Fe), Av. Fernando Abril Martorell, 106, Torre A, 46026 Valencia, Spain
2. IVF Laboratory, IVIRMA Roma, Via Federico Calabresi, 11, 00169 Rome, Italy
3. Andrology Laboratory and Sperm Bank, IVIRMA Valencia, Plaza de la Policia Local 3, 46015 Valencia, Spain
* Correspondence: ana.navarro@ivirma.com
† These authors contributed equally to this work.
‡ These authors contributed equally to this work.

Abstract: Background: Concomitant with delays in childbearing, concerns have been raised of whether advanced paternal age is associated with adverse reproductive outcomes, but the evidence is controversial in part due to the uncertain threshold in which to consider advanced paternal age and confounding maternal factors. This retrospective study aimed to evaluate the effect of paternal age on reproductive outcomes related to the pregnancy and perinatal health of the offspring. Methods: We retrospectively evaluated 16,268 cases of patients who underwent IVF or ICSI (using autologous sperm and donated oocytes, between January 2008 and March 2020, at Spanish IVIRMA clinics. Patients were divided based on paternal age at conception [≤30 (n = 204), 31–40 (n = 5752), and >40 years (n = 10,312)], and the differences in obstetrical and perinatal outcomes were analyzed by descriptive analysis, followed by univariate and multivariate analysis. Results: Fathers 31–40 and >40 years old were associated with lower odds of caesarean delivery [AOR 0.63 (95% CI, 0.44–0.90); p = 0.012) and AOR 0.61 (95% CI, 0.41–0.91; p = 0.017), respectively] and longer pregnancies [ARC 5.09 (95% CI, 2.39–7.79; p < 0.001) and ARC 4.54 (95% CI, 1.51–7.58; p = 0.003), respectively] with respect to fathers ≤30 years old. Furthermore, fathers aged 31–40 years old had lower odds of having a female infant (AOR, 0.70; 95% CI, 0.49–0.99; p = 0.045) than those ≤30. The rest of obstetrical and perinatal outcomes, which we deemed more medically-relevant as they were considered serious for health, were comparable between groups with our adjusted model. Conclusions: Despite this hopeful message to fathers of advanced paternal age, future studies should consider the short- and long-term outcomes of the offspring and try to better elucidate the associations of advanced paternal age with reproductive outcomes and the molecular mechanisms underlying the observed associations.

Keywords: paternal age; assisted reproductive technology (ART); obstetrical outcomes; perinatal outcomes; donated oocytes; pregnancy; offspring's health

1. Introduction

In recent years, delays in childbearing have increased the average maternal and paternal age at which the first child is conceived [1,2]. These delays are due to various sociocultural factors including educational, professional, economic, and personal changes, increased life expectancy, improved contraception, advanced age at marriage, and the availability of assisted reproductive technologies (ARTs). In this regard, studying the possible effect(s) of age on reproductive outcomes is becoming increasingly relevant [3–9].

While the influence of advanced maternal age (>35 years) on reproductive outcomes, pregnancy, and offspring health has been extensively characterized [10–13], it has been difficult to establish a similar cut-off in men (although it has been proposed as >40 [14–16]), since the evidence on the effects of advanced paternal age is currently limited. With the considerable reduction in fertility and elevated chromosomal aneuploidy (notably augmenting the risk of Down syndrome, among other disorders) correlated with advanced maternal age, concerns have been raised of whether advanced paternal age may also be associated with adverse reproductive outcomes, or potential obstetrical or perinatal risks.

Among the few studies that have evaluated the consequence(s) of advanced paternal age on male fertility potential, reproductive success, pregnancy, and offspring health, the findings are controversial, and the study designs were not appropriate [5,6,17–20]. Although some studies have not found associations [21,22], others have agreed that advanced paternal age affects reproductive hormones, testicular function, and spermatogenesis, altering clinical semen parameters (measured with basic semen analysis), molecular markers related to fertility (e.g., reactive oxygen species, telomeres, and DNA integrity), and offspring genetics (through aneuploidy, epigenetics, and de novo mutations), ultimately resulting in infertility and/or adverse reproductive outcomes [3,5,14,19,23–25]. Recently, several studies have pointed out the potential involvement of the increase in paternal age in a wide range of adverse outcomes related to the pregnancy and health of the offspring. In this regard, advanced paternal age has been associated with an increased risk of spontaneous miscarriage [15], stillbirth [26], premature birth, low birth weight [27,28], low Apgar score [29], gestational diabetes, and caesarean section [14,24]. However, not all studies have found such associations between any of these variables and increased paternal age, so the results are controversial [20,30,31]. Offspring pathologies that have been associated with advanced paternal age include several cancers (e.g., pediatric brain cancers, retinoblastoma, acute lymphoblastic leukemia, and non-Hodgkin lymphoma [32,33]; and adult breast, prostate, and nervous system cancers [34]), orofacial clefts (i.e., cleft lip and palate) [14,23,34], achondroplasia [26], and Apert syndrome [35], along with congenital heart defects [34,36,37]. Indeed, Fang et al. found that compared to fathers aged 25–29, fathers $\geq$40 years old could increase the risk of cardiovascular abnormalities, facial deformities, urogenital abnormalities, and chromosome disorders in the offspring [38]. Additionally, the prevalence of Down syndrome, autism spectrum disorders [39], schizophrenia [40], and bipolar disorders [41] is also postulated to be augmented in association with advanced paternal age [14]. Finally, while some studies have found an increase in embryo chromosomal aneuploidy with advanced paternal age [42,43], others have not [6,7]. Taken together, this evidence suggests that paternal age could be associated with reproductive risks related to pregnancy and offspring health, however, further research is necessary.

As advanced paternal age is often accompanied by advanced maternal age, which may also contribute to negative obstetric and perinatal outcomes [12], studies using donated oocytes can, to some extent, standardize and homogenize the female factors [44,45] to more confidently study the effects of the male factors. In this regard, two novelties of this current study were the use of donated oocytes and the consideration of maternal age in the adjusted analysis to more confidently evaluate the possible association(s) of paternal age with greater risks of problems related to the pregnancy and offspring health.

The present study aimed to evaluate the effect of paternal age on the reproductive outcomes related to the pregnancy and offspring health in couples undergoing in vitro fertilization (IVF) or intracytoplasmic sperm injection (ICSI) using donated oocytes and autologous sperm in a large population of patients in order to control the female contribution to the main outcomes evaluated.

2. Materials and Methods

2.1. Study Design

This retrospective, observational, multicentric cohort study evaluated the reproductive outcomes of couples that underwent at least one IVF or ICSI cycle (using the father's own sperm and donated oocytes) between January 2008 and March 2020 at a Spanish IVIRMA clinic, and had clinical follow-up during and after the pregnancy. Cases in which the semen samples were obtained from testicular biopsy or epididymis aspirate were excluded. We also excluded IVF/ICSI cycles in which half of the oocytes were inseminated by IVF and the other half by ICSI. Only singleton deliveries were included, and only the first delivery of each patient was considered. We included couples when a pregnancy was achieved whether they had a live birth or not.

Patients included in the study had different female and male etiologies for infertility, or did not have any. Teratozoospermia, oligozoospermia, or karyotype alteration were some of the male etiologies for infertility. Regarding female etiologies, some of them included karyotype alteration, endometriosis, low ovarian reserve, maternal age, premature ovarian failure, or polycystic ovarian syndrome.

Relevant clinical outcomes were extracted from the electronic medical records of the patients, and compiled into a database to filter erroneous or incomplete data and analyze the study variables.

2.2. Assisted Reproductive Technologies

Ejaculated semen samples were liquefied for 30 min at 37 °C and 5% CO_2, and standard semen analysis was used to evaluate several macroscopic (i.e., volume, pH, and viscosity) and microscopic parameters (i.e., concentration, motility, and morphology). Sperm was capacitated using the swim-up technique [46] or density gradients [47].

Oocyte donors and recipients underwent controlled ovarian stimulation and endometrial preparation, respectively, as previously described [48,49]. Oocytes were retrieved from donors, decumulated, and inseminated by conventional IVF or ICSI [50]. The resulting embryos were cultured, and embryo development was evaluated [47]. If clinically indicated, embryos were biopsied for preimplantation genetic testing (PGT) [51]. Finally, embryos were transferred, and a clinical follow-up was conducted to assess the reproductive outcomes of the couple.

2.3. Outcome Measures

The outcome measures of the following study included several obstetrical and perinatal outcomes. In terms of obstetrical outcomes, we considered type of delivery (caesarean versus vaginal), preterm birth (<37 weeks), gestational diabetes, anemia, hypertension, pre-eclampsia (presence of hypertension and proteinuria after 20 weeks of gestation), and premature rupture of membranes (PROM; before week 37). Regarding the perinatal outcomes, we evaluated the neonate's gestational age, sex, weight (low birth weight was defined as <2500 g), length, cranial perimeter, Apgar score (1, 5, and 10 min), and admission to the neonatal intensive care unit (NICU). We also measured the gestational results in terms of fetal death, perinatal death, live birth, and premature live birth. Data export was conducted to obtain the clinical database followed by the filtering of the data and the statistical analysis.

2.4. Statistical Analysis

We first conducted a descriptive analysis, followed by univariate and multivariate model analysis using the youngest group of men ($\leq$30 years) as a reference for the models. In the descriptive analysis, ANOVAs were used to compare the continuous variables, while Chi-squares were employed for the categorical variables. For the univariate model analysis, generalized linear models were applied for the categorical variables and linear models were applied for the continuous variables. Multivariate analysis was performed adjusting for maternal age, maternal body mass index (BMI), paternal age, fresh sperm sample concentration and progressive motility, insemination technique, cycle type, gestational age, transfer on day 5, and type of delivery (when appropriate).

All analyses were carried out in R (version 4.0.3). In all cases, $p < 0.05$ was considered statistically significant.

3. Results

3.1. Baseline Patient and ART Characteristics

A total of 16,268 couples (with fathers aged 21–54 years old) were included in the study. Patients were arbitrarily divided into three groups, based on paternal age at conception [≤30 (n = 204), 31–40 (n = 5752), and >40 years old (n = 10,312)]. The clinical characteristics of the participants in each group including the patient, cycle, and semen characteristics are presented in Table 1. Patients included in the study had different female and male etiologies for infertility, or did not have any.

Table 1. Baseline characteristics and ART details of the study population.

	≤30	31–40	>40	p
Number of patients	204	5752	10,312	
Paternal age (years)	28.71 (28.48–28.95)	37.42 (37.36–37.48)	43.93 (43.88–43.97)	<0.001 *
Paternal BMI (kg/m^2)	23.66 (23.10–24.22)	23.03 (22.93–23.12)	23.48 (23.41–23.56)	<0.001 *
Maternal age (years)	28.47 (28.21–28.72)	37.14 (37.08–37.21)	43.58 (43.54–43.63)	<0.001 *
Maternal BMI (kg/m^2)	23.60 (23.06–24.14)	23.02 (22.93–23.12)	23.47 (23.40–23.54)	<0.001 *
Oocyte donor age (years)	24.95 (24.37–25.52)	25.44 (25.33–25.55)	25.42 (25.33–25.50)	0.254
Sperm concentration (million/mL)	47.06 (41.76–52.36)	42.66 (41.78–43.53)	44.29 (43.61–44.96)	0.006 *
Progressive motility of sperm	28.79 (25.35–32.23)	32.62 (32.04–33.21)	31.32 (30.90–31.74)	<0.001 *
Number of oocytes	13.10 (12.56–13.65)	12.96 (12.86–13.06)	12.78 (12.71–12.86)	0.013 *
Insemination technique				<0.001 *
IVF	8.82% (5.31–13.59)	3.46% (3.00–3.96)	3.44% (3.10–3.81)	
ICSI	91.18% (86.41–94.69)	96.54% (96.04–97.00)	96.56% (96.19–96.90)	
Oocyte state				<0.001 *
Fresh	51.60% (44.21–58.93)	57.92% (56.61–59.23)	55.10% (54.11–56.08)	
Vitrified	46.81% (39.51–54.21)	40.20% (38.90–41.50)	43.76% (42.78–44.74)	
Mixed	1.60% (0.33–4.59)	1.88% (1.54–2.27)	1.14% (0.94–1.37)	
Cycle type				<0.001 *
Stimulated	1.49% (0.31–4.28)	0.62% (0.43–0.86)	0.38% (0.27–0.52)	
Natural	4.46% (2.06–8.29)	8.22% (7.52–8.97)	6.22% (5.76–6.71)	
Substituted	94.06% (89.85–96.89)	91.16% (90.39–91.89)	93.39% (92.89–93.87)	
Capacitation method				0.019 *
Density gradient	51.47% (44.39–58.51)	56.43% (55.14–57.72)	56.74% (55.78–57.70)	
Swim-up	41.67% (34.82–48.76)	35.34% (34.11–36.60)	35.04% (34.12–35.97)	
Only washed	1.96% (0.54–4.94)	2.54% (2.15–2.98)	3.29% (2.95–3.65)	
Embryo transfer				<0.001 *
Prior to day 5	31.37% (25.07–38.22)	26.73% (25.59–27.89)	22.29% (21.49–23.10)	
On or after day 5	68.63% (61.78–74.93)	73.27% (72.11–74.41)	77.71% (76.90–78.51)	

Results are presented as a proportion (for categorical variables) or mean (for continuous variables) with corresponding 95% confidence intervals and p value of the comparisons between age groups. BMI, body mass index; ICSI, intracytoplasmic sperm injection; IVF, in vitro fertilization. * $p < 0.05$.

3.2. Association of Paternal Age and Obstetrical Outcomes

Paternal age (i.e., ≤30, 31–40, and >40 years old) had no significant effect on the comparison of gestational results between groups in terms of fetal death [0.00% (95% CI, 0.00–1.79), 0.03% (95% CI, 0.00–0.13), and 0.07% (95% CI, 0.03–0.14), respectively], perinatal death [0.00% (95% CI, 0.00–1.79), 0.14% (95% CI, 0.06–0.27), and 0.07% (95% CI, 0.03–0.14), respectively], live birth [97.55% (95% CI, 94.37–99.20), 99.04% (95% CI, 98.76–99.28), and 99.02% (95% CI, 98.81–99.20), respectively], or premature live birth [2.45% (95% CI, 0.80–5.63), 0.78% (95% CI, 0.57–1.05), and 0.84% (95% CI, 0.68–1.04), respectively] over the total number of pregnancies.

Significant differences were found between the age groups in terms of gestational diabetes, hypertension, pre-eclampsia, PROM, and type of delivery, but not for anemia or preterm birth (Table 2).

Table 2. Obstetrical outcomes associated with paternal age following in vitro fertilization or intracytoplasmic sperm injection using autologous sperm and donated oocytes.

	Proportion (95% CI)	p	OR (95% CI)	p	AOR (95% CI)	Adjusted p
Gestational diabetes		<0.001 *				
≤30	6.49% (2.14–14.51)		Reference	-	Reference	-
31–40	9.80% (8.68–11.01)		1.56 (0.63–3.91)	0.338	1.11 (0.38–3.23)	0.845
>40	12.80% (11.84–13.80)		2.11 (0.85–5.25)	0.107	1.04 (0.33–3.21)	0.953
Anemia		0.167				
≤30	3.95% (0.82–11.11)		Reference	-	Reference	-
31–40	10.70% (9.53–11.95)		2.92 (0.91–9.31)	0.071	3.47 (0.82–14.69)	0.092
>40	10.51% (9.63–11.44)		2.86 (0.90–9.10)	0.076	3.43 (0.77–15.35)	0.107
Hypertension		<0.001 *				
≤30	22.67% (13.79–33.79)		Reference	-	Reference	-
31–40	10.49% (9.33–11.75)		0.40 (0.23–0.70)	0.001 *	0.53 (0.25–1.10)	0.089
>40	12.77% (11.80–13.79)		0.50 (0.29–0.86)	0.013 *	0.58 (0.25–1.35)	0.206
Preeclampsia		0.029 *				
≤30	7.58% (2.51–16.80)		Reference	-	Reference	-
31–40	3.04% (2.39–3.81)		0.38 (0.15–0.98)	0.045 *	0.42 (0.12–1.42)	0.162
>40	4.04% (3.47–4.69)		0.51 (0.20–1.30)	0.158	0.48 (0.12–1.99)	0.314
PROM		0.016 *				
≤30	10.81% (4.78–20.20)		Reference	-	Reference	-
31–40	4.25% (3.50–5.11)		0.37 (0.17–0.78)	0.009 *	0.81 (0.22–3.00)	0.756
>40	4.06% (3.50–4.68)		0.35 (0.17–0.74)	0.006 *	1.15 (0.26–5.17)	0.851
Preterm birth		0.132				
≤30	15.92% (11.15–21.73)		Reference	-	Reference	-
31–40	11.64% (10.82–12.49)		0.70 (0.47–1.02)	0.065	0.64 (0.40–1.02)	0.063
>40	11.39% (10.78–12.02)		0.68 (0.46–1.00)	0.047 *	0.61 (0.35–1.06)	0.079
Delivery by cesarian section [a]		<0.001 *				
≤30	47.31% (39.96–54.75)		Reference	-	Reference	-
31–40	50.95% (49.60–52.29)		1.16 (0.86–1.55)	0.33	0.63 (0.44–0.90)	0.012 *
>40	64.04% (63.06–65.00)		1.98 (1.48–2.65)	<0.001 *	0.61 (0.41–0.91)	0.017 *

Men were divided according to their age at conception (i.e., ≤30, 31–40, or >40 years old). Results are presented as a percentage with 95% confidence intervals (CI), odds ratio (OR) with 95% CI and p value of the comparison, and adjusted OR (AOR) and adjusted p value. PROM, premature rupture of membranes (prior to 37 weeks). * $p < 0.05$.
[a] Proportion/probability of caesarean section (rather than vaginal) delivery.

The partners of men ≤30 years old had a significantly increased risk of developing hypertension than the partners of men aged 31–40 (OR, 0.40; 95% CI, 0.23–0.70; $p = 0.001$) or >40 years old (OR, 0.50; 95% CI, 0.29–0.86; $p = 0.013$); experiencing preeclampsia than partners of men 31–40 years old (OR, 0.38; 95% CI, 0.15–0.98; $p = 0.045$); PROM than the partners of men 31–40 (OR, 0.37; 95% CI, 0.17–0.78; $p = 0.009$) or >40 years old (OR, 0.35; 95% CI, 0.17–0.74; $p = 0.006$); and having a preterm birth than the partners of men >40 years old (OR, 0.68; 95% CI, 0.46–1.00; $p = 0.047$). Furthermore, fathers >40 years old were associated with a significantly increased risk of caesarean delivery (OR, 1.98; 95% CI, 1.48–2.65; $p < 0.001$) (Table 2).

Given the retrospective nature of our study and the possibility to have relevant variables related to the outcomes differently distributed among groups, to avoid potential biases derived from the difference between the groups, the statistical differences we observed among our groups (Table 1) were accounted for in subsequent statistical modeling. Specifically, we adjusted for maternal age and BMI, paternal age, fresh sperm sample concentration and progressive motility, insemination technique, cycle type, gestational age, embryo transfer on day 5, and type of delivery (when appropriate). Considering these potential confounders, paternal age did not significantly affect gestational diabetes, anemia, hypertension, preeclampsia, PROM, or preterm birth. However, paternal age ≤30 years old was found to significantly increase the risk of having a caesarean delivery, with respect to fathers that were 31–40 (AOR, 0.63; 95% CI, 0.44–0.90; $p = 0.012$) and >40 years old (AOR, 0.61; 95% CI, 0.41–0.91; $p = 0.017$), assuming all other covariates were at the baseline (Table 2).

3.3. Association of Paternal Age and Perinatal Outcomes

Among the 16,244 deliveries that resulted in a live birth, 204 were from fathers ≤30 years old; 5742 were from fathers 31–40 years old; and 10,298 were from fathers >40 years old. Comparing the different age groups, we found significant differences related to gestational age (in days; $p < 0.001$), infant length ($p = 0.010$), and cranial perimeter ($p = 0.012$). However, paternal age was not significantly related to infant sex ($p = 0.11$), weight ($p = 0.535$), low birth weight ($p = 0.279$), NICU admission ($p = 0.063$), or Apgar score at 1, 5, and 10 min ($p = 0.256$, $p = 0.478$, and $p = 0.112$, respectively) (Table 3).

Table 3. Perinatal outcomes associated with paternal age following in vitro fertilization or intracytoplasmic sperm injection using autologous sperm and donated oocytes.

	Proportion (%)/Mean (95% CI)	p	OR/RC (95% CI)	p	AOR/ARC (95% CI)	Adjusted p Value
Gestational age (days)		<0.001 *				
≤30	270.11 (267.39–272.84)		Reference	-	Reference	-
31–40	273.60 (273.18–274.02)		3.49 (1.23–5.74)	0.002 *	5.09 (2.39–7.79)	<0.001 *
>40	271.80 (271.50–272.11)		1.69 (−0.55–3.93)	0.139	4.54 (1.51–7.58)	0.003 *
Sex [a]		0.11				
≤30	54.97% (47.63–62.16)		Reference	-	Reference	-
31–40	47.81% (46.47–49.15)		0.75 (0.56–1.00)	0.052	0.70 (0.49–0.99)	0.045 *
>40	48.72% (47.72–49.72)		0.78 (0.58–1.04)	0.088	0.75 (0.50–1.11)	0.153
Birth weight		0.535				
≤30	3118.60 (3010.19–3227.02)		Reference	-	Reference	-
31–40	3166.93 (3148.48–3185.38)		48.33 (−51.13–147.79)	0.341	63.75 (−25.13–152.64)	0.16
>40	3172.08 (3158.36–3185.80)		53.48 (−45.29–152.24)	0.289	81.96 (−18.31–182.23)	0.109
Low birth weight		0.279				
≤30	12.32% (7.34–18.99)		Reference	-	Reference	-
31–40	10.90% (9.95–11.90)		0.87 (0.52–1.46)	0.599	0.95 (0.41–2.19)	0.898
>40	10.04% (9.34–10.78)		0.79 (0.48–1.33)	0.38	0.92 (0.35–2.41)	0.865
Length at birth		0.010 *				
≤30	48.89 (48.16–49.63)		Reference	-	Reference	-
31–40	49.71 (49.62–49.81)		0.82 (0.27–1.37)	0.003 *	0.38 (−0.14–0.90)	0.156
>40	49.73 (49.66–49.80)		0.84 (0.30–1.39)	0.002 *	0.50 (−0.08–1.08)	0.09
Cranial perimeter		0.012 *				
≤30	34.00 (33.43–34.57)		Reference	-	Reference	-
31–40	34.38 (34.28–34.47)		0.38 (−0.17–0.92)	0.179	−0.02 (−0.55–0.52)	0.948
>40	34.52 (34.45–34.59)		0.52 (−0.02–1.06)	0.061	0.03 (−0.56–0.62)	0.922
Apgar score 1		0.256				
≤30	9.00 (8.65–9.35)		Reference	-	Reference	-
31–40	8.77 (8.71–8.83)		−0.23 (−0.56–0.09)	0.163	−0.33 (−0.70–0.05)	0.085
>40	8.81 (8.76–8.85)		−0.20 (−0.52–0.13)	0.24	−0.28 (−0.69–0.14)	0.187
Apgar score 5		0.478				
≤30	9.72 (9.56–9.88)		Reference	-	Reference	-
31–40	9.60 (9.56–9.64)		−0.12 (−0.34–0.10)	0.28	−0.21 (−0.47–0.05)	0.107
>40	9.62 (9.59–9.64)		−0.11 (−0.32–0.11)	0.346	−0.20 (−0.48–0.08)	0.164
Apgar score 10		0.112				
≤30	9.75 (9.49–10.01)		Reference	-	Reference	-
31–40	9.76 (9.70–9.82)		0.01 (−0.29–0.30)	0.97	−0.21 (−0.55–0.13)	0.229
>40	9.82 (9.79–9.86)		0.07 (−0.22–0.37)	0.625	−0.20 (−0.57–0.18)	0.309
NICU admission		0.063				
≤30	19.54% (11.81–29.43)		Reference	-	Reference	-
31–40	11.55% (10.44–12.73)		0.54 (0.31–0.92)	0.025 *	0.74 (0.35–1.54)	0.418
>40	11.42% (10.60–12.28)		0.53 (0.31–0.91)	0.021 *	0.83 (0.36–1.93)	0.661

Men were divided according to their age at conception (i.e., ≤30, 31–40, or >40 years old). Results are presented as a proportion or mean with corresponding 95% confidence intervals (CI) and computed p values of the comparison between the three groups; odds ratio (OR) or regression coefficient (RC) with corresponding 95% CI and a p value of the comparisons, and adjusted OR (AOR) or adjusted RC (ARC) and adjusted p value. * $p < 0.05$. NICU, neonatal intensive care unit. [a] Percentage of live female births over the total number of live births.

Using the group of fathers ≤30 years old as the reference, partners of fathers 31–40 years old had significantly longer gestations (RC 3.49; 95% CI, 1.23–5.74; $p = 0.002$), and infants born to fathers 31–40 and >40 years old were significantly longer (RC 0.82 [95% CI, 0.27–1.37; $p = 0.003$] and RC 0.84 [95% CI, 0.30–1.39; $p = 0.002$], respectively), and had significantly lower odds of being admitted to the NICU (OR 0.54 [95% CI, 0.31–0.92; $p = 0.025$] and

OR 0.53 [95% CI, 0.31–0.91; p = 0.021], respectively). No significant differences were found among the remaining variables analyzed (Table 3). Notably, after adjusting for the potential confounding variables, the effect of paternal age on the duration of the pregnancy was even more pronounced, with an ARC of 5.09 (95% CI, 2.39–7.79; p < 0.001) for the fathers aged 31–40, and ARC of 4.54 (95% CI, 1.51–7.58; p = 0.003) for fathers >40. Fathers aged 31–40 had 30% lower odds of having a female infant (AOR, 0.70; 95% CI, 0.49–0.99; p = 0.045) than those ≤30. As for the remaining perinatal outcomes, no significant associations were found (Table 3).

4. Discussion

The present retrospective study aimed to evaluate the effect(s) of paternal age on obstetrical and perinatal outcomes, following IVF or ICSI using autologous sperm and donated oocytes, in a nationwide-population cohort. Using donated oocytes allowed us to adequately model male contributions to the reproductive outcomes by removing, to some extent, the female biases (e.g., advanced maternal age) [44,45]. Indeed, our findings demonstrated that maternal and paternal age were positively correlated (Table 1), but the mean oocyte donor age was comparable between all groups (24.95 for ≤30 vs. 25.44 for 31–40 vs. 25.42 for >40; p = 0.254).

While several studies have pointed out the potential involvement of the increase in paternal age in a wide range of adverse outcomes related to pregnancy and the offspring's health [14,24,26–29], the evidence remains controversial [20,30,31]. Our study did initially find statistically significant differences for a few obstetrical and perinatal outcomes between men aged 31–40 and >40 with those ≤30 years. However after accounting for several confounding variables (i.e., maternal age and BMI, paternal age, fresh sperm sample concentration and progressive motility, insemination technique, cycle type, gestational age, embryo transfer on day 5, and type of delivery [when appropriate]), advanced paternal age at conception was only associated with a minor risk of having a caesarean delivery, a longer pregnancy, and lower odds of having a female infant, which, sometimes has more to do with personal rather than medical decisions, in the case of caesarean, or that have limited clinical relevance as for having a female newborn or having relatively higher gestational age. Indeed, the outcomes that we considered to have more medical relevance (as they were considered serious for the health of the mother or newborn) were found to be comparable by our adjusted model. Nevertheless, due to the evident delays in childbearing highlighted by this study (with 35.36% of participants between 31 and 40 and 63.39% >40 years old), the effects of advanced paternal age merit further evaluation with future prospective studies that consider the short- and/or long-term outcomes of the offspring, and preclinical models that try to elucidate the molecular mechanisms underlying the observed differences [5].

Regarding obstetrical complications, our initial comparisons revealed that anemia more than doubled when the paternal age was >40 rather than ≤30 (10.51% vs. 3.95%, respectively), which corresponded with the AOR of 3.43 (95% CI, 0.77–15.35) we found between these two groups, however, these results were not significant. Similarly, our initial comparisons revealed that the risk of gestational diabetes doubled with paternal age >40 compared to ≤30 (12.80% vs. 6.49%, respectively), and our univariate and multivariate models confirmed this finding with an OR of 2.11 (95% CI, 0.85–5.25) and an AOR of 1.04 (95% CI, 0.33–3.21), but there were no significant differences. Interestingly, Khandwala et al. also reported a higher OR of gestational diabetes when the father was aged older than 45 [14,24], however, their study did not involve ART nor oocyte donation. On the other hand, after accounting for maternal age and other risk factors, Hurley and DeFranco did not find that increased paternal age was associated with a significant increase in the rates of preeclampsia, preterm birth, or NICU admission [20,30,31], as was the case with our multivariate analysis.

Although our findings support those of Chen et al., in that advanced paternal age (>40 years) was not a risk factor for adverse outcomes in the offspring [20,30,31], there was a discord with other previous studies with regard to the perinatal outcomes.

Specifically, we found no significant difference between the mean Apgar scores (1, 5, and 10) of infants born to fathers aged 31–40 or >40 years compared to ≤30, which contradicts a study from Sun et al., who found a modest effect of advanced paternal age on the Apgar score [29]. Furthermore, our univariate and multivariate analyses indicated that paternal age was not significantly associated with birth weight or low birth weight (<2500 g), in contrast to the study by Chung et al., who found that paternal age, among others, was significantly associated with low birth weight in the univariate and multivariate analysis [28], and to the study by Goisis et al., who also found an association between paternal age and low birth weight [27].

In some countries, advanced maternal age is a limitation for the access to, efficacy, and success of ART, but such limitations do not currently exist for men, mainly because there is no consensus on what is considered to be advanced paternal age, and the effects it may have on reproductive outcomes remain controversial. We acknowledge that the different cut-offs used for the paternal age classes in each study can influence the interpretation of the results and impede the discovery of possible associations. In this regard, establishing and standardizing a threshold age for men where fertility decreases and reproductive risks increase (comparable to the one established for women at 35 years of age) can dually aid in personal family planning and clinical decision-making, especially in the context of reproductive medicine counselling and fertility care. Moreover, it should also be considered if studies used oocyte donation or adjusted for maternal age to control for this important confounding factor. Furthermore, although several investigations have examined the possible association between the increase in paternal age and reproductive variables, there is still a need to better clarify the molecular mechanisms that can cause these associations [5].

Finally, due to the retrospective nature of this study, there were some clinical biases and there was some missing data (i.e., incomplete patient histories) limiting the sample size, but statistical power was still achieved by evaluating a nationwide-population cohort. It must be noticed that the major strength of this study was the use of oocyte donation standardizing female factors (to some extent).

5. Conclusions

Due to the evident delays in fatherhood, concerns have been raised of whether advanced paternal age can be associated with adverse reproductive outcomes, and studies focusing on this topic are increasing, although evidence on this matter remains controversial. Our study revealed some statistically significant associations between the increase in paternal age and obstetrical and perinatal outcomes following IVF or ICSI using autologous sperm and donated oocytes. Specifically, we found that fathers >30 years old were associated with a decreased risk of caesarean delivery and longer gestations, and fathers 31–40 years old had lower odds of having a female infant than men ≤30. Although these findings were interesting, we considered them to be of less clinical relevance than the other outcomes we evaluated, and within this context, our study sends a hopeful message to fathers of advanced paternal age. Nonetheless, future perspectives comprise the need for further well-defined preclinical and prospective clinical studies to respectively better elucidate the associations of advanced paternal age with reproductive outcomes and the molecular mechanisms underlying the observed associations, and improve reproductive counselling and fertility care. Finally, the consideration of oocyte donation treatments standardizing female factors (to some extent) and the large sample size should be emphasized as important points of the study.

Author Contributions: Conceptualization, A.N.-G., M.G.J., I.H., L.M., R.R.-E. and N.G.; Methodology, A.N.-G., M.G.J., I.H., L.M., R.R.-E. and N.G; Investigation, A.N.-G., M.G.J., I.H. and L.M.; Data curation, A.N.-G., M.G.J., I.H. and L.M.; Writing—original draft preparation, A.N.-G. and N.G.; Writing—review and editing, R.R.-E. and N.G.; Supervision, N.G.; Project administration, N.G. All authors have read and agreed to the published version of the manuscript.

Funding: A.N.-G. is supported by the Spanish Ministry of Science, Innovation, and Universities (FPU19/06126). M.G.J. is supported by the Instituto de Salud Carlos III (FI19/00051 2019/0172).

Institutional Review Board Statement: This retrospective study was approved by the Research Ethics Committee of the University and Polytechnic Hospital La Fe in Valencia, Spain (project code 2011-FIVI−092-NG and date of approval 2 December 2020).

Informed Consent Statement: Patient consent was waived due to the retrospective nature of this study.

Data Availability Statement: Not applicable.

Acknowledgments: The authors would like to acknowledge Juan Manuel Mascarós, statistician at the IVI Foundation, for his technical assistance during the statistical analysis. The authors would also like to thank all the clinicians and technicians of the Spanish IVIRMA clinics for their cooperation in recording the reproductive variables that made this study possible.

Conflicts of Interest: The authors declare no conflict of interest.

References

1. Matthews, T.J.; Hamilton, B.E. Delayed Childbearing: More Women Are Having Their First Child Later in Life. *NCHS Data Brief* **2009**, 1–8. Available online: https://pubmed.ncbi.nlm.nih.gov/19674536/ (accessed on 13 July 2022).
2. Khandwala, Y.S.; Zhang, C.A.; Lu, Y.; Eisenberg, M.L. The Age of Fathers in the USA Is Rising: An Analysis of 168,867,480 Births from 1972 to 2015. *Hum. Reprod.* **2017**, *32*, 2110–2116. [CrossRef] [PubMed]
3. Kühnert, B.; Nieschlag, E. Reproductive Functions of the Ageing Male. *Hum. Reprod. Update* **2004**, *10*, 327–339. [CrossRef] [PubMed]
4. Bray, I.; Gunnell, D.; Smith, G.D. Advanced Paternal Age: How Old Is Too Old? *J. Epidemiol. Community Health* **2006**, *60*, 851–853. [CrossRef]
5. Sharma, R.; Agarwal, A.; Rohra, V.K.; Assidi, M.; Abu-Elmagd, M.; Turki, R.F. Effects of Increased Paternal Age on Sperm Quality, Reproductive Outcome and Associated Epigenetic Risks to Offspring. *Reprod. Biol. Endocrinol.* **2015**, *13*, 35. [CrossRef] [PubMed]
6. Carrasquillo, R.J.; Kohn, T.P.; Cinnioglu, C.; Rubio, C.; Simon, C.; Ramasamy, R.; Al-Asmar, N. Advanced Paternal Age Does Not Affect Embryo Aneuploidy Following Blastocyst Biopsy in Egg Donor Cycles. *J. Assist. Reprod. Genet.* **2019**, *36*, 2039–2045. [CrossRef] [PubMed]
7. Dviri, M.; Madjunkova, S.; Koziarz, A.; Antes, R.; Abramov, R.; Mashiach, J.; Moskovtsev, S.; Kuznyetsova, I.; Librach, C. Is There a Correlation between Paternal Age and Aneuploidy Rate? An Analysis of 3,118 Embryos Derived from Young Egg Donors. *Fertil. Steril.* **2020**, *114*, 293–300. [CrossRef] [PubMed]
8. Sigman, M. Introduction: What to Do with Older Prospective Fathers: The Risks of Advanced Paternal Age. *Fertil. Steril.* **2017**, *107*, 299–300. [CrossRef]
9. Jennings, M.O.; Owen, R.C.; Keefe, D.; Kim, E.D. Management and Counseling of the Male with Advanced Paternal Age. *Fertil. Steril.* **2017**, *107*, 324–328. [CrossRef]
10. Ogawa, K.; Urayama, K.Y.; Tanigaki, S.; Sago, H.; Sato, S.; Saito, S.; Morisaki, N. Association between Very Advanced Maternal Age and Adverse Pregnancy Outcomes: A Cross Sectional Japanese Study. *BMC Pregnancy Childbirth* **2017**, *17*, 349. [CrossRef]
11. Londero, A.P.; Rossetti, E.; Pittini, C.; Cagnacci, A.; Driul, L. Maternal Age and the Risk of Adverse Pregnancy Outcomes: A Retrospective Cohort Study. *BMC Pregnancy Childbirth* **2019**, *19*, 261. [CrossRef]
12. Li, H.; Nawsherwan; Fan, C.; Mubarik, S.; Nabi, G.; Ping, Y.X. The Trend in Delayed Childbearing and Its Potential Consequences on Pregnancy Outcomes: A Single Center 9-Years Retrospective Cohort Study in Hubei, China. *BMC Pregnancy Childbirth* **2022**, *22*, 514. [CrossRef] [PubMed]
13. Saccone, G.; Gragnano, E.; Ilardi, B.; Marrone, V.; Strina, I.; Venturella, R.; Berghella, V.; Zullo, F. Maternal and Perinatal Complications According to Maternal Age: A Systematic Review and Meta-Analysis. *Int. J. Gynecol. Obstet.* **2022**, *159*, 43–55. [CrossRef] [PubMed]
14. Oldereid, N.B.; Wennerholm, U.B.; Pinborg, A.; Loft, A.; Laivuori, H.; Petzold, M.; Romundstad, L.B.; Söderström-Anttila, V.; Bergh, C. The Effect of Paternal Factors on Perinatal and Paediatric Outcomes: A Systematic Review and Meta-Analysis. *Hum. Reprod. Update* **2018**, *24*, 320–389. [CrossRef] [PubMed]
15. du Fossé, N.A.; van der Hoorn, M.L.P.; van Lith, J.M.M.; le Cessie, S.; Lashley, E.E.L.O. Advanced Paternal Age Is Associated with an Increased Risk of Spontaneous Miscarriage: A Systematic Review and Meta-Analysis. *Hum. Reprod. Update* **2020**, *26*, 650–669. [CrossRef]
16. Barsky, M.; Blesson, C.S. Should We Be Worried about Advanced Paternal Age? *Fertil. Steril.* **2020**, *114*, 259–260. [CrossRef]
17. Beguería, R.; García, D.; Obradors, A.; Poisot, F.; Vassena, R.; Vernaeve, V. Paternal Age and Assisted Reproductive Outcomes in ICSI Donor Oocytes: Is There an Effect of Older Fathers? *Hum. Reprod.* **2014**, *29*, 2114–2122. [CrossRef]
18. Wu, Y.; Kang, X.; Zheng, H.; Liu, H.; Huang, Q.; Liu, J. Effect of Paternal Age on Reproductive Outcomes of Intracytoplasmic Sperm Injection. *PLoS ONE* **2016**, *11*, e0149867. [CrossRef]
19. Mazur, D.J.; Lipshultz, L.I. Infertility in the Aging Male. *Curr. Urol. Rep.* **2018**, *19*, 54. [CrossRef]

20. Hurley, E.G.; DeFranco, E.A. Influence of Paternal Age on Perinatal Outcomes. *Am. J. Obstet. Gynecol.* **2017**, *217*, 566.e1–566.e6. [CrossRef]
21. Bellver, J.; Garrido, N.; Remohí, J.; Pellicer, A.; Meseguer, M. Influence of Paternal Age on Assisted Reproduction Outcome. *Reprod. Biomed. Online* **2008**, *17*, 595–604. [CrossRef]
22. Gallardo, E.; Simon, C.; Levy, M.; Guanes, P.P.; Remohi, J.; Pellicer, A. Effect of Age on Sperm Fertility Potential: Oocyte Donation as a Model. *Fertil. Steril.* **1996**, *66*, 260–264. [CrossRef] [PubMed]
23. Herati, A.S.; Zhelyazkova, B.H.; Butler, P.R.; Lamb, D.J. Age-Related Alterations in the Genetics and Genomics of the Male Germ Line. *Fertil. Steril.* **2017**, *107*, 319–323. [CrossRef] [PubMed]
24. Khandwala, Y.S.; Baker, V.L.; Shaw, G.M.; Stevenson, D.K.; Lu, Y.; Eisenberg, M.L. Association of Paternal Age with Perinatal Outcomes between 2007 and 2016 in the United States: Population Based Cohort Study. *BMJ* **2018**, *363*, k4372. [CrossRef]
25. Kidd, S.A.; Eskenazi, B.; Wyrobek, A.J. Effects of Male Age on Semen Quality and Fertility: A Review of the Literature. *Fertil. Steril.* **2001**, *75*, 237–248. [CrossRef] [PubMed]
26. Lawson, G.; Fletcher, R. Delayed Fatherhood. *J. Fam. Plan. Reprod. Health Care* **2014**, *40*, 283–288. [CrossRef]
27. Goisis, A.; Remes, H.; Barclay, K.; Martikainen, P.; Myrskylä, M. Paternal Age and the Risk of Low Birth Weight and Preterm Delivery: A Finnish Register-Based Study. *J. Epidemiol. Community Health* **2018**, *72*, 1104–1109. [CrossRef]
28. Chung, Y.H.; Hwang, I.S.; Jung, G.; Ko, H.S. Advanced Parental Age Is an Independent Risk Factor for Term Low Birth Weight and Macrosomia. *Medicine* **2022**, *26*, e29846. [CrossRef]
29. Sun, Y.; Vestergaard, M.; Zhu, J.L.; Madsen, K.M.; Olsen, J. Paternal Age and Apgar Scores of Newborn Infants. *Epidemiology* **2006**, *17*, 473–474. [CrossRef]
30. Chen, X.K.; Wen, S.W.; Smith, G.; Leader, A.; Sutandar, M.; Yang, Q.; Walker, M. Maternal Age, Paternal Age and New-Onset Hypertension in Late Pregnancy. *Hypertens. Pregnancy* **2006**, *25*, 217–227. [CrossRef]
31. Chen, X.K.; Wen, S.W.; Krewski, D.; Fleming, N.; Yang, Q.; Walker, M.C. Paternal Age and Adverse Birth Outcomes: Teenager or 40+, Who Is at Risk? *Hum. Reprod.* **2008**, *23*, 1290–1296. [CrossRef]
32. Larfors, G.; Hallböök, H.; Simonsson, B. Parental Age, Family Size, and Offspring's Risk of Childhood and Adult Acute Leukemia. *Cancer Epidemiol. Biomark. Prev.* **2012**, *21*, 1185–1190. [CrossRef] [PubMed]
33. Domingues, A.; Moore, K.J.; Sample, J.; Kharoud, H.; Marcotte, E.L.; Spector, L.G. Parental Age and Childhood Lymphoma and Solid Tumor Risk: A Literature Review and Meta-Analysis. *JNCI Cancer Spectr.* **2022**, *6*, pkac040. [CrossRef] [PubMed]
34. Materna-Kiryluk, A.; Wiśniewska, K.; Badura-Stronka, M.; Mejnartowicz, J.; Więckowska, B.; Balcar-Boroń, A.; Czerwionka-Szaflarska, M.; Gajewska, E.; Godula-Stuglik, U.; Krawczyński, M.; et al. Parental Age as a Risk Factor for Isolated Congenital Malformations in a Polish Population. *Paediatr. Perinat. Epidemiol.* **2009**, *23*, 29–40. [CrossRef] [PubMed]
35. Yoon, S.; Qin, J.; Glaser, R.L.; Jabs, E.W.; Wexler, N.S.; Sokol, R.; Arnheim, N.; Calabrese, P. The Ups and Downs of Mutation Frequencies during Aging Can Account for the Apert Syndrome Paternal Age Effect. *PLoS Genet.* **2009**, *5*, e1000558. [CrossRef]
36. Olshan, A.F.; Schnitzer, P.G.; Baird, P.A. Paternal Age and the Risk of Congenital Heart Defects. *Teratology* **1994**, *50*, 80–84. [CrossRef]
37. Joinau-Zoulovits, F.; Bertille, N.; Cohen, J.F.; Khoshnood, B. Association between Advanced Paternal Age and Congenital Heart Defects: A Systematic Review and Meta-Analysis. *Hum. Reprod.* **2020**, *35*, 2113–2123. [CrossRef]
38. Fang, Y.; Wang, Y.; Peng, M.; Xu, J.; Fan, Z.; Liu, C.; Zhao, K.; Zhang, H. Effect of Paternal Age on Offspring Birth Defects: A Systematic Review and Meta-Analysis. *Aging* **2020**, *12*, 25373–25394. [CrossRef]
39. Reichenberg, A.; Gross, R.; Weiser, M.; Bresnahan, M.; Silverman, J.; Harlap, S.; Rabinowitz, J.; Shulman, C.; Malaspina, D.; Lubin, G.; et al. Advancing Paternal Age and Autism. *Arch. Gen. Psychiatry* **2006**, *63*, 1026–1032. [CrossRef]
40. Khachadourian, V.; Zaks, N.; Lin, E.; Reichenberg, A.; Janecka, M. Advanced Paternal Age and Risk of Schizophrenia in Offspring—Review of Epidemiological Findings and Potential Mechanisms. *Schizophr. Res.* **2021**, *233*, 72–79. [CrossRef] [PubMed]
41. Weiser, M.; Fenchel, D.; Frenkel, O.; Fruchter, E.; Burshtein, S.; Ben Yehuda, A.; Yoffe, R.; Bergman-Levi, T.; Reichenberg, A.; Davidson, M.; et al. Understanding the Association between Advanced Paternal Age and Schizophrenia and Bipolar Disorder. *Psychol. Med.* **2020**, *50*, 431–437. [CrossRef]
42. García-Ferreyra, J.; Hilario, R.; Dueñas, J. High Percentages of Embryos with 21, 18 or 13 Trisomy Are Related to Advanced Paternal Age in Donor Egg Cycles. *J. Bras. Reprod. Assist.* **2018**, *22*, 26–34. [CrossRef]
43. Kasman, A.M.; Li, S.; Zhao, Q.; Behr, B.; Eisenberg, M.L. Relationship between Male Age, Semen Parameters and Assisted Reproductive Technology Outcomes. *Andrology* **2021**, *9*, 245–252. [CrossRef]
44. Hervás, I.; Pacheco, A.; Gil Julia, M.; Rivera-Egea, R.; Navarro-Gomezlechon, A.; Garrido, N. Sperm Deoxyribonucleic Acid Fragmentation (by Terminal Deoxynucleotidyl Transferase Biotin DUTP Nick End Labeling Assay) Does Not Impair Reproductive Success Measured as Cumulative Live Birth Rates per Donor Metaphase II Oocyte Used. *Fertil. Steril.* **2022**, *118*, 79–89. [CrossRef] [PubMed]
45. Gil Juliá, M.; Hervás, I.; Navarro-Gomezlechon, A.; Quintana, F.; Amorós, D.; Pacheco, A.; González-Ravina, C.; Rivera-Egea, R.; Garrido, N. Cumulative Live Birth Rates in Donor Oocyte ICSI Cycles Are Not Improved by Magnetic-Activated Cell Sorting Sperm Selection. *Reprod. Biomed. Online* **2022**, *44*, 677–684. [CrossRef] [PubMed]
46. Romany, L.; Garrido, N.; Motato, Y.; Aparicio, B.; Remohí, J.; Meseguer, M. Removal of Annexin V-Positive Sperm Cells for Intracytoplasmic Sperm Injection in Ovum Donation Cycles Does Not Improve Reproductive Outcome: A Controlled and Randomized Trial in Unselected Males. *Fertil. Steril.* **2014**, *102*, 1567–1575.e1. [CrossRef] [PubMed]

47. Esbert, M.; Pacheco, A.; Soares, S.R.; Amorós, D.; Florensa, M.; Ballesteros, A.; Meseguer, M. High Sperm DNA Fragmentation Delays Human Embryo Kinetics When Oocytes from Young and Healthy Donors Are Microinjected. *Andrology* **2018**, *6*, 697–706. [CrossRef] [PubMed]
48. Bellver, J.; Melo, M.A.B.; Bosch, E.; Serra, V.; Remohí, J.; Pellicer, A. Obesity and Poor Reproductive Outcome: The Potential Role of the Endometrium. *Fertil. Steril.* **2007**, *88*, 446–451. [CrossRef]
49. Cobo, A.; Meseguer, M.; Remohí, J.; Pellicer, A. Use of Cryo-Banked Oocytes in an Ovum Donation Programme: A Prospective, Randomized, Controlled, Clinical Trial. *Hum. Reprod.* **2010**, *25*, 2239–2246. [CrossRef]
50. Cobo, A.; Garrido, N.; Pellicer, A.; Remohí, J. Six Years' Experience in Ovum Donation Using Vitrified Oocytes: Report of Cumulative Outcomes, Impact of Storage Time, and Development of a Predictive Model for Oocyte Survival Rate. *Fertil. Steril.* **2015**, *104*, 1426–1434.e8. [CrossRef]
51. de Los Santos, M.J.; Diez Juan, A.; Mifsud, A.; Mercader, A.; Meseguer, M.; Rubio, C.; Pellicer, A. Variables Associated with Mitochondrial Copy Number in Human Blastocysts: What Can We Learn from Trophectoderm Biopsies? *Fertil. Steril.* **2018**, *109*, 110–117. [CrossRef]

Disclaimer/Publisher's Note: The statements, opinions and data contained in all publications are solely those of the individual author(s) and contributor(s) and not of MDPI and/or the editor(s). MDPI and/or the editor(s) disclaim responsibility for any injury to people or property resulting from any ideas, methods, instructions or products referred to in the content.

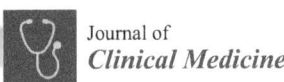

Article

The Impact of Endometrioma on Embryo Quality in In Vitro Fertilization: A Retrospective Cohort Study

Houjin Dongye [1,2,3,4,5], Yizheng Tian [1,2,3,4,5], Dan Qi [1,2,3,4,5], Yanbo Du [1,2,3,4,5],* and Lei Yan [1,2,3,4,5],*

1. Center for Reproductive Medicine, Shandong University, Jinan 250012, China
2. Key Laboratory of Reproductive Endocrinology of Ministry of Education, Shandong University, Jinan 250012, China
3. Shandong Key Laboratory of Reproductive Medicine, Jinan 250012, China
4. Shandong Provincial Clinical Research Center for Reproductive Health, Jinan 250012, China
5. National Research Center for Assisted Reproductive Technology and Reproductive Genetics, Shandong University, Jinan 250012, China
* Correspondence: 13011734515@163.com (Y.D.); yanlei@sdu.edu.cn (L.Y.)

Abstract: The influence of endometrioma on oocyte and embryo competence is inconclusive. Furthermore, the benefits of surgical treatment remain uncertain. This study aimed to investigate the effect of endometrioma on oocyte and embryo quality from a morphological perspective and further explore whether surgery could contribute to improving oocyte and embryo competence. A total of 664 IVF cycles with endometrioma (538 cycles underwent surgeries) and 3133 IVF cycles from the control group were included. The propensity score matching was used to balance the baseline differences between groups. There was a lower MII oocyte rate (85.0% versus 87.8%, $p < 0.001$; 84.9% versus 87.6%, $p = 0.001$) and a similar good-quality embryos rate in women with endometrioma (and those who underwent surgeries) compared with control group. For women with endometrioma, the rates of blastocyst development (67.1% versus 60.2%; $p = 0.013$) and good blastocyst development (40.7% versus 35.2%; $p = 0.049$) were significantly higher in those who had undergone surgical treatment compared with those who had not, but the rates of MII oocytes (79.9% versus 87.7%; $p < 0.001$) and normal fertilization (55.2% versus 66.2%; $p < 0.001$) were lower. The study indicates that endometrioma, including its surgical treatment, compromises the oocyte maturity not the embryo quality at the cleavage stage; however, the surgery seems to contribute to improving blastocyst development.

Keywords: endometrioma; oocyte quality; embryo quality; IVF

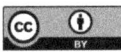

1. Introduction

Endometriosis is a common gynecological disease characterized by the presence of endometrial glands and stroma outside the uterine cavity, increasingly considered a chronic inflammatory condition [1,2]. This affects 5–10% of reproductive aged women and up to 50% of infertile women [3,4]. Endometrioma, the most common pathotype of endometriosis, is present at 17–44% of patients [5]. Numerous studies have demonstrated the negative effect of endometriosis, especially endometrioma, on female fertility [6–8]. It is estimated that 30–50% of patients are afflicted with infertility [9]. A meta-analysis by Harb et al., pooling the results from 27 observational studies, a total of 8984 patients, showed a lower implantation rate and clinical pregnancy rate in women with stage III/IV endometriosis compared with women without endometriosis [10]. Opøien et al. reported a significantly decreased live birth rate in women with endometriomas by classifying women with stage III/IV endometriosis into groups with and without endometriomas [11]. However, the exact pathogenic mechanisms of endometrioma-related infertility remain unclear. Several factors have been proposed to account for this problem such as distorted tubo-ovarian anatomy, mechanical stretching, alteration in follicular microenvironment, impaired endometrial receptivity, chronic inflammatory changes in the pelvic cavity, and reduced oocyte and embryo competence [12–15].

It is already acknowledged that oocyte and embryo quality is vital to a successful outcome of in vitro fertilization (IVF). At present, a number of criteria for evaluating oocyte and embryo quality mainly based on morphological characteristics have been established to select high-quality oocytes and embryos for improving subsequent pregnancy outcomes. In recent years, the issue that the influence of endometrioma on oocyte and embryo competence has raised growing attention; nevertheless, the results of these studies are inconclusive. González-Foruria et al. indicated that the number of oocytes retrieved and metaphase stage II (MII) oocytes was lower in 101 women with endometriomas in comparison with 822 women with infertility factors other than endometriosis [7]. Conversely, Reinblatt et al. failed to find this significant difference in the number of retrieved oocytes and MII oocytes between women with bilateral endometriomas and those who had undergone IVF due to tubal or malefactor infertility [16]. Moreover, Filippi et al. conducted a prospective cohort study, and the result showed the oocytes quality and the rate of high-quality embryos were comparable between affected and intact ovaries in women with unoperated unilateral endometrioma [17]. Surgery is the major treatment modality for endometrioma when intervention is required, however, the benefits of surgery remain uncertain, including whether surgery would damage an ovarian reserve or improve oocyte and embryo competence.

This study aims to investigate the effect of endometrioma on oocyte and embryo quality from the morphological perspective and further explore whether surgery could contribute to improving the oocyte and embryo competence.

2. Materials and Methods

2.1. Study Design and Population

This retrospective cohort study analyzed IVF data from the Reproductive Hospital Affiliated to Shandong University between January 2013 and December 2019. The study population was patients with endometrioma diagnosed by ultrasonography. All patients from the endometrioma with surgery group had undergone cystectomy by laparoscopy or laparotomy. The control group consisted of women with infertility due to tubal factors during the same period. The inclusion criteria were as follows: age ≤ 40 years; women without non-endometriotic ovarian cyst; control population had not undergone surgery for ovary; normal sperm (concentration $\geq 15 \times 10^6$/mL, total motility $\geq 40\%$, normal morphology $\geq 4\%$) in the male according to the fifth edition of World Health Organization (WHO) guidelines. The exclusion criteria included: intracytoplasmic sperm injection (ICSI), preimplantation genetic testing (PGT), hydrosalpinx, pelvic adhesions, polycystic ovarian syndrome (PCOS), primary ovarian insufficiency (POI), premature ovarian failure (POF), decreased ovarian reserve, hyperprolactinemia, hyperthyroidism, hypothyroidism, adrenal disease, adenomyosis, and cycles with donated oocytes or sperm. This research was approved by the Institutional Review Board (IRB) of Reproductive Hospital affiliated to Shandong University (2020-14).

2.2. IVF Procedures

Controlled ovarian hyperstimulation, oocyte retrieval, fertilization, embryo culture, and evaluation were in line with our center's standard protocols as previously reported [18]. In brief, the ovarian stimulation protocol was determined based on the patient's infertility cause, ovarian function, age, and menstrual cycle. Several commonly used stimulation protocols included long gonadotropin releasing hormone (GnRH) agonist protocol, short GnRH agonist protocol, ultra-long GnRH agonist protocol, and GnRH antagonist protocol, whilst other unconventional protocols included a mild stimulation protocol and natural cycle protocol, but the above stimulation protocols were previously described in detail [19]. The gonadotropin dose was adjusted depending on the follicular growth monitored by transvaginal ultrasound (TVUS) scan and serum sex steroids tests. In our hospital, recombinant follicle stimulating hormone was administered during controlled ovarian hyperstimulation and human menopausal gonadotropin could be added at the discretion of different doctors. The final oocyte maturation was triggered with human chorionic gonadotropin (hCG) at a dose of 4000–10,000 IU when at least two follicles measured 18 mm or more in mean diameter. Oocyte retrieval guided by TVUS was performed 34–36 h after hCG administration. IVF was carried out according to the semen parameters approximately 4–6 h after follicular aspiration. Embryo development was assessed by morphologic criteria at our center. The cleavage stage embryos were scored by Puissant criteria on the basis of the number and size of blastomeres as well as the percentage of anucleate fragments [20]. The blastocysts were graded by Gardner criteria on the basis of the degree of blastocyst expansion as well as the development of the inner cell mass (ICM) and trophectoderm (TE) [21]. Fresh embryo transfer could be cancelled in some cases such as ovarian hyperstimulation syndrome (OHSS), early elevated progesterone level, no viable oocytes or embryos, and thin endometrium.

2.3. Study Outcomes

The primary outcome was a good-quality embryo rate which was defined as the proportion of good-quality embryos over normally fertilized oocytes. The good-quality embryos were defined as 7–10 cells without multinucleation, ≥ 3 points, and cultured from normal zygotes on Day 3. The second outcomes were the number of oocytes retrieved, rates of MII oocytes, normal fertilization, embryo development (Day2, Day3), blastocyst development, and good blastocyst development. The good blastocysts were considered embryos with an expansion score ≥ 3, without C in the development of ICM and TE on Day 5 and Day 6. The detailed definitions of the above study outcomes were in accordance with the Vienna consensus [22].

2.4. Statistical Analysis

The normality of data was assessed using the Shapiro–Wilk test. Continuous variables were represented as median (interquartile range), with the Mann–Whitney U test for between-group differences. Categorical data were expressed as frequency and percentage, and the differences between groups were examined via Pearson chi-square test or Fisher's exact test. A p value < 0.05 was considered statistically significant. To reduce the impact of selection bias and confounding factors, propensity score matching (PSM) was used. The propensity score model was built using the multivariable logistic regression analysis that included all baseline characteristics. A 1:1 matching was performed using nearest neighbor matching with a caliper width of 0.02, and without replacement. The standardized mean difference (SMD) was calculated to assess the between-group balance of baseline characteristics before and after matching. An absolute value of SMD less than 0.1 was interpreted as comparability. All statistical analyses were conducted with the use of R programming language (version 4.1.2, R Core Team 2021, Vienna, Austria) and Statistical Package for the Social Sciences (SPSS) software (version 26.0, IBM, Chicago, IL, USA).

3. Results

3.1. Basal Characteristics between Groups

A total of 664 IVF cycles with endometrioma, among which 538 cycles underwent endometrioma-related surgeries, and 3133 IVF cycles from control group were included in the analysis. No differences were observed only in sperm concentration and total motility, the proportion of short GnRH agonist protocol, days of ovarian stimulation, and gonadotrophin initiating dose of all 19 baseline variables between endometrioma and control group. After matching, 532 pairs of cycles were included, and all baseline characteristics were comparable between groups (Table 1). For subgroup analysis, before matching, the absolute value of SMD for all baseline variables was more than 0.1 except for sperm concentration and total motility, the proportion of short GnRH agonist protocol, days of ovarian stimulation, gonadotrophin initiating dose, and endometrial thickness on the hCG trigger day between the endometrioma with surgery and control groups. After matching, the two comparison groups were balanced, and 441 pairs of cycles were included (Table S1). For endometrioma with and without surgery, before matching, there were significant differences in the 13 baseline characteristics between endometrioma with and without surgery. After matching, 109 pairs of cycles were included, and the between-group differences were not significant (Table S2).

Table 1. Baseline characteristics of the women with endometrioma and control group before and after PSM.

Characteristic	Before Matching			After Matching		
	Endometrioma Group (n = 664)	Control Group (n = 3133)	SMD	Endometrioma Group (n = 532)	Control Group (n = 532)	SMD
Age (years)	31 (28–34)	32 (29–35)	0.212	31 (29–34)	31 (28–35)	0.013
BMI (kg/m^2)	22.33 (20.36–24.22)	23.3 (21.22–25.88)	0.367	22.5 (20.66–24.68)	22.23 (20.11–25.01)	0.024
Type of infertility						
Primary	367 (55.3)	940 (30.0)	0.508	263 (49.4)	256 (48.1)	0.026
Secondary	297 (44.7)	2193 (70.0)	0.508	269 (50.6)	276 (51.9)	0.026
Basal FSH (IU/L)	7.23 (5.99–8.91)	6.55 (5.6–7.81)	0.283	7.21 (6.00–8.55)	7 (5.91–8.48)	0.006
Basal LH (IU/L)	4.84 (3.73–6.17)	4.5 (3.36–5.88)	0.122	4.76 (3.58–5.97)	4.52 (3.40–6.09)	0.010
Basal oestradiol (pg/mL)	37.8 (27.03–52.38)	33.8 (25.72–45)	0.195	36.90 (26.05–50.78)	35.60 (25.33–49.08)	0.007
AMH	1.91 (0.92–3.75)	2.5 (1.35–4.26)	0.199	1.99 (0.98–3.88)	2.09 (1.03–3.73)	0.027
AFC	9 (6–13)	12 (9–17)	0.629	9 (7–14)	10 (7–13)	0.020
Sperm concentration ($\times 10^6$/mL)	60.45 (40.23–84.58)	59 (39.3–86.1)	0.030	60.25 (40.33–82.5)	61.1 (38.70–85.30)	0.012
Sperm motility (%)	66.90 (56.13–79.4)	67.10 (55.9–78.3)	0.028	66.55 (56.63–78.65)	68.75 (56.90–79.10)	0.059
Sperm normal morphology (%)	5.91 (4.85–7.41)	6.00 (4.95–7.56)	0.122	5.91 (4.88–7.34)	5.91 (4.89–7.39)	0.020
Ovarian stimulation regimen						
Long GnRH agonist protocol	192 (28.9)	1512 (48.3)	0.427	188 (35.3)	186 (35.0)	0.008
Ultra-long GnRH agonist protocol	154 (23.2)	174 (5.6)	0.418	77 (14.5)	83 (15.6)	0.027
Short GnRH agonist protocol	169 (25.5)	826 (26.4)	0.021	150 (28.2)	144 (27.1)	0.026
GnRH antagonist protocol	79 (11.9)	511 (16.3)	0.136	73 (13.7)	79 (14.8)	0.035
Other	70 (10.5)	110 (3.5)	0.229	44 (8.3)	40 (7.5)	0.024
Days of ovarian stimulation	10 (9–12)	10 (9–11)	0.069	10 (9–12)	10 (9–12)	0.027
Gonadotrophin starting dose (IU)	187.5 (150–225)	150 (150–225)	0.091	175 (150–225)	175 (150–225)	0.003
Total gonadotropin dose (IU)	2100 (1500–2913)	1800 (1356–2475)	0.194	2000 (1500–2769)	2025 (1500–2700)	0.010
Endometrial thickness on HCG trigger day (cm)	1.10 (1.00–1.25)	1.00 (0.90–1.20)	0.148	1.10 (0.95–1.25)	1.10 (0.95–1.20)	0.021
LH level on HCG trigger day (IU)	2.67 (1.43–5.08)	2.66 (1.65–4.35)	0.155	2.71 (1.52–4.82)	2.73 (1.57–4.92)	0.020
Oestradiol level on HCG trigger day (pg/mL)	2341 (1421–3425)	2825 (1802–4169)	0.266	2416 (1492–3559)	2364 (1450–3583)	0.010
Progesterone level on HCG trigger day (ng/mL)	0.81 (0.55–1.14)	0.67 (0.46–0.97)	0.136	0.80 (0.52–1.11)	0.68 (0.46–1.00)	0.035

Values are presented as median (interquartile range) or n (%). BMI: Body mass index; FSH: Follicle-stimulating hormone; LH: Luteinizing hormone; AMH: Anti-Müllerian hormone; AFC: Antral follicle count; GnRH: Gonadotropin releasing hormone; HCG: Human chorionic gonadotropin; PSM: Propensity score matching; SMD: Standardized mean difference. SMD values of less than 0.1 were considered no statistical significance.

3.2. Outcomes

The MII oocytes rate was significantly lower in the endometrioma group than in the control group (85.0% versus 87.8%; $p < 0.001$). Additionally, there was a trend toward a lower good-quality embryos rate in the endometrioma group compared with control group, although the difference did not reach statistical significance. In addition, other outcomes such as the number of oocytes retrieved, the rates of normal fertilization, embryo development (Day 2, Day 3), blastocyst development, and good blastocyst development were similar between the two groups. There were no significant differences in the rates of clinical pregnancy, miscarriage, and live birth (Table 2).

Table 2. Outcomes of the women with endometrioma and control group after PSM.

Outcome	Endometrioma Group (n = 532)	Control Group (n = 532)	p Value
No. of oocytes retrieved	7 (4–12)	8 (4–12)	0.336
MII oocytes rate	3787/4455 (85.0)	3996/4550 (87.8)	<0.001
Normal fertilization rate	2724/4455 (61.1)	2851/4550 (62.7)	0.139
Embryo development rate on Day 2	1905/2724 (69.9)	2023/2851 (71.0)	0.402
Embryo development rate on Day 3	1061/2724 (39.0)	1121/2851 (39.3)	0.778
Good-quality embryos rate on Day 3	1482/2724 (54.4)	1601/2851 (56.2)	0.189
Blastocyst development rate	1721/2724 (63.2)	1747/2851 (61.3)	0.143
Good blastocyst development rate	1004/2724 (36.9)	1005/2851 (35.3)	0.212
Cycles cancellation rate	199/532 (27.2)	167/532 (23.9)	0.149
Clinical pregnancy rate	178/333 (53.5)	191/365 (52.3)	0.766
Miscarriage rate	21/178 (11.8)	19/191 (9.9)	0.568
Live birth rate	152/333 (45.6)	166/365 (45.5)	0.965

Values are presented as median (interquartile range) or n (%). MII: metaphase stage II; PSM: propensity score matching.

The good-quality embryos rate appeared to be higher in endometrioma with surgery than in the control group, however, the difference was not statistically significant. The cycles of endometrioma with surgery was associated with lower MII oocytes rate than the control group (84.9% versus 87.6%; $p = 0.001$). Beyond that, other outcomes including pregnancy outcomes did not differ significantly between comparison groups (Table 3).

Table 3. Outcomes of the women with endometrioma who received surgery and the control group after PSM.

Outcome	Endometrioma with Surgery (n = 441)	Control Group (n = 441)	p Value
No. of oocytes retrieved	7 (4–11)	7 (4–12)	0.657
MII oocytes rate	3140/3700 (84.9)	3255/3717 (87.6)	0.001
Normal fertilization rate	2224/3700 (60.1)	2298/3717 (61.8)	0.130
Embryo development rate on Day 2	1552/2224 (69.8)	1615/2298 (70.3)	0.717
Embryo development rate on Day 3	877/2224 (39.4)	877/2298 (38.2)	0.381
Good-quality embryos rate on Day 3	1239/2224 (55.7)	1239/2298 (53.9)	0.226
Blastocyst development rate	1399/2224 (62.9)	1425/2298 (62)	0.535
Good blastocyst development rate	830/2224 (37.3)	864/2298 (37.6)	0.847
Cycles cancellation rate	161/441 (26.7)	165/441 (27.2)	0.850
Clinical pregnancy rate	148/280 (52.9)	156/276 (56.5)	0.385
Miscarriage rate	17/148 (11.5)	14/156 (9.0)	0.469
Live birth rate	125/280 (44.6)	141/276 (51.1)	0.128

Values are presented as median (interquartile range) or n (%). MII: metaphase stage II; PSM: propensity score matching.

For endometrioma with and without surgery, the MII oocytes rate was significantly lower in the endometrioma group with surgery (79.9% versus 87.7%; $p < 0.001$), while the good-quality embryos rate was comparable between groups. The surgery for endometrioma may result in a lower normal fertilization rate (55.2% versus 66.2%; $p < 0.001$). Nevertheless, there were higher rates of blastocyst development and good blastocyst development in the endometrioma group with surgery (67.1% versus 60.2%, $p = 0.013$; 40.7% versus 35.2%, $p = 0.049$). As for other outcomes including pregnancy outcomes, no significant between-group differences were found (Table 4).

Table 4. Outcomes of the endometrioma women with and without surgery after PSM.

Outcome	Endometrioma with Surgery (n = 109)	Endometrioma without Surgery (n = 109)	p Value
No. of oocytes retrieved	8 (5–13)	8 (5–12)	0.950
MII oocytes rate	811/1015 (79.9)	880/1003 (87.7)	<0.001
Normal fertilization rate	560/1015 (55.2)	664/1003 (66.2)	<0.001
Embryo development rate on Day 2	405/560 (72.3)	453/664 (68.2)	0.119
Embryo development rate on Day 3	237/560 (42.3)	273/664 (41.1)	0.670
Good-quality embryos rate on Day 3	310/560 (55.4)	361/664 (54.4)	0.729
Blastocyst development rate	376/560 (67.1)	400/664 (60.2)	0.013
Good blastocyst development rate	228/560 (40.7)	234/664 (35.2)	0.049
Cycles cancellation rate	44/109 (28.8)	36/109 (24.8)	0.444
Clinical pregnancy rate	33/65 (50.8)	45/73 (61.6)	0.198
Miscarriage rate	2/33 (6.1)	4/45 (8.9)	0.974
Live birth rate	30/65 (46.2)	40/73 (54.8)	0.311

Values are presented as median (interquartile range) or n (%). MII: metaphase stage II; PSM: propensity score matching.

4. Discussion

The study demonstrated that there was a lower MII oocytes rate and a similar good-quality embryos rate in women with endometrioma (as well as those who underwent surgical treatment) compared with the control group, other outcomes were comparable. For women with endometrioma, the rates of blastocyst development and good blastocyst development were significantly higher in those that had prior surgical treatment compared with those who had not; however, the rates of normal fertilization and MII oocytes were lower. Moreover, other outcomes including good-quality embryos rate did not significantly differ between the two groups.

A growing number of cohort studies have investigated the effect of endometrioma on oocyte and embryo quality in IVF/ICSI, but there was substantial heterogeneity across these studies whether in study design or results. Benaglia et al. included 39 women with unoperated bilateral endometriomas and 78 control subjects by 1:2 matching, and reported a comparable number of high-quality embryos but a significantly lower number of oocytes retrieved and suitable oocytes which included MII oocytes and type 1 cumulus-oocyte complex in the endometriomas group [23]. Similarly, Suzuki et al. failed to detect a difference in the rate of good-quality embryos between 80 IVF cycles with endometrioma and 283 cycles with tubal factor infertility, and they found a lower number of oocytes retrieved in the study group, but the MII oocytes rate was not shown [24]. Notably, these studies were all small sample sizes. In contrast, a large retrospective cohort study conducted by Wu et al. indicated a significantly lower number of top-quality embryos and blastocyst rates, in addition to a decreased number of oocytes retrieved and oocyte maturation rate in endometrioma group compared with control group [25]. Furthermore, a meta-analysis by Yang et al., pooling the results from nine studies, reported a similar number of good-quality embryos but a lower number of MII oocytes in endometrioma group, they also made comparisons in unilateral endometrioma, but no difference was found in the number of MII oocytes and embryos formed between ovaries affected and contralateral normal ovaries [26]. There are many underlying mechanisms for the negative effect of endometrioma on oocytes quality. It has been proposed that the altered follicular microenvironment such as excessive reactive oxygen species and free radicals production and high expression of inflammatory cytokines would lead to DNA damage and meiotic spindle disorganization; thus, the oocytes quality is compromised [27–29]. However, the exact pathophysiology remains to be elucidated.

The surgical management of endometrioma prior to IVF/ICSI is a point deserving attention, with increasing evidence questioning the benefits of surgery. More recent studies have observed the decreased ovarian reserve after cystectomy, and the damage may be due to the removal of the normal ovarian tissue or electrocoagulation injury during operation [30,31]. Our research indicated that surgery for endometrioma had no negative impact on embryos quality on Day 3, but was associated with compromised oocytes maturity. Furthermore, the blastocysts quality was found to be improved in this population, and this finding would contribute to patient counselling and clinical practice as the blastocyst-stage embryo transfer—especially the frozen single blastocyst transfer—strategy is becoming increasingly popular [32]. In line with our results, Li et al. reported a comparable high-quality embryo rate per oocyte retrieved and a lower number of MII oocytes in women with endometrioma having undergone cystectomy compared with those who underwent aspiration, whereas the difference in the viable blastocyst rate was not observed [33]. At present, only one randomized controlled trial on this issue was published, enrolling a total of 99 women with endometriomas measuring 3–6 cm in diameter, which demonstrated that surgery for endometrioma resulted in a reduced number of retrieved mature oocytes while the embryonic development was ignored [34]. Additionally, in a recent meta-analysis, Hamdan et al. extracted data from 33 eligible studies, in which the synthetic results showed there were no differences in the number of oocytes retrieved between women with endometrioma who received prior surgical treatment and those who did not [35]. In general, the effect of endometrioma, especially its surgical treatment, on embryo quality, is still poorly investigated, as most existing literature focuses on its effect on oocyte quantity and quality. More research on this aspect is needed to draw a definite conclusion. The latest guideline on endometriosis developed by the European Society of Human Reproduction and Embryology (ESHRE) does not recommend the routine performance of surgery for endometrioma prior to IVF/ICSI, considering its negative impact on ovarian reserve, but it can be performed to improve the accessibility of follicles at the time of oocyte retrieval [36]. In practice, clinicians should comprehensively evaluate various clinical variables such as previous interventions, ovarian reserve, pain symptoms, bilaterality, sonographic feature of malignancy, growth, and size to determine whether the benefits of surgery for endometriomas outweigh its potential risk [37].

The strengths of this study include the large sample size and detailed baseline characteristics that enhance statistical power. Beyond that, the indicators for evaluating oocyte and embryo quality, as recommended by the Vienna consensus, are comprehensive and systematic. Currently, in other studies of this field, the indexes used to assess embryo quality do not cover the entire process of embryonic development. More importantly, the use of PSM to balance baseline differences between groups, combined with the incorporation of all variables into the propensity score model due to the large sample size, makes the analysis more statistically efficient and robust, thus reinforcing the persuasiveness of the results.

There are also some limitations to be noted in this study. Firstly, the diagnosis of endometrioma is made by ultrasonography instead of pathology, which could result in the selection bias of the study population. This is also a common limitation in the field investigating the impact of endometrioma on IVF/ICSI cycle outcomes. It is estimated that the TVUS has good accuracy for endometrioma with a sensitivity and specificity of 93% and 96%, which makes this technology more practical [38]. Secondly, the evaluation for embryo quality is based on morphological criteria in this study, however, the embryos retrieved from women with endometrioma may be intrinsically changed, which would not translate into morphological alterations. At present, the dominant laboratory performance indicators for assessing embryo quality are based on morphological features, although some other methods such as the analysis of morphokinetics by time-lapse imaging have been applied. Thirdly, the non-homogeneity of the stimulation protocols is another problem of note. Admittedly, many different stimulation protocols have been used in this retrospective study which could negatively impact the statistical data. However, the proportions of different stimulation protocols are not significantly different between the comparison groups with the use of PSM, although many different stimulation protocols have been used. Finally, both the study and control populations are confined to IVF cycles, meaning that the results cannot be extrapolated to other populations.

5. Conclusions

To conclude, our results suggest that endometrioma, including the corresponding surgical treatment, compromises the oocyte maturity not the embryo quality at the cleavage stage; however, surgery does not significantly influence the live birth rate, although the surgery seems to contribute to improving the blastocyst development. Furthermore, more high-quality evidence is required to elucidate the effect of endometrioma, especially its surgical treatment on embryo competence.

Supplementary Materials: The following supporting information can be downloaded at: https://www.mdpi.com/article/10.3390/jcm12062416/s1, Table S1: Baseline characteristics of the women with endometrioma who received surgery and the control group before and after PSM; Table S2: Baseline characteristics of the endometrioma women with and without surgery before and after PSM.

Author Contributions: Conceptualization, L.Y.; Methodology, H.D.; Validation, Y.D.; Formal Analysis, H.D.; Investigation, Y.T.; Resources, D.Q.; Data Curation, Y.T.; Writing—Original Draft Preparation, H.D.; Writing—Review and Editing, L.Y. and Y.D.; Visualization, D.Q.; Supervision, Y.D.; Project Administration, L.Y.; Funding Acquisition, L.Y. and Y.D. All authors have read and agreed to the published version of the manuscript.

Funding: This study was supported by the National Key Research and Development Program of China (2022YFC2704002) and the Shandong Natural Science Youth Foundation (ZR2020QH058).

Institutional Review Board Statement: This research was approved by the Institutional Review Board (IRB) of Reproductive Hospital affiliated to Shandong University (protocol code: 2020-14, data of approval: 23 March 2020).

Informed Consent Statement: Not applicable.

Data Availability Statement: Not applicable.

Acknowledgments: The authors thank Lin Zhang, from Maternal and Child Health Care of Shandong Province for providing statistical help.

Conflicts of Interest: The authors declare no conflict of interest.

References

1. Tomassetti, C.; Johnson, N.P.; Petrozza, J.; Abrao, M.S.; Einarsson, J.I.; Horne, A.W.; Lee, T.T.; Missmer, S.; Vermeulen, N.; Zondervan, K.T.; et al. An International Terminology for Endometriosis, 2021. *J. Minim. Invasive Gynecol.* **2021**, *28*, 1849–1859. [CrossRef]
2. Johnson, N.P.; Hummelshoj, L.; Adamson, G.D.; Keckstein, J.; Taylor, H.S.; Abrao, M.S.; Bush, D.; Kiesel, L.; Tamimi, R.; Sharpe-Timms, K.; et al. World Endometriosis Society consensus on the classification of endometriosis. *Hum. Reprod.* **2017**, *32*, 315–324. [CrossRef]
3. Taylor, H.S.; Kotlyar, A.M.; Flores, V.A. Endometriosis is a chronic systemic disease: Clinical challenges and novel innovations. *Lancet* **2021**, *397*, 839–852. [CrossRef]
4. Zondervan, K.T.; Becker, C.M.; Missmer, S.A. Endometriosis. *N. Engl. J. Med.* **2020**, *382*, 1244–1256. [CrossRef]
5. Busacca, M.; Vignali, M. Ovarian endometriosis: From pathogenesis to surgical treatment. *Curr. Opin. Obstet. Gynecol.* **2003**, *15*, 321–326. [CrossRef]
6. Senapati, S.; Sammel, M.D.; Morse, C.; Barnhart, K.T. Impact of endometriosis on in vitro fertilization outcomes: An evaluation of the Society for Assisted Reproductive Technologies Database. *Fertil. Steril.* **2016**, *106*, 164–171.e1. [CrossRef] [PubMed]
7. González-Foruria, I.; Soldevila, P.B.; Rodríguez, I.; Rodríguez-Purata, J.; Pardos, C.; García, S.; Pascual, M.; Barri, P.N.; Polyzos, N.P. Do ovarian endometriomas affect ovarian response to ovarian stimulation for IVF/ICSI? *Reprod. Biomed. Online* **2020**, *41*, 37–43. [CrossRef]
8. Kasapoglu, I.; Ata, B.; Uyaniklar, O.; Seyhan, A.; Orhan, A.; Yildiz Oguz, S.; Uncu, G. Endometrioma-related reduction in ovarian reserve (ERROR): A prospective longitudinal study. *Fertil. Steril.* **2018**, *110*, 122–127. [CrossRef] [PubMed]
9. Muteshi, C.M.; Ohuma, E.O.; Child, T.; Becker, C.M. The effect of endometriosis on live birth rate and other reproductive outcomes in ART cycles: A cohort study. *Hum. Reprod. Open* **2018**, *2018*, hoy016. [CrossRef] [PubMed]
10. Harb, H.M.; Gallos, I.D.; Chu, J.; Harb, M.; Coomarasamy, A. The effect of endometriosis on in vitro fertilisation outcome: A systematic review and meta-analysis. *BJOG* **2013**, *120*, 1308–1320. [CrossRef]
11. Opøien, H.K.; Fedorcsak, P.; Omland, A.K.; Abyholm, T.; Bjercke, S.; Ertzeid, G.; Oldereid, N.; Mellembakken, J.R.; Tanbo, T. In vitro fertilization is a successful treatment in endometriosis-associated infertility. *Fertil. Steril.* **2012**, *97*, 912–918. [CrossRef]

12. Corachán, A.; Pellicer, N.; Pellicer, A.; Ferrero, H. Novel therapeutic targets to improve IVF outcomes in endometriosis patients: A review and future prospects. *Hum. Reprod. Update* **2021**, *27*, 923–972. [CrossRef] [PubMed]
13. Lin, X.; Dai, Y.; Tong, X.; Xu, W.; Huang, Q.; Jin, X.; Li, C.; Zhou, F.; Zhou, H.; Lin, X.; et al. Excessive oxidative stress in cumulus granulosa cells induced cell senescence contributes to endometriosis-associated infertility. *Redox Biol.* **2020**, *30*, 101431. [CrossRef] [PubMed]
14. Ferrero, H.; Corachán, A.; Aguilar, A.; Quiñonero, A.; Carbajo-García, M.C.; Alamá, P.; Tejera, A.; Taboas, E.; Muñoz, E.; Pellicer, A.; et al. Single-cell RNA sequencing of oocytes from ovarian endometriosis patients reveals a differential transcriptomic profile associated with lower quality. *Hum. Reprod.* **2019**, *34*, 1302–1312. [CrossRef] [PubMed]
15. Sanchez, A.M.; Viganò, P.; Somigliana, E.; Panina-Bordignon, P.; Vercellini, P.; Candiani, M. The distinguishing cellular and molecular features of the endometriotic ovarian cyst: From pathophysiology to the potential endometrioma-mediated damage to the ovary. *Hum. Reprod. Update* **2014**, *20*, 217–230. [CrossRef]
16. Reinblatt, S.L.; Ishai, L.; Shehata, F.; Son, W.Y.; Tulandi, T.; Almog, B. Effects of ovarian endometrioma on embryo quality. *Fertil. Steril.* **2011**, *95*, 2700–2702. [CrossRef]
17. Filippi, F.; Benaglia, L.; Paffoni, A.; Restelli, L.; Vercellini, P.; Somigliana, E.; Fedele, L. Ovarian endometriomas and oocyte quality: Insights from in vitro fertilization cycles. *Fertil. Steril.* **2014**, *101*, 988–993.e1. [CrossRef]
18. Wei, D.; Sun, Y.; Liu, J.; Liang, X.; Zhu, Y.; Shi, Y.; Chen, Z.J. Live birth after fresh versus frozen single blastocyst transfer (Frefro-blastocyst): Study protocol for a randomized controlled trial. *Trials* **2017**, *18*, 253. [CrossRef]
19. Guo, Z.; Xu, X.; Zhang, L.; Zhang, L.; Yan, L.; Ma, J. Endometrial thickness is associated with incidence of small-for-gestational-age infants in fresh in vitro fertilization-intracytoplasmic sperm injection and embryo transfer cycles. *Fertil. Steril.* **2020**, *113*, 745–752. [CrossRef]
20. Puissant, F.; Van Rysselberge, M.; Barlow, P.; Deweze, J.; Leroy, F. Embryo scoring as a prognostic tool in IVF treatment. *Hum. Reprod.* **1987**, *2*, 705–708. [CrossRef]
21. Gardner, D.K.; Lane, M.; Stevens, J.; Schlenker, T.; Schoolcraft, W.B. Blastocyst score affects implantation and pregnancy outcome: Towards a single blastocyst transfer. *Fertil. Steril.* **2000**, *73*, 1155–1158. [CrossRef]
22. ESHRE Special Interest Group of Embryology and Alpha Scientists in Reproductive Medicine. The Vienna consensus: Report of an expert meeting on the development of ART laboratory performance indicators. *Reprod. Biomed. Online* **2017**, *35*, 494–510. [CrossRef]
23. Benaglia, L.; Bermejo, A.; Somigliana, E.; Faulisi, S.; Ragni, G.; Fedele, L.; Garcia-Velasco, J.A. In vitro fertilization outcome in women with unoperated bilateral endometriomas. *Fertil. Steril.* **2013**, *99*, 1714–1719. [CrossRef]
24. Suzuki, T.; Izumi, S.I.; Matsubayashi, H.; Awaji, H.; Yoshikata, K.; Makino, T. Impact of ovarian endometrioma on oocytes and pregnancy outcome in in vitro fertilization. *Fertil. Steril.* **2005**, *83*, 908–913. [CrossRef]
25. Wu, Y.; Yang, R.; Lan, J.; Lin, H.; Jiao, X.; Zhang, Q. Ovarian Endometrioma Negatively Impacts Oocyte Quality and Quantity But Not Pregnancy Outcomes in Women Undergoing IVF/ICSI Treatment: A Retrospective Cohort Study. *Front. Endocrinol. (Lausanne)* **2021**, *12*, 739228. [CrossRef] [PubMed]
26. Yang, C.; Geng, Y.; Li, Y.; Chen, C.; Gao, Y. Impact of ovarian endometrioma on ovarian responsiveness and IVF: A systematic review and meta-analysis. *Reprod. Biomed. Online* **2015**, *31*, 9–19. [CrossRef] [PubMed]
27. Simopoulou, M.; Rapani, A.; Grigoriadis, S.; Pantou, A.; Tsioulou, P.; Maziotis, E.; Tzanakaki, D.; Triantafyllidou, O.; Kalampokas, T.; Siristatidis, C.; et al. Getting to Know Endometriosis-Related Infertility Better: A Review on How Endometriosis Affects Oocyte Quality and Embryo Development. *Biomedicines* **2021**, *9*, 273. [CrossRef] [PubMed]
28. Yland, J.; Pina Carvalho, L.F.; Beste, M.; Bailey, A.; Thomas, C.; Abrao, M.S.; Racowsky, C.; Griffith, L.; Missmer, S.A. Endometrioma, the follicular fluid inflammatory network and its association with oocyte and embryo characteristics. *Reprod. Biomed. Online* **2020**, *40*, 399–408. [CrossRef]
29. Opøien, H.K.; Fedorcsak, P.; Polec, A.; Stensen, M.H.; Åbyholm, T.; Tanbo, T. Do endometriomas induce an inflammatory reaction in nearby follicles? *Hum. Reprod.* **2013**, *28*, 1837–1845. [CrossRef]
30. Goodman, L.R.; Goldberg, J.M.; Flyckt, R.L.; Gupta, M.; Harwalker, J.; Falcone, T. Effect of surgery on ovarian reserve in women with endometriomas, endometriosis and controls. *Am. J. Obstet. Gynecol.* **2016**, *215*, 589.e1–589.e6. [CrossRef]
31. Uncu, G.; Kasapoglu, I.; Ozerkan, K.; Seyhan, A.; Oral Yilmaztepe, A.; Ata, B. Prospective assessment of the impact of endometriomas and their removal on ovarian reserve and determinants of the rate of decline in ovarian reserve. *Hum. Reprod.* **2013**, *28*, 2140–2145. [CrossRef] [PubMed]
32. Wei, D.; Liu, J.Y.; Sun, Y.; Shi, Y.; Zhang, B.; Liu, J.Q.; Tan, J.; Liang, X.; Cao, Y.; Wang, Z.; et al. Frozen versus fresh single blastocyst transfer in ovulatory women: A multicentre, randomised controlled trial. *Lancet* **2019**, *393*, 1310–1318. [CrossRef] [PubMed]
33. Li, A.; Zhang, J.; Kuang, Y.; Yu, C. Analysis of IVF/ICSI-FET Outcomes in Women With Advanced Endometriosis: Influence on Ovarian Response and Oocyte Competence. *Front. Endocrinol.* **2020**, *11*, 427. [CrossRef]
34. Demirol, A.; Guven, S.; Baykal, C.; Gurgan, T. Effect of endometrioma cystectomy on IVF outcome: A prospective randomized study. *Reprod. Biomed. Online* **2006**, *12*, 639–643. [CrossRef]
35. Hamdan, M.; Dunselman, G.; Li, T.C.; Cheong, Y. The impact of endometrioma on IVF/ICSI outcomes: A systematic review and meta-analysis. *Hum. Reprod. Update* **2015**, *21*, 809–825. [CrossRef] [PubMed]
36. Becker, C.M.; Bokor, A.; Heikinheimo, O.; Horne, A.; Jansen, F.; Kiesel, L.; King, K.; Kvaskoff, M.; Nap, A.; Petersen, K.; et al. ESHRE guideline: Endometriosis. *Hum. Reprod. Open* **2022**, *2022*, hoac009. [CrossRef]

37. Garcia-Velasco, J.A.; Somigliana, E. Management of endometriomas in women requiring IVF: To touch or not to touch. *Hum. Reprod.* **2009**, *24*, 496–501. [CrossRef]
38. Nisenblat, V.; Bossuyt, P.M.; Farquhar, C.; Johnson, N.; Hull, M.L. Imaging modalities for the non-invasive diagnosis of endometriosis. *Cochrane Database Syst. Rev.* **2016**, *2*, CD009591. [CrossRef] [PubMed]

Disclaimer/Publisher's Note: The statements, opinions and data contained in all publications are solely those of the individual author(s) and contributor(s) and not of MDPI and/or the editor(s). MDPI and/or the editor(s) disclaim responsibility for any injury to people or property resulting from any ideas, methods, instructions or products referred to in the content.

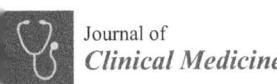

Article

Novel Time-Lapse Parameters Correlate with Embryo Ploidy and Suggest an Improvement in Non-Invasive Embryo Selection

Clara Serrano-Novillo *, Laia Uroz and Carmen Márquez

Gravida, Hospital de Barcelona, 08034 Barcelona, Spain
* Correspondence: cserrano@gravidabcn.com; Tel.: +34-93-206-64-89

Abstract: Selecting the best embryo for transfer is key to success in assisted reproduction. The use of algorithms or artificial intelligence can already predict blastulation or implantation with good results. However, ploidy predictions still rely on invasive techniques. Embryologists are still essential, and improving their evaluation tools can enhance clinical outcomes. This study analyzed 374 blastocysts from preimplantation genetic testing cycles. Embryos were cultured in time-lapse incubators and tested for aneuploidies; images were then studied for morphokinetic parameters. We present a new parameter, "st_2, start of t_2", detected at the beginning of the first cell cleavage, as strongly implicated in ploidy status. We describe specific cytoplasmic movement patterns associated with ploidy status. Aneuploid embryos also present slower developmental rates (t_3, t_5, t_{5B}, t_B, cc3, and t_5-t_2). Our analysis demonstrates a positive correlation among them for euploid embryos, while aneuploids present non-sequential behaviors. A logistic regression study confirmed the implications of the described parameters, showing a ROC value of 0.69 for ploidy prediction (95% confidence interval (CI), 0.62 to 0.76). Our results show that optimizing the relevant indicators to select the most suitable blastocyst, such as by including st_2, could reduce the time until the pregnancy of a euploid baby while avoiding invasive and expensive methods.

Keywords: embryo quality; preimplantation genetic testing; morphokinetics; time-lapse; ploidy

1. Introduction

The selection of the best embryo for transfer is key to success in in vitro fertilization (IVF) treatments. Identifying the embryo with the greatest potential for producing an evolutive pregnancy results in better clinical outcomes while minimizing the associated risks, multiple gestations, and potential complications, both maternal and fetal [1,2]. Embryo evaluation is mainly based on morphological criteria, such as fragmentation, multinucleation or cell size and number, following common grading methods [3]. Major advances in assisted reproductive technologies, especially regarding embryo culture, have allowed for the extension of long-term cultures up to the blastocyst stage, enabling better embryo scoring parameters [4–6].

However, while these techniques have been useful for more than 30 years, there is an evident lack of information considering that embryonic development follows a sequence of timed and coordinated events, which require specific developmental rates. Time-lapse (TL) technology solved the problem of static observations and opened new horizons for the study of these dynamic processes. Since the introduction of TL technology, new kinetic markers have been identified and are associated with higher implantation rates. Using this non-invasive scoring method, several studies have found an association between human embryo ploidy and morphokinetics: slower progression, delayed blastulation, and specific cleavage times, such as t3 or the interval t5-t2, have previously been associated with chromosomal aberrations [7–10].

Nevertheless, clinical pregnancy rates remain at ≈30% [11], a relatively low figure. Clinicians and embryologists urge to find new approaches to improve the selection method and raise these rates without increasing the number of embryos transferred. Genetic screening of embryos may seem a promising solution for this issue, as several studies demonstrate chromosomal alterations to be one of the most common causes of abnormal embryos in IVF (and, thus, of poor clinical outcomes) [12–14]. Aneuploid embryos, which often present apparently good development and morphology, are associated with implantation failure, miscarriage, and congenital defects [15].

Preimplantation genetic testing (PGT) for aneuploidies allows for the selection of chromosomally normal embryos. This can raise implantation rates up to 70% when transferring an euploid embryo [16]. However, PGT is not always possible or indicated. Some risks are associated with the technique, as it is an invasive methodology and not completely reliable. The possibility of misdiagnosis, an embryo lacking a diagnosis, or inconclusive results should be considered. Furthermore, the financial cost of embryo testing is elevated; there may be social reasons to discard the embryos, and some clinics do not have the advanced technology required. Therefore, new non-invasive embryo selection methods need to be studied. The search for an association between morphokinetic variables and aneuploidy has recently gained attention, with researchers seeking to find models or algorithms that could help to predict embryo ploidy status, most recently with the help of artificial intelligence (AI). Most authors agree on the importance of early cleavages and also associate delayed blastulation with chromosomal abnormalities, but they apply different pivotal parameters in their predicting models [17–19]. In this context, risk models are often not applicable to all TL devices and clinics and depend on the subjectivity or working methodology of each team. The use of AI is promising and can already predict blastulation and implantation with good results, but it cannot yet predict ploidy. Moreover, AI presents some other limitations at present (i.e., the software needs to be trained and often corrected by embryologists, embryos with aberrant development are often miss-annotated, it represents an expensive investment for small clinics, etc.). Therefore, embryologists are still essential for embryo evaluation and the selection of the best embryos for transfer.

The aim of this study is to understand the implications and relation of several classic and novel morphokinetic markers to embryo behavior and to elucidate their ploidy prediction potential, incorporating this information as a key selection tool that is accessible to all. We describe a strategy for predicting the ploidy status of an embryo while avoiding invasive methods and establish the best indicators to select the most suitable blastocyst to achieve a pregnancy with a euploid baby.

2. Materials and Methods

2.1. Study Design

This retrospective study was conducted at the Gravida Fertilitat Avançada center in Barcelona, Spain. The cohort of the study was drawn from a total of 85 treatments of 73 patients, including 374 blastocysts fertilized using both conventional in vitro fertilization (IVF) ($n = 202$) and intracytoplasmic sperm injection (ICSI) ($n = 172$) in cycles from January 2018 to February 2020. Owing to its retrospective nature and the absence of a priori intervention, the present study did not require the approval of an external review board. The data collection is part of the routine clinical procedure, is not sensitive, and is de-identified; therefore, this observational study posed no risk in terms of compromising the identity or safety of the studied individuals. Among the cases included in the study, with a total of 674 embryos fertilized, 374 (55.5%) of the embryos developed to the blastocyst stage and were able to be biopsied and therefore analyzed by PGT for aneuploidies on the fifth or sixth day of culture (D5 or D6). The annotation of morphokinetic characteristics was performed on all available and analyzed embryos, and the study was blinded to ploidy. Embryos with incomplete annotations failed amplification, and/or abnormal or no fertilization were excluded from the analysis.

This study included patients undergoing PGT due to recurrent miscarriage, repeated implantation failure, advanced maternal age, altered karyotype, and also those doing so electively. A minimum number of embryos to proceed with PGT was not set. The female age ranged from 26 to 45 years (mean ± standard deviation, 38.0 ± 3.9).

2.2. Ovarian Stimulation

The ovarian stimulation protocol was based on the patient's age, hormone levels, antral follicle counts, and prior treatments. Briefly, recombinant alpha or beta FSH (with or without urinary menotropins) were used for ovarian stimulation, ranging from 150 to 375 IU, according to the patient type and ovarian reserve (Gonal F® (Merck, Darmstadt, Germany) or Menopur® (Ferring, Kastrup, Denmark)). To prevent ovulation before egg collection, GnRH antagonists (Orgalutran® (Organon, Amsterdam, The Netherlands) were administered daily starting on day 5 or 6 after FSH administration. Final follicular maturation was triggered with hCG and/or a GnRH agonist (Ovitrelle® (Merck, Darmstadt, Germany) and Decapeptyl® (Ipsen, Boulogne-Billancourt, France), respectively). GnRH agonist was used when patients had ≥10 follicles over 14 mm or estradiol levels ≥2500 pg/mL. If lower levels of follicles were found, a combination of hCG and GnRH was administered.

2.3. Oocyte Retrieval and Embryo Culture

Oocytes were retrieved 36 h after the follicular maturation trigger using a transvaginal ultrasound-guided needle. The procedure was performed with the patients under sedation. Oocytes were incubated for around 3 h in Global for Fertilization® medium (LifeGlobal, Guilford, USA) under an oil overlay (Ovoil™, Vitrolife, Gothenburg, Sweden) at 37 °C and 6.6% CO_2 and 5% O_2 (previously equilibrated overnight). For ICSI samples, cumulus cells surrounding the oocytes were removed enzymatically with hyaluronidase (HYASE™, Vitrolife) and by pipetting, and ICSI was performed on metaphase II oocytes, which were placed on individual microwells of Geri® (Merck) TL or conventional culture plates, depending on the case. For conventional IVF, oocyte–cumulus complexes were coincubated with sperm overnight. Fertilization was checked 16–18 h post-insemination. Normally fertilized oocytes from IVF were also placed in individual multiwells of the Geri® or conventional culture plates and loaded into the Geri® system or conventional incubator, respectively. Both culture methods were performed in Global Total LP® medium (Vitrolife) covered in mineral oil for up to 6 days at 37 °C with 6–6.7% CO_2 and 5% O_2. The culture was briefly interrupted on day 3 in order to perform the assisted hatching and ensure that all embryos were able to hatch prior to the biopsy.

For the TL technology embryos, images of each fertilized oocyte were acquired automatically every 5 min through 11 focal planes. These time-lapse images were used for the assessment of the embryo's development and to identify the precise timing of developmental events as they were assessed by the embryologists studying the images.

2.4. Trophectoderm Biopsy and PGT

Biopsy was performed on day 5/6 of development in all high-quality blastocytes, including grading A and B for the inner cell mass (ICM) and trophoectoderm (TE). Briefly, a combination of laser pulses and mechanical separation was performed to achieve 5–10 TE cells to be used for genetic screening. The biopsied cells were washed and collected in sterile PCR tubes. After the TE biopsy, the embryos were vitrified according to the manufacturer's instructions (Kitazato, Shizuoka, Japan).

Biopsied cells were diagnosed using whole-genome amplification (NGS, Next Generation Sequencing) by an external genetic analysis laboratory. The NGS platform was used to detect 24-chromosome aneuploidies from a single whole-genome sample. The copy-number values were determined to identify deviations (positive for gains and negative for losses). Each chromosome region was classified as euploid (<30% aneuploidy) or aneuploid (≥30% aneuploidy). Euploid embryos were those showing euploid values for all chromosomes.

2.5. Time-Lapse Analysis and Recording of Kinetic and Morphological Parameters

Time-lapse images acquired during the culture period to the point of the biopsy were used for the assessment of the embryo's development. The time of insemination by ICSI or the hour when the conventional IVF was performed was programmed into the Geri System when the slide was loaded. Embryologists studying time-lapse images annotated the precise timing of the developmental events observed using the viewer. All times were recorded in hours and normalized to the pronuclei fading time (using t_{PNf} as t_0) to enable us to study the embryos from IVF and ICSI together. Table S1 shows definitions of the dynamic events studied. Morphological features were also tracked, including the morphology of the cells, fragmentation, multinucleation at the 2- or 4-cell stage, pronuclei morphology, direct and reverse cleavage, and the compaction process. Strict guidelines were established for the annotation of video footage. Embryo grading was performed following the recommendations of Alikani et al. [20], the Gardner classification [4], and ESHRE and ASRM guidance [8,21].

A novel parameter is described and studied (start of t2, st_2), corresponding to the first cytoplasmic movements prior to the first cytokinesis (Video S1). The cytoplasmic movements were divided into 3 groups depending on their observed phenotype: Pattern 0 for no detectable movements at the microscope level (Video S2); Pattern 1 for non-patterned movements (Video S3); and Pattern 2 for circular movements (Video S4). The initial detection of all these movements in groups 1 and 2 were labeled as st_2 for each embryo. Group 0 embryos lack st_2 annotation. Thus, st_2 annotation corresponds to the first detectable frame of the following movements: halo disappearance, cytoplasmic waves (which usually lead to anarchic blebbing), or circling cytoplasm movements. Specific membrane movements, such as pseudo-furrows or rubbing movements, among others, were not considered, as st_2 refers only to cytoplasmic movements. All annotations were blinded to ploidy.

2.6. Statistical Analysis

Continuous data are expressed as means with standard deviations, and categorical data are expressed as percentages. The relationship between the various parameters studied and the chromosomal dotation was assessed. Categorical data and proportions were analyzed using Chi-square tests. The normality of continuous data was assessed, and a T-test was used for continuous variables. Univariate and multivariate logistic regression analyses were used to create a model for enhanced selection based on aneuploidy, and the odds ratio (OR) was expressed in terms of the 95% confidence interval (95% CI) and significance. Receiver operating characteristic (ROC) curves were used to test the predictive value of all variables included in the model with respect to chromosomal normality. Statistical analysis was performed using GraphPad software. $p < 0.05$ was considered statistically significant.

3. Results

In this study, 374 embryos from 85 IVF/ICSI cycles were studied for aneuploidy. The mean age of the female partners was 38.0 years, ranging from 22 to 45 years. The patient demographics, indications for performing genetic testing on the embryos, and cycle characteristics are summarized in Table S2. A total of 158 embryos were diagnosed as euploid, resulting in a 42.2% global euploidy rate (38.3% per cycle). No differences were observed in this rate when comparing embryos from different fertilization techniques (conventional IVF (38.1%) or ICSI (47.1%)).

Several morphokinetic parameters showed a high association with ploidy status (Table 1). Euploid embryos appear to be faster in their development, reaching specific division times (st_2, t_3, t_5) and blastocyst formation moments (t_{SB}, t_B) earlier than the aneuploid group. Similarly, some intervals also appear to be shorter in the euploid group (cc3, t_5–t_2). The mean times for these parameters for euploid and aneuploidy embryos, respectively, are as follows: st_2: 1.5 ± 0.9 vs. 1.6 ± 0.7; t_3: 12.9 ± 3.4 vs. 13.6 ± 2.6; t_5: 25.5 ± 6.1 vs. 27.1 ± 4.5; t_{SB}: 73.8 ± 7.0 vs. 76.3 ± 7.5; t_B: 83.6 ± 7.4 vs. 86.2 ± 7.6; cc3:

12.5 ± 4.8 vs. 13.6 ± 2.9; t_5-t_2: 22.9 ± 6.2 vs. 24.4 ± 4.7. Data from the euploid group are distributed more equally, while the aneuploid population tends to be more dispersed, especially above the median.

Table 1. Annotations for morphokinetic parameters were analyzed using time-lapse technology.

	Euploid Embryos		Aneuploid Embryos		p-Value
	Mean (h) ± 95% CI	n	Mean (h) ± 95% CI	n	
st_2	1.5 ± 0.9	128	1.6 ± 0.7	157	0.03
t_2	2.6 ± 0.5	156	2.7 ± 0.6	216	ns
t_3	12.9 ± 3.4	157	13.6 ± 2.6	215	0.05
t_4	14.4 ± 2.4	155	14.6 ± 2.2	213	ns
t_5	25.5 ± 6.1	156	27.1 ± 4.5	215	0.004
t_8	34.8 ± 7.4	154	35.2 ± 7.3	213	ns
t_{SC}	54.2 ± 11.5	156	54.7 ± 11.3	216	ns
t_{SB}	73.8 ± 7.0	158	76.3 ± 7.5	216	0.001
t_B	83.6 ± 7.4	151	86.2 ± 7.6	212	0.001
t_2–st_2	1.2 ± 0.9	128	1.1 ± 0.8	157	ns
cc2 (t_3–t_2)	10.4 ± 3.4	156	10.8 ± 2.9	215	ns
cc3 (t_5–t_3)	12.5 ± 4.8	156	13.6 ± 2.9	215	0.006
t_5–t_2	22.9 ± 6.2	156	24.4 ± 4.7	215	0.008
s2 (t_4–t_3)	1.5 ± 1.0	155	1.2 ± 1.3	213	ns
s3 (t_8–t_5)	9.2 ± 3.7	154	8.3 ± 3.6	213	ns
t_{SC}–t_8	19.6 ± 5.5	154	19.5 ± 5.8	213	ns
t_B–t_{SB}	9.9 ± 2.6	151	10.0 ± 2.9	212	ns

ns: not significant.

St_2, a novel and poorly studied parameter, was shown to be highly discrepant between euploid and aneuploid blastocysts. St_2 was considered to be the initial cytoplasmatic movement that embryos present prior to the first cell cleavage. These phenomena presented different expressions, divided into three corresponding groups. Some of the embryos (Pattern 0) did not present any detectable movements when observed under the microscope. These embryos did not present halo dissolution or redistribution of the cytoplasmic material, either towards the cortex (as commonly described) or in any other textural change. A small group of embryos lacking a flare or halo, in addition to not showing any other cytoplasmic reorganization, are included in this group. The cleavage to the two-cell stage was smooth (Video S2). Pattern 1 includes embryos with cytoplasmic or peripheral (adjacent to the membrane) vibration-like movements prior to the first cell division. These movements do not follow any identifiable pattern and have a random appearance. Movements annotated in this group include halo disappearance (Video S3A), cytoplasmic polarization, or random waves (Video S3B,C), which usually lead to anarchic blebbing. However, specific membrane movements, such as pseudo-furrows or rubbing movements, among others, were not considered; we only focused on cytoplasmic movements. Commonly, these start after the PN breakdown, but we also detected them immediately prior to the pronuclei disappearance (referring specifically to halo fading). When this was the case, st_2 was annotated and, accordingly, adopted negative values after the PN fading correction was applied. Pattern 2 embryos present clear circular wave movements at the cytoplasm (Video S4). Circular movements are often repeated, and most of the embryos presenting this cortical rotation exhibit at least 2–3 complete rotations before cell cleavage. The occurrence of each pattern is shown in Table 2 and shows a clear correlation with chromosomal dotation

(p value < 0.0001). Pattern 2 was highly associated with euploid embryos: 90% of the embryos with circular movements were diagnosed as euploid. In contrast, Pattern 0 was more frequently observed in aneuploid embryos compared to euploid blastocysts (66.3% vs. 33.7%, respectively).

Table 2. Occurrence of the different cytoplasmic patterns of st_2 in euploid and aneuploid embryos.

	Euploid Embryos	Aneuploid Embryos	p-Value
Pattern 0	30 (33.7%)	59 (66.3%)	
Pattern 1	110 (41.5%)	155 (58.5%)	<0.0001
Pattern 2	18 (90.0%)	2 (10.0%)	

Regarding the morphological variables visible with TL technology, we studied multinucleation, direct or reverse cleavage, the size and symmetry of pronuclei, the presence of exclusion cells, and the compaction process. None of these parameters appear to be significantly associated with the ploidy status.

The correlation between the various morphokinetic timings and intervals studied is represented in a correlation matrix. For euploid embryos, especially in the case of intervals (Figure 1), we found a positive correlation for most of them. Initial divisions, as well as the blastulation process, appear to be significantly involved in chromosomal dotation, with early cleavages presenting a clear correlation with blastulation time. On the contrary, aneuploid embryos showed null or insignificant correlations, with r values that were not statistically different from 0.

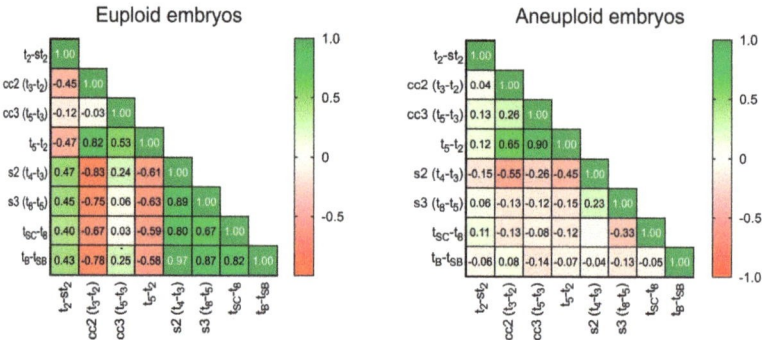

Figure 1. Correlation matrix of the studied interval parameters. The left panel shows the matrix obtained for euploid embryos; the right shows that obtained for aneuploid embryos. Numbers inside cells show r values. The color legend shows the degree of correlation: green (1.0), positive correlation; red (−1.0), negative correlation; 0, no correlation.

Using univariate logistic regression models, we confirmed the parameters that most strongly affect the ploidy status (Table 3). We filtered the most relevant parameters according to all of our results, controlled the data for egg age (as it is a known confounder), and performed a multivariate logistic regression study to develop a model using the Odds ratios (Table 4). The area under the ROC curve was AUC = 0.69, with a 95% confidence interval (0.62 to 0.76), which suggests an existing but moderate predictive ability. Using this system, we were able to identify 49.5% of euploid embryos. However, 80.6% of aneuploid embryos were correctly classified. When looking at the specific weight of each parameter on the model, only the st_2 pattern significantly affected the outcome as an independent predictive factor.

Table 3. Univariate logistic regression analysis.

Parameter	Odds Ratio	95% IC	p-Value
st_2	0.763	1.017–1.936	0.04
t_2	1.265	0.887–1.844	ns
t_3	1.061	0.990–1.138	ns
t_4	1.014	0.926–1.110	ns
t_5	1.058	0.017–0.097	0.005
t_8	1.008	0.980–10.37	ns
t_{SC}	1.005	0.988–1.023	ns
t_{SB}	1.051	1.021–1.083	<0.001
t_B	1.049	1.020–1.081	<0.001
t_2-st_2	0.715	0.537–0.899	<0.0001
cc2 (t_3-t_2)	1.043	0.976–1.115	ns
cc3 (t_5-t_3)	1.080	1.022–1.146	0.006
t_5-t_2	1.053	1.013–1.096	0.008
s2 (t_4-t_3)	0.931	0.845–1.023	ns
s3 (t_8-t_5)	0.983	0.955–1.013	ns
$t_{SC}-t_8$	1.000	0.983–1.017	ns
t_B-t_{SB}	1.006	0.961–1.056	ns
st_2 pattern	0.635	0.468–0.845	0.001

ns: not significant.

Table 4. Multivariate logistic regression analysis.

Parameter	Odds Ratio	95% IC	p-Value
st_2	0.979	0.642–1.493	ns
t_5	0.655	0.362–1.143	ns
t_{SB}	0.968	0.899–1.044	ns
t_B	0.984	0.916–1.052	ns
cc3 (t_5-t_3)	1.380	0.820–2.398	ns
(t_5-t_2)	1.012	0.8725–1.167	ns
st_2 pattern	1.648	1.088–2.539	0.02

ns: not significant.

4. Discussion

This study retrospectively analyzed the relationship between embryo development data and chromosomal dotation, and the results show that morphokinetics of embryo development are related to embryo ploidy. Embryonic aneuploidies may affect the development and cleavage behavior of embryos. By using time-lapse culture systems, we were able to monitor and identify those kinetic events and transient morphological attributes that can help us better select embryos for transfer by predicting embryo ploidy without using PGT. While an improvement in clinical outcomes has been seen over recent years when using TL incubators, meta-analyses comparing these studies show little to no evidence of the improvement of embryo selection when using TL embryo selection software compared to conventional assessments [22]. Therefore, it is necessary to refine TL embryo evaluation systems.

We found no differences between embryos from conventional IVF versus ICSI, either in fertilization or in euploidy rates. The majority of published studies focus on ICSI cycles. We believe that neglecting conventional IVF in these studies is a mistake, as it is an optimal technique for many couples, especially in cases with non-male-factor infertility. Additionally, while ICSI used to be mandatory before PGT studies to avoid sperm DNA contamination, by switching from a D3 to a TE biopsy, this potential risk can be overlooked [23]. By including IVF cycles in our study, we are able to apply the results obtained to all our patients, regardless of the fertilization technique that is suitable for them. We did find differences in maternal age between the euploid and aneuploid groups. While oocyte age is one of the main known factors affecting euploidy, we applied corrections to our prediction models to discard age as a confounding factor.

It is worth mentioning that PGT-A does not increase cumulative pregnancy rates. The probability of achieving a successful pregnancy after transferring a euploid embryo is significantly higher compared to the results of transferring an embryo without genetic analysis. However, it does not have superior outcomes for a whole embryo pool. Focusing on individual embryo transfers and not on cumulative outcomes falsely suggests that PGT-A improves outcomes, but it actually shortens the time and transferences required to achieve these results [24,25]. IVF treatments can be onerous and tedious for patients with fertility problems; they are associated with stress, and they represent a significant economic burden for the patients. Reducing the time and attempts needed for the whole process is a benefit in and of itself, so the advantages of PGT-A for specific patients are undeniable. However, questions continue to be raised regarding the invasiveness of the technique and the question of whether only a specific subset of patients truly benefit more from its usage (e.g., in cases with advanced maternal age or previous miscarriages).

Novel techniques for identifying euploid embryos without the technical and economic drawbacks of invasive and non-invasive preimplantation screening must be found. Reducing transfer failures could lead to fewer patients discontinuing treatment. Nowadays, new approaches for diagnosing embryo ploidy using novel, less invasive techniques are being developed, such as non-invasive preimplantation genetic testing, which is based on the analysis of DNA found within the blastocoel fluid of blastocysts and in spent media culture (niPGT) [26–28]. However, despite the significant potential of niPGT, we are a long way from making those procedures accessible to all patients, both because problems related to complexity, technical complications, and limitations remain unsolved and also because of the high economic cost such procedures can entail despite not being diagnostic methods but giving a "recommendation" result instead. A polar body biopsy is also an alternative. This technique is less invasive than TE biopsy, it does not affect embryo morphokinetics, and it has no negative impact on implantation events. However, only maternal genetic information is obtained. Although 90% of human aneuploidies at birth are of maternal origin, the possibility of paternal aneuploidies cannot be dismissed [29].

Meanwhile, the use of algorithms and grading systems based on morphokinetic parameters to predict ploidy can be of great help when selecting embryos for transfer. Even for those patients who do not have a medical recommendation to perform PGT-A, we could increase the success rates of IVF treatments by increasing the probability of transferring euploid embryos. Our results, in line with previously published studies [10,30], show that high-quality embryos also present aneuploidies at a considerable rate (50.3% of AA blastocysts are aneuploidy in our study). Thus, we need more than a static grading system based on quality, from which we can predict the genetic content of the embryo. AI prediction models are, in this sense, promising. However, they are still in the development phases and do not reach the same level of specificity as PGT.

Regarding the morphological markers observed thanks to TL, including pronuclei morphology, multinucleation, chaotic cleavages, or the compaction process, none of the studied variables appeared to be related to the embryo's ploidy status. These markers were previously identified as critical parameters for blastocyst formation [31–33]. However, some seem to also be clearly related to ploidy abnormalities, such as an aberrant number of cell nuclei. Two main hypotheses can explain this fact. First, defective markers are highly associated with bad blastulation, and we only analyze high-quality blastocysts for the PGT study. Those embryos presenting altered parameters affecting blastocyst formation would not reach the optimal stage to be biopsied and, thus, would not have been included in this study. During preimplantation development, there is a progressive loss of abnormal embryos caused by growth arrest or degeneration. Accordingly, the sample size for these variables was extremely small in most of the cases. Second, embryos may present "self-correction" systems for some of these parameters. For example, while excluded cells may be associated with chromosomal defects, this may be the reason that these particular cells are excluded from the blastocyst [34]. It has also been noted that multinucleated cells have the potential for self-correction during the first cleavages and develop euploid blastocysts [35].

Similarly, some studies report that around 20% of trisomies in cleavage-stage embryos are self-corrected and lead to euploid blastocysts [36]. However, in all of these self-correcting cases, there can exist collateral abnormalities such as uniparental disomies.

Focusing on kinetic markers, we found seven timings to be particularly strongly associated with chromosomal status: st_2, t_3, t_5, t_{SB}, t_B, $cc3$, and t_5–t_2. These key markers demonstrate that there are critical steps throughout the whole embryo development process. Our results agree with those of previous studies, which described synchronized and early cleavages, as well as early blastulation, as being valuable for ploidy prognosis [17–19]. Furthermore, we performed a test to identify outliers prior to the study. Interestingly, more extreme values were found in the aneuploid population. Thus, abnormal or aberrant behaviors are often related to altered chromosomal content. In most of the studies published, slower blastocyst formation is associated with poorer embryo viability [37]. We also obtained similar results, whereby delayed timings are associated with aberrant embryos. The sooner and shorter those changes are, the higher the probability of euploidy. This delay in development could be explained by the abnormal activation of the spindle assembly checkpoint [38] in those cells presenting aneuploidy, as the aneuploid chromosome encounters difficulties in aligning with the metaphase plate. Additionally, a defective or lax checkpoint during embryonic development may lead to further development with chaotic or aberrant divisions [39].

Curiously, we found higher aneuploidy rates to be associated with delayed blastulation, but we found no difference in the ploidy status between D5 and D6 biopsied embryos. A consistent conclusion has not yet been reached in this ongoing debate. Some authors suggest better clinical outcomes for D5 embryos [40,41], whereas other studies find no differences associated with the embryo transfer day [42–44]. A common explanation for lower pregnancy outcomes for D6 transfer is the discordance between the patient endometrium and the embryo stage. Particularly in fresh cycles, when the implantation window is advanced after ovarian stimulation, we face an embryo–endometrium desynchronization scenario, especially in D6 transfers. When only high-quality embryos in fresh transfers were considered, no differences were found between D5 and D6 blastocysts [45]. Low-quality embryos could present with slower development and also be associated with chromosomal anomalies that could impair their viability and the implantation potential of those fresh D6 blastocysts. Again, only high-quality embryos are candidates for embryo biopsy and PGT-A in our clinic, excluding those potentially altered embryos. Moreover, we normalize our study times to the disappearance of PN, suggesting that the impact of D5 vs. D6 potential may not rely on pure timings themselves but rather on the way they progress from one stage to another (especially because we include conventional IVF cycles). Delayed fertilization followed by a chronological and punctual division can result in a euploid and viable D6 blastocyst, while early fertilization followed by decompensated or delayed division steps can be associated with a D5 embryo with a poor prognosis. Thus, delayed blastulation refers to the embryonic inner time spent until the start of or complete blastulation, but it does not directly correlate to "our" D5 or D6.

We found a poorly studied parameter that is of special importance in this context: st_2. St_2 refers to the initial cytoplasmic macroscopic observable movements that precede the first cytokinesis. We demonstrated that the start of the t_2 division is key to the ploidy outcome, as delayed times for this first movement are associated with a higher likelihood of aneuploidy and affect the following cleavages. There are molecular steps required for cell division (maturation, chromosome division, protein machinery, etc.) that can translate into these ooplasmic movements. This organelle reorganization, which prepares the cell to divide, could be more important than the time spent in proper cytokinesis itself. For example, halo disappearance is related to the microtubule-mediated withdrawal of mitochondria and other cytoplasmic components of perinuclear regions, and mitochondrial activity is highly involved in cell cycle regulation [46]. Fertilization cytoplasmic dynamics have been described in detail in relation to the PN appearance, alignment, and fading events and can predict clinical outcomes [47]. Fast cleavage is related to good blastocyst formation with regard to membrane ruffling [48]. St$_2$, meanwhile, is an ooplasmic event prior to the first cell cleavage that could also be used in embryo evaluation, as we found it to be related to ploidy. Based on our results, embryos presenting early st$_2$ movements are more likely to present euploid complements, while membrane blebbing is usually observed later. Additionally, the nature of the cortex dynamics is important, as we describe three types of movement. A lack of movement is associated with poor blastulation prognosis [49], and we see a tendency towards aneuploidy. Embryos diagnosed as aneuploid in Pattern 0 are almost twice as numerous as the euploid group. While cytoplasmic movements are found in both euploid and aneuploid populations, circular waves, in particular, appear to be a characteristic of euploid embryos. All of the embryos presenting this rotation, except two, were diagnosed as euploid. However, while the statistical power of these results is strong, the proportion of Pattern 2 embryos is small compared to the total sample of embryos studied. A bigger study could be valuable in further corroborating these results.

We also found an interesting correlation between most of the kinetic markers exclusively in euploid embryos. This confirms that aneuploid embryos present altered cleavage and developmental times, not only promoting delayed blastulation but also desynchronizing most of the sequential steps and division without a clear pattern. This chaotic behavior in aneuploid embryos is reinforced by the conventional grading system, as these embryos present oscillating gradings throughout their development. Our correlation matrix reveals that synchronic even cleavages (which lead to even numbers of cells, e.g., t_4–t_3) positively condition blastulation time. In contrast, synchronized and sequential odd cleavages (which lead to odd numbers of cells, e.g., t_3–t_2) inversely affect blastocyst formation and are a good prognostic for normal chromosomal content. The logistic regression model derived from this study presents an AUC = 0.69 and can help us to discard aneuploid embryos in 80.6% of cases. This can be useful when trying to select the best embryo for transfer, by rejecting those with a higher probability of aneuploidy. As mentioned above, machine learning algorithms and AI are promising tools, but they are still not fully reliable for ploidy selection. In this study, we tested our embryo populations retrospectively using AI to obtain a score and ranking of ploidy prediction. The present embryo evaluation system based on morphokinetic parameters, including st$_2$, obtains slightly better results than the use of AI-integrated predictors (AUC 0.69 vs. 0.64, respectively) [50]. While it was a small study, together, these results suggest the potential benefit of adding the novel markers described here to embryo selection systems.

Several algorithms and models have been developed to predict embryo ploidy [18,51]. However, some studies found no correlation in distinguishing euploidy [52]. Not only that, but some authors applied published models and failed to obtain accurate predictions for their cohort of blastocysts [53]. Considering all these discrepancies, it is imperative that all TL embryologists are meticulously trained to identify all of the developmental markers equally. Not only may the annotation vary slightly from one center to another (where slight variation is enough to invalidate a given model), but external factors may also bias the developmental morphokinetics (e.g., ovarian stimulation, temperature, pH, or culture media, among others). Therefore, we contend that it is useful not to apply an external model but to identify key markers that may condition every cohort independently of the center and laboratory. When using AI, the decision-making process of machine learning models is a black box. We cannot overlook the fact that AI could be taking into account parameters still unknown to embryologists, such as st$_2$. Thus, it is crucial that we decipher these parameters and optimize evaluation systems, both to improve embryologists' work and to optimize future artificial systems.

While none of these promising methods are fully developed, we can (or must) improve embryologists' grading tools for selecting the best embryos for transfer. Embryologists remain essential for embryo selection. While it could be helpful to have software helping them to decide, it is crucial that we understand what is behind these decisions. Identifying novel developmental events can help us to better understand AI models and ploidy implications. We present st$_2$ as an improvement tool to include in evaluation systems, paying special attention to the movement type (circular, not patterned or absent). This study has some limitations due to the sample size in some variables or groups and the retrospective nature of the analysis. Future studies, including large prospective RCTs, could be useful in maximizing time-lapse technology embryo assessments as a non-invasive, cost-effective alternative to PGT-A.

5. Conclusions

Morphokinetic analysis is not able to detect aneuploid embryos as accurately as PGT does, but it has the potential to identify the most suitable embryos and reduce the time to pregnancy. We have found two potential tools that can help to select the best embryo for transfer. (i) Our study demonstrates the importance of the relation between a wider group of developmental stages instead of focusing on one or two markers. By paying close attention to the correlation between crucial markers, especially the synchronicity and sequentially of the cleavages, we can discard potentially aneuploid embryos. (ii) We describe st_2 as a novel parameter that strongly influences the developmental progress of the following steps and which is strongly associated with chromosomal status. Specific cytoplasmic waving patterns correlate with ploidy diagnosis, with circling movements being the most strongly correlated with euploidy. Including this marker in conventional grading systems, as well as in selection models and algorithms, will lead to better results by improving embryo selection.

Supplementary Materials: The following supporting information can be downloaded at: https://www.mdpi.com/article/10.3390/jcm12082983/s1, Table S1: Nomenclature of morphokinetic dynamic events; Table S2: Baseline characteristics of patients involved in the study; Video S1: Start of t_2 (st_2); Video S2: Pattern 0 embryo examples; Video S3: Pattern 1 embryo examples; Video S4: Pattern 2 embryo examples.

Author Contributions: Conceptualization, C.S.-N. and C.M.; Methodology, C.S.-N.; Data collection: C.S.-N.; Formal Analysis, C.S.-N.; Statistical analysis: C.S.-N.; Writing the article: C.S.-N.; Critical revision of the article: C.S.-N., L.U. and C.M., Final approval of the article: C.S.-N., L.U. and C.M. All authors have read and agreed to the published version of the manuscript.

Funding: This research received no external funding.

Institutional Review Board Statement: Ethical review and approval were waived for this study due to its retrospective nature and absence of a priori intervention. The data collection is part of the routine clinical procedure, is not sensitive and is de-identified. Therefore this observational study has no risk of compromising the identity or safety of the individual.

Informed Consent Statement: Patient consent was waived due to the retrospective and observational nature of this study.

Data Availability Statement: Not applicable.

Conflicts of Interest: The authors declare no conflict of interest.

References

1. Dayan, N.; Joseph, K.S.; Fell, D.B.; Laskin, C.A.; Basso, O.; Park, A.L.; Luo, J.; Guan, J.; Ray, J.G. Infertility treatment and risk of severe maternal morbidity: A propensity score-matched cohort study. *Can. Med. Assoc. J.* **2019**, *191*, E118–E127. [CrossRef] [PubMed]
2. Kulkarni, A.D.; Jamieson, D.J.; Jones, H.W., Jr.; Kissin, D.M.; Gallo, M.F.; Macaluso, M.; Adashi, E.Y. Fertility treatments and multiple births in the United States. *N. Engl. J. Med.* **2013**, *369*, 2218–2225. [CrossRef] [PubMed]
3. Machtinger, R.; Racowsky, C. Morphological systems of human embryo assessment and clinical evidence. *Reprod. Biomed. Online* **2013**, *26*, 210–221. [CrossRef]
4. Gardner, D.; Schoolcraft, W. In vitro culture of human blastocysts. In *Towards Reproductive Certainty*; CRC Press: Boca Raton, FL, USA, 1999; pp. 378–388.
5. Gardner, D.K.; Lane, M.; Stevens, J.; Schlenker, T.; Schoolcraft, W.B. Blastocyst score affects implantation and pregnancy outcome: Towards a single blastocyst transfer. *Fertil. Steril.* **2000**, *73*, 1155–1158. [CrossRef]
6. Gardner, D.K.; Schoolcraft, W.B. Culture and transfer of human blastocysts. *Curr. Opin. Obstet. Gynecol.* **1999**, *11*, 307–311. [CrossRef] [PubMed]

7. Del Carmen Nogales, M.; Bronet, F.; Basile, N.; Martinez, E.M.; Linan, A.; Rodrigo, L.; Meseguer, M. Type of chromosome abnormality affects embryo morphology dynamics. *Fertil. Steril.* **2017**, *107*, 229–235.e222. [CrossRef]
8. ESHRE Working Group on Time-Lapse Technology; Apter, S.; Ebner, T.; Freour, T.; Guns, Y.; Kovacic, B.; Le Clef, N.; Marques, M.; Meseguer, M.; Montjean, D.; et al. Good practice recommendations for the use of time-lapse technology. *Hum. Reprod. Open* **2020**, *2020*, 8. [CrossRef]
9. Minasi, M.G.; Colasante, A.; Riccio, T.; Ruberti, A.; Casciani, V.; Scarselli, F.; Spinella, F.; Fiorentino, F.; Varricchio, M.T.; Greco, E. Correlation between aneuploidy, standard morphology evaluation and morphokinetic development in 1730 biopsied blastocysts: A consecutive case series study. *Hum. Reprod.* **2016**, *31*, 2245–2254. [CrossRef]
10. Zaninovic, N.; Irani, M.; Meseguer, M. Assessment of embryo morphology and developmental dynamics by time-lapse microscopy: Is there a relation to implantation and ploidy? *Fertil. Steril.* **2017**, *108*, 722–729. [CrossRef]
11. ESHRE. European pregnancy rates from IVF and ICSI 'appear to have reached a peak'. In Proceedings of the 35th ESHRE Annual Meeting, Vienna, Austria, 23–26 June 2019.
12. Munne, S. Chromosome abnormalities and their relationship to morphology and development of human embryos. *Reprod. Biomed. Online* **2006**, *12*, 234–253. [CrossRef]
13. Phan, V.; Littman, E.; Harris, D.; Severino, M.; La, A. Correlation between aneuploidy and blastocyst quality. *Fertil. Steril.* **2013**, *100*, S525–S526. [CrossRef]
14. Savio Figueira Rde, C.; Setti, A.S.; Braga, D.P.; Iaconelli, A., Jr.; Borges, E., Jr. Blastocyst Morphology Holds Clues Concerning the Chromosomal Status of The Embryo. *Int. J. Fertil. Steril.* **2015**, *9*, 215–220. [CrossRef] [PubMed]
15. Shahbazi, M.N.; Wang, T.; Tao, X.; Weatherbee, B.A.T.; Sun, L.; Zhan, Y.; Keller, L.; Smith, G.D.; Pellicer, A.; Scott, R.T., Jr.; et al. Developmental potential of aneuploid human embryos cultured beyond implantation. *Nat. Commun.* **2020**, *11*, 3987. [CrossRef]
16. Pirtea, P.; De Ziegler, D.; Tao, X.; Sun, L.; Zhan, Y.; Ayoubi, J.M.; Seli, E.; Franasiak, J.M.; Scott, R.T., Jr. Rate of true recurrent implantation failure is low: Results of three successive frozen euploid single embryo transfers. *Fertil. Steril.* **2021**, *115*, 45–53. [CrossRef]
17. Basile, N.; Nogales Mdel, C.; Bronet, F.; Florensa, M.; Riqueiros, M.; Rodrigo, L.; Garcia-Velasco, J.; Meseguer, M. Increasing the probability of selecting chromosomally normal embryos by time-lapse morphokinetics analysis. *Fertil. Steril.* **2014**, *101*, 699–704. [CrossRef]
18. Campbell, A.; Fishel, S.; Bowman, N.; Duffy, S.; Sedler, M.; Hickman, C.F. Modelling a risk classification of aneuploidy in human embryos using non-invasive morphokinetics. *Reprod. Biomed. Online* **2013**, *26*, 477–485. [CrossRef] [PubMed]
19. Swain, J.E. Could time-lapse embryo imaging reduce the need for biopsy and PGS? *J. Assist. Reprod. Genet.* **2013**, *30*, 1081–1090. [CrossRef] [PubMed]
20. Alikani, M.; Cohen, J.; Tomkin, G.; Garrisi, G.J.; Mack, C.; Scott, R.T. Human embryo fragmentation in vitro and its implications for pregnancy and implantation. *Fertil. Steril.* **1999**, *71*, 836–842. [CrossRef]
21. Alpha Scientists in Reproductive Medicine; ESHRE Special Interest Group of Embryology. The Istanbul consensus workshop on embryo assessment: Proceedings of an expert meeting. *Hum. Reprod.* **2011**, *26*, 1270–1283. [CrossRef]
22. Armstrong, S.; Bhide, P.; Jordan, V.; Pacey, A.; Marjoribanks, J.; Farquhar, C. Time-lapse systems for embryo incubation and assessment in assisted reproduction. *Cochrane Database Syst. Rev.* **2019**, *29*, CD011320. [CrossRef]
23. Feldman, B.; Aizer, A.; Brengauz, M.; Dotan, K.; Levron, J.; Schiff, E.; Orvieto, R. Pre-implantation genetic diagnosis-should we use ICSI for all? *J. Assist. Reprod. Genet.* **2017**, *34*, 1179–1183. [CrossRef] [PubMed]
24. Kemper, J.M.; Wang, R.; Rolnik, D.L.; Mol, B.W. Preimplantation genetic testing for aneuploidy: Are we examining the correct outcomes? *Hum. Reprod.* **2020**, *35*, 2408–2412. [CrossRef] [PubMed]
25. Murphy, L.A.; Seidler, E.A.; Vaughan, D.A.; Resetkova, N.; Penzias, A.S.; Toth, T.L.; Thornton, K.L.; Sakkas, D. To test or not to test? A framework for counselling patients on preimplantation genetic testing for aneuploidy (PGT-A). *Hum. Reprod.* **2018**, *34*, 268–275. [CrossRef] [PubMed]
26. Palini, S.; Galluzzi, L.; De Stefani, S.; Bianchi, M.; Wells, D.; Magnani, M.; Bulletti, C. Genomic DNA in human blastocoele fluid. *Reprod. Biomed. Online* **2013**, *26*, 603–610. [CrossRef]
27. Stigliani, S.; Persico, L.; Lagazio, C.; Anserini, P.; Venturini, P.L.; Scaruffi, P. Mitochondrial DNA in Day 3 embryo culture medium is a novel, non-invasive biomarker of blastocyst potential and implantation outcome. *Mol. Hum. Reprod.* **2014**, *20*, 1238–1246. [CrossRef] [PubMed]
28. Xu, J.; Fang, R.; Chen, L.; Chen, D.; Xiao, J.P.; Yang, W.; Wang, H.; Song, X.; Ma, T.; Bo, S.; et al. Noninvasive chromosome screening of human embryos by genome sequencing of embryo culture medium for in vitro fertilization. *Proc. Natl. Acad. Sci. USA* **2016**, *113*, 11907–11912. [CrossRef]
29. Schenk, M.; Groselj-Strele, A.; Eberhard, K.; Feldmeier, E.; Kastelic, D.; Cerk, S.; Weiss, G. Impact of polar body biopsy on embryo morphokinetics—Back to the roots in preimplantation genetic testing? *J. Assist. Reprod. Genet.* **2018**, *35*, 1521–1528. [CrossRef]
30. Alfarawati, S.; Fragouli, E.; Colls, P.; Stevens, J.; Gutiérrez-Mateo, C.; Schoolcraft, W.B.; Katz-Jaffe, M.G.; Wells, D. The relationship between blastocyst morphology, chromosomal abnormality, and embryo gender. *Fertil. Steril.* **2011**, *95*, 520–524. [CrossRef]
31. Gamiz, P.; Rubio, C.; de los Santos, M.J.; Mercader, A.; Simon, C.; Remohi, J.; Pellicer, A. The effect of pronuclear morphology on early development and chromosomal abnormalities in cleavage-stage embryos. *Hum. Reprod.* **2003**, *18*, 2413–2419. [CrossRef]
32. Nasiri, N.; Eftekhari-Yazdi, P. An overview of the available methods for morphological scoring of pre-implantation embryos in in vitro fertilization. *Cell J.* **2015**, *16*, 392–405. [CrossRef]

33. Sjoblom, P.; Menezes, J.; Cummins, L.; Mathiyalagan, B.; Costello, M.F. Prediction of embryo developmental potential and pregnancy based on early stage morphological characteristics. *Fertil. Steril.* **2006**, *86*, 848–861. [CrossRef] [PubMed]
34. Lagalla, C.; Tarozzi, N.; Sciajno, R.; Wells, D.; Di Santo, M.; Nadalini, M.; Distratis, V.; Borini, A. Embryos with morphokinetic abnormalities may develop into euploid blastocysts. *Reprod. Biomed. Online* **2017**, *34*, 137–146. [CrossRef]
35. Balakier, H.; Sojecki, A.; Motamedi, G.; Librach, C. Impact of multinucleated blastomeres on embryo developmental competence, morphokinetics, and aneuploidy. *Fertil. Steril.* **2016**, *106*, 608–614.e2. [CrossRef] [PubMed]
36. Capalbo, A.; Bono, S.; Spizzichino, L.; Biricik, A.; Baldi, M.; Colamaria, S.; Ubaldi, F.M.; Rienzi, L.; Fiorentino, F. Sequential comprehensive chromosome analysis on polar bodies, blastomeres and trophoblast: Insights into female meiotic errors and chromosomal segregation in the preimplantation window of embryo development. *Hum. Reprod.* **2013**, *28*, 509–518. [CrossRef] [PubMed]
37. Sciorio, R.; Thong, K.J.; Pickering, S.J. Increased pregnancy outcome after day 5 versus day 6 transfers of human vitrified-warmed blastocysts. *Zygote* **2019**, *27*, 279–284. [CrossRef]
38. Stukenberg, P.T.; Burke, D.J. Connecting the microtubule attachment status of each kinetochore to cell cycle arrest through the spindle assembly checkpoint. *Chromosoma* **2015**, *124*, 463–480. [CrossRef]
39. Jacobs, K.; Van de Velde, H.; De Paepe, C.; Sermon, K.; Spits, C. Mitotic spindle disruption in human preimplantation embryos activates the spindle assembly checkpoint but not apoptosis until Day 5 of development. *Mol. Hum. Reprod.* **2017**, *23*, 321–329. [CrossRef]
40. Mesut, N.; Ciray, H.N.; Mesut, A.; Aksoy, T.; Bahceci, M. Cryopreservation of blastocysts is the most feasible strategy in good responder patients. *Fertil. Steril.* **2011**, *96*, 1121–1125.e1. [CrossRef]
41. Xing, W.; Cai, L.; Sun, L.; Ou, J. Comparison of Pregnancy Outcomes of High-Quality D5- and D6-Blastocyst Transfer in Hormone-Replacement Frozen-Thawed Cycles. *Int. J. Clin. Med.* **2017**, *8*, 565–571. [CrossRef]
42. Hashimoto, S.; Amo, A.; Hama, S.; Ito, K.; Nakaoka, Y.; Morimoto, Y. Growth retardation in human blastocysts increases the incidence of abnormal spindles and decreases implantation potential after vitrification. *Hum. Reprod.* **2013**, *28*, 1528–1535. [CrossRef]
43. Sunkara, S.K.; Siozos, A.; Bolton, V.N.; Khalaf, Y.; Braude, P.R.; El-Toukhy, T. The influence of delayed blastocyst formation on the outcome of frozen-thawed blastocyst transfer: A systematic review and meta-analysis. *Hum. Reprod.* **2010**, *25*, 1906–1915. [CrossRef] [PubMed]
44. Xu, H.; Qiu, S.; Chen, X.; Zhu, S.; Sun, Y.; Zheng, B. D6 blastocyst transfer on day 6 in frozen-thawed cycles should be avoided: A retrospective cohort study. *BMC Pregnancy Childbirth* **2020**, *20*, 519. [CrossRef] [PubMed]
45. Yang, H.; Yang, Q.; Dai, S.; Li, G.; Jin, H.; Yao, G.; Sun, Y. Comparison of differences in development potentials between frozen-thawed D5 and D6 blastocysts and their relationship with pregnancy outcomes. *J. Assist. Reprod. Genet.* **2016**, *33*, 865–872. [CrossRef] [PubMed]
46. Van Blerkom, J.; Davis, P.; Alexander, S. Differential mitochondrial distribution in human pronuclear embryos leads to disproportionate inheritance between blastomeres: Relationship to microtubular organization, ATP content and competence. *Hum. Reprod.* **2000**, *15*, 2621–2633. [CrossRef] [PubMed]
47. Coticchio, G.; Mignini Renzini, M.; Novara, P.V.; Lain, M.; De Ponti, E.; Turchi, D.; Fadini, R.; Dal Canto, M. Focused time-lapse analysis reveals novel aspects of human fertilization and suggests new parameters of embryo viability. *Hum. Reprod.* **2018**, *33*, 23–31. [CrossRef]
48. Wong, C.C.; Loewke, K.E.; Bossert, N.L.; Behr, B.; De Jonge, C.J.; Baer, T.M.; Reijo Pera, R.A. Non-invasive imaging of human embryos before embryonic genome activation predicts development to the blastocyst stage. *Nat. Biotechnol.* **2010**, *28*, 1115–1121. [CrossRef]
49. Ezoe, K.; Miki, T.; Okimura, T.; Uchiyama, K.; Yabuuchi, A.; Kobayashi, T.; Kato, K. Characteristics of the cytoplasmic halo during fertilisation correlate with the live birth rate after fresh cleaved embryo transfer on day 2 in minimal ovarian stimulation cycles: A retrospective observational study. *Reprod. Biol. Endocrinol.* **2021**, *19*, 172. [CrossRef]
50. Serrano-Novillo, C. Automatic assessment of Time-Lapse videos using CHLOE-EQ can automate KPI assessment to validate the operational performance of an IVF Clinic. In Proceedings of the ALPHA Biennial Conference, Sevilla, Spain, 6–9 October 2022.
51. Campbell, A.; Fishel, S.; Bowman, N.; Duffy, S.; Sedler, M.; Thornton, S. Retrospective analysis of outcomes after IVF using an aneuploidy risk model derived from time-lapse imaging without PGS. *Reprod. Biomed. Online* **2013**, *27*, 140–146. [CrossRef]
52. Rienzi, L.; Capalbo, A.; Stoppa, M.; Romano, S.; Maggiulli, R.; Albricci, L.; Scarica, C.; Farcomeni, A.; Vajta, G.; Ubaldi, F.M. No evidence of association between blastocyst aneuploidy and morphokinetic assessment in a selected population of poor-prognosis patients: A longitudinal cohort study. *Reprod. Biomed. Online* **2015**, *30*, 57–66. [CrossRef]
53. Kramer, Y.G.; Kofinas, J.D.; Melzer, K.; Noyes, N.; McCaffrey, C.; Buldo-Licciardi, J.; McCulloh, D.H.; Grifo, J.A. Assessing morphokinetic parameters via time lapse microscopy (TLM) to predict euploidy: Are aneuploidy risk classification models universal? *J. Assist. Reprod. Genet.* **2014**, *31*, 1231–1242. [CrossRef]

Disclaimer/Publisher's Note: The statements, opinions and data contained in all publications are solely those of the individual author(s) and contributor(s) and not of MDPI and/or the editor(s). MDPI and/or the editor(s) disclaim responsibility for any injury to people or property resulting from any ideas, methods, instructions or products referred to in the content.

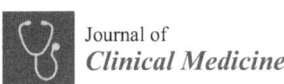

Review

Adverse Pregnancy Outcomes and Maternal Periodontal Disease: An Overview on Meta-Analytic and Methodological Quality

Vanessa Machado [1,2,*], Madalena Ferreira [1], Luísa Lopes [1], José João Mendes [1,2] and João Botelho [1,2]

1. Clinical Research Unit (CRU), Egas Moniz Center for Interdisciplinary Research, Egas Moniz School of Health and Science, 2829-511 Caparica, Portugal
2. Evidence-Based Hub, Egas Moniz Center for Interdisciplinary Research, Egas Moniz School of Health and Science, 2829-511 Almada, Portugal
* Correspondence: vmachado@egasmoniz.edu.pt

Abstract: This umbrella review aims to appraise the methodological quality and strength of evidence on the association between maternal periodontitis and adverse pregnancy outcomes (APOs). PubMed, CENTRAL, Web-of-Science, LILACS, and Clinical Trials were searched until February 2023, without date or language restrictions. Two authors independently screened studies, extracted data, performed the risk-of-bias analysis, and estimated the meta-analytic strengths and validity and the fail-safe number (FSN). A total of 43 SRs were identified, of which 34 conducted meta-analyses. Of the 28 APOs, periodontitis had a strong association with preterm birth (PTB), low birth weight (LBW), and gestational diabetes mellitus (GDM), PTB and LBW showed all levels of strength, and pre-eclampsia showed only suggestive and weak strength. Regarding the consistency of the significant estimates, only 8.7% were likely to change in the future. The impact of periodontal treatment on APOs was examined in 15 SRs, 11 of which conducted meta-analyses. Forty-one meta-analyses were included and showed that periodontal treatment did not have a strong association with APOs, although PTB revealed all levels of strength and LBW showed only suggestive and weak evidence. Strong and highly suggestive evidence from observational studies supports an association of periodontitis with a higher risk of PTB, LBW, GDM, and pre-eclampsia. The effect of periodontal treatment on the prevention of APOs is still uncertain and requires future studies to draw definitive and robust conclusions.

Keywords: adverse pregnancy outcomes; oral health; periodontitis; umbrella review

1. Introduction

Periodontitis is a chronic disease characterized by persistent inflammation that progressively damages the tissues surrounding the teeth [1,2]. The homeostasis disruption results in a host immune and inflammatory response in the periodontium with tissue destruction, gingival bleeding, and systemic inflammatory repercussions [1,2]. Among the several systemic conditions linked to periodontitis, adverse pregnancy outcomes (APOs) stand out [3–5] with their impact on maternal and infant health.

Approximately 40% of pregnant women worldwide are estimated to suffer from periodontitis [3,6]. During pregnancy, hormonal changes promote vascular permeability, which increases the likelihood of gingival inflammation [5,7]. The oral microbiome of pregnant women is a relatively stable community [8], but it can shift to distinct compositions [9–11] that may increase the risk of periodontitis [7] and, consequently, the association withother maternal complications such as gestational diabetes mellitus (GDM) [12]. Yet, prenatal dental care effectively reduces the carriage of oral pathogens (such as *Streptococcus mutans*) [8].

Since Offenbacher et al. in 1996 first reported a possible association between periodontal disease and preterm birth (PTB) [13], a new series of studies in periodontal medicine has linked maternal periodontitis to APOs, namely PTB, low birth weight (LBW), pre-eclampsia, GDM, and miscarriage/stillbirth (M/SB) [4,14].

With the exponential increase in clinical studies, a large number of systematic reviews regarding this association have emerged. In the light of current knowledge, five previous umbrella reviews summarized the available evidence and identified gaps in this association [15–19]. Nevertheless, none of the latter explored the statistical consistency of the estimates in the context of the available research. Therefore, an umbrella review assessing the methodological quality and strength of evidence on the association between maternal periodontitis and APOs was deemed timely.

2. Materials and Methods

This umbrella review was defined a priori by all authors, published online in the PROSPERO platform (ID: CRD42022358842), and conducted according to the Preferred Reporting Items for Systematic Reviews and Meta-Analysis (PRISMA) guidelines (Supplementary Data S1) [20].

2.1. Focused Question and Eligibility Criteria

The following focused PI(E)CO questions were addressed: "Do women with periodontitis have an increased risk of APOs compared to women without periodontitis?" (Population: Pregnant women; Exposure: Periodontitis; Comparison: Non-periodontitis; Outcomes: APOs) and "Does periodontal treatment reduce the risk of APOs?" (Population: Pregnant women; Intervention: Periodontal treatment; Comparison: No periodontal treatment; Outcomes: APOs).

Studies were eligible for inclusion based on the following criteria: (1) systematic reviews with or without meta-analysis; (2) retrieved data from human studies; (3) evaluated the association between APOs and periodontal disease (either observational or interventional). There were no restrictions regarding the year or language of publication. Exclusion criteria were as follows: (1) systematic reviews of systematic reviews (umbrella reviews); (2) commentaries, abstracts, letters to the editor, or consensus; (3) unsuitable inclusion criteria; and (4) inclusion of animal studies in the meta-analysis.

2.2. Study Selection

We conducted a comprehensive search of the following five electronic databases: PubMed (via MEDLINE), Cochrane Database of Systematic Reviews, Web of Science (WOS), Latin-American Scientific Literature in Health Sciences (LILACS), and Clinical Trials.gov, from the earliest data available up to February 2023. We merged keywords and subject headings according to the thesaurus of each database: #1: (periodontal diseases[MeSH]) OR (gingivitis[MeSH]) OR (gingival inflammation) OR (periodontal health) OR (root planing[MeSH]) OR (periodontal therapy) OR (periodontal treatment) OR (scaling and root planing) OR (supragingival and subgingival scaling); #2: (Pregnant Women[MeSH]) OR (Pregnancy[MeSH]) OR (Parturition[MeSH]); #3: (pregnancy outcome[MeSH])) OR (pregnancy complications[MeSH]) OR (premature birth[MeSH]) OR (low birth weight) OR (gestational Age[MeSH]) OR (Diabetes, Gestational[MeSH]) OR (Abortion, Spontaneous[MeSH]); #3: (systematic review) OR (meta-analysis) OR (metaanalysis); #1 AND #2 AND #3. The search was adapted according to each database, using the same keywords and word combinations. Additional relevant literature was included after a manual search of six periodontology- and gynecology-specific journals (namely, Obstetrics and Gynecology, British Journal of Obstetrics and Gynecology, American Journal of Obstetrics and Gynecology, Journal of Periodontal Research, Journal of Clinical Periodontology, and Journal of Periodontology). The grey literature was searched using the OpenGrey portal (http://www.opengrey.eu/ (accessed on 23 February 2023)). The electronic search was performed by two researchers (M.F. and V.M.) who independently screened the titles and abstracts of all the retrieved articles and excluded duplicates and unrelated studies. Any disagreements were resolved by discussion with a third reviewer (J.B.).

2.3. Data Items and Data Collection Process

A predefined table was used to extract the necessary data from each eligible study, including study identification (authors, publication year, country of origin), search period, number and type of the included studies, population size, periodontal case definition and clinical measures, obstetric complication outcomes, methodological quality tool used, effect size and 95% CI, and funding information. All information was extracted by two independent researchers (M.F. and V.M.), and any disagreements were resolved by discussion with a third researcher (J.B.). Intra- and inter-examiner agreement was assessed using Cohen's Kappa statistic (0.89; 95% CI: 0.87–0.90). Corresponding authors were contacted, when necessary to clarify data or obtain missing information.

2.4. Methodological Quality Appraisal

The included systematic reviews were independently assessed by two reviewers (M.F. and V.M.) using the A MeaSurement Tool to Assess Systematic Reviews (AMSTAR 2) [21]. AMSTAR 2 is a comprehensive 16-item tool that rates the overall confidence in the results of the review. According to the AMSTAR 2 guidelines, systematic reviews are categorized as: High ("zero or one non-critical weakness"); Moderate ("more than one non-critical weakness"); Low ("one critical flaw with or without non-critical weaknesses"); and Critically Low ("more than one critical flaw with or without non-critical weaknesses").

2.5. Meta-Analytical Estimates Strengths and Validity

Data were processed and managed using Excel from MS Office 365 to calculate inferential statistical analyses. To grade meta-analyses, we used a previously defined methodology by Papadimitrou et al. (2021) [22]. Therefore, associations were defined into four levels of evidence: strong, highly suggestive, suggestive, and weak evidence [22,23], as follows:

- Strong evidence: >1000 cases included in the meta-analysis, based on a threshold that ensured 80% power for hazard ratios ≥ 1.20 ($\alpha = 0.05$) 38; p-value $\leq 10^{-6}$ of statistical significance in meta-analysis 50–52; heterogeneity (I^2) below 50%; the null value was excluded by the 95% prediction interval; and no evidence of small study effects or excess significance bias.
- Highly suggestive: >1000 cases were included in the meta-analysis; p-value $\leq 10^{-6}$, and the largest study in the meta-analysis was statistically significant.
- Suggestive evidence: >1000 cases were included in the meta-analysis, and random effects $\leq 10^{-3}$ 50–52 was categorized.
- Weak evidence: if the latter conditions were not verified.

The fail-safe number (FSN) for statistically significant meta-analyses was then calculated using Rosenberg's FSN [24], followed by the median and range for each evidence grade (strong, highly suggestive, suggestive, and weak).

2.6. Overlap

Total overlap according to the association of periodontal disease with APOs or the effect of periodontal therapy on APOs was determined using the formula proposed by Pieper et al. [25]. The results were expressed as percentages and corrected covered area (CCA) values between 0 and 15. A CCA value of 0–5 indicates low overlap, 6–10 moderate overlap, 11–15 high overlap, and >15 very high overlap.

3. Results

3.1. Study Selection and Systematic Reviews Characteristics

The search strategy yielded a total of 678 potentially relevant studies (Figure 1). After removing duplicates (n = 119), a total of 559 records were screened for eligibility criteria by title and abstract, and 487 records were excluded. After full-paper assessment, 29 were excluded with the respective reasons for exclusion detailed in Supplementary Data S2. As a result, 43 systematic reviews met all of the eligibility criteria and were included for qualitative synthesis and 19 for quantitative analyses.

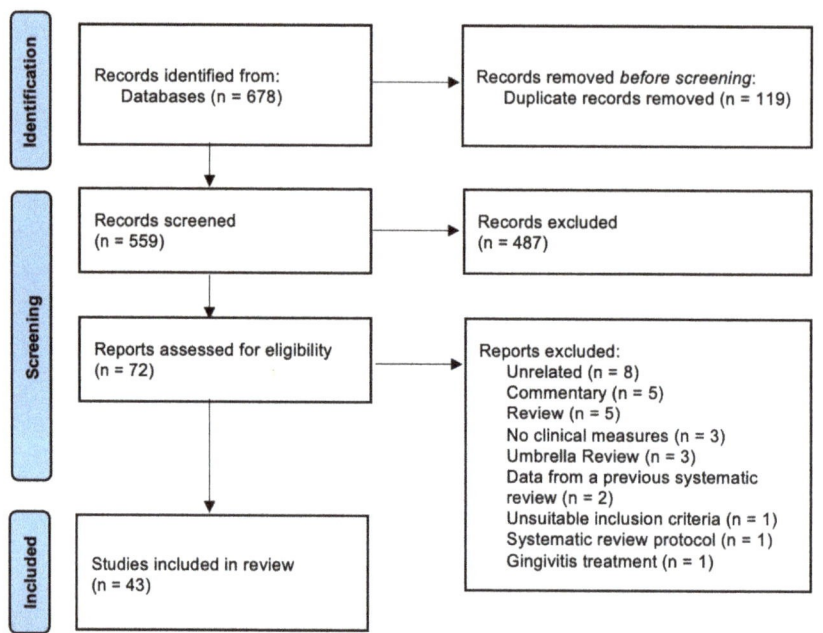

Figure 1. PRISMA flowchart showing the exclusion and inclusion process of the literature review.

Overall, we included 34 and 9 systematic reviews with and without meta-analysis, respectively (Supplementary Data S3). Of the 43 articles analyzed, 37.2% (n = 16) were published in dental journals, 32.6% (n = 14) in obstetrics and gynecology journals, and 30.2% (n = 13) in general medical journals. Almost 40% (n = 17) of all the included articles were published between 2010 and 2013. Regarding study type, 16 systematic reviews included only controlled trials, 20 included only observational studies, and 7 included both. Twenty-eight systematic reviews addressed the association between maternal periodontal status and the risk of APOs, while the other 15 studies aimed to evaluate the impact of periodontal treatment during pregnancy on perinatal outcomes. The majority followed the PRISMA guidelines (39.5%, n = 17), although 39.5% (n = 17) did not prepare the review process according to any standardized guideline (Supplementary Data S3). Regarding methodological quality assessment, Cochrane tools (27.9%, n = 12) and the Newcastle-Ottawa scale (23.3%, n = 10) were the most commonly used instruments.

3.2. Methodological Quality Assessment

Good inter-examiner reliability was found for the AMSTAR 2 screening (Cohen Kappa score = 0.84; 95% CI: 0.81–0.88). Overall, 35 studies were judged to be of critically low quality, 2 as of low quality, 1 as of moderate quality and 5 of high methodological quality (Supplementary Data S3, Figure 2 and detailed in Supplementary Data S4). Of those of high quality, 2 studies explored the association of periodontal disease with APOs and the remaining 3 studies investigated the effect of periodontal treatment on APOs. Only one of the included systematic reviews fully met the AMSTAR-2 checklist. Regarding language restriction, 7 systematic reviews did not report this characteristic, 18 applied a language restriction, and the remaining 18 studies had no language restrictions. Furthermore, most systematic reviews failed to report the sources of funding for the studies included in the review (90.7%, n = 39), to search for grey literature (86.0%, n = 37), to specify a plan to investigate causes of heterogeneity (65.1%, n = 28), to search trial and/or study registries (58.1%, n = 25), and to provide a list of excluded studies with justification (53.5%, n = 23). Study selection and data extraction in duplicates were not performed in 20.9% (n = 9) and 32.6% (n = 14), respectively. In addition, the definition of the review methods a priori was considered in only 5 studies (11.6%) for all included systematic reviews.

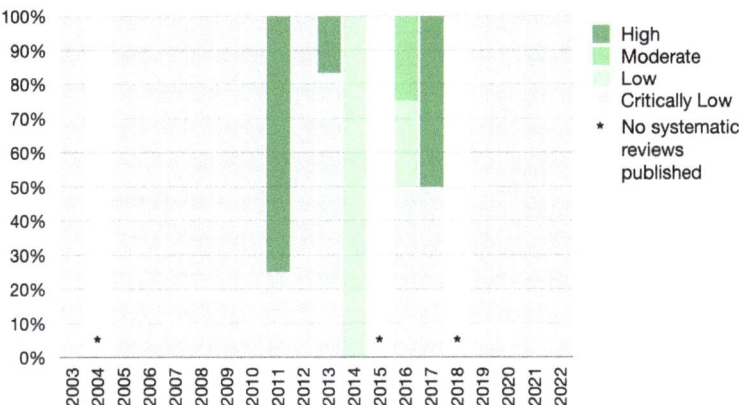

Figure 2. Diagram showing results from the methodological quality assessment of included systematic reviews.

3.3. The Association of Periodontal Disease with APOs

Overall, 28 systematic reviews analyzed the association of periodontal disease with APOs, of which 14 systematic reviews conducted meta-analyses (53.8%). A total of 28 meta-analytical estimates were conducted and analyzed below. The overlap observed was 58.7% with a CCA of 5.74% (Supplementary Data S5).

3.3.1. Meta-Analytic Strength of Estimates

Of the twenty-eight estimates, periodontal disease had a strong association with three APOs: PTB (less than 37 weeks), LBW (less than 2500 g), and gestational diabetes mellitus (Figure 3). PTB (less than 37 weeks) and LBW (less than 2500 g) showed all the remaining levels of strength, yet pre-eclampsia showed suggestive and weak evidence. In addition, highly suggestive evidence was found for the combination PTB/LBW (n = 3). Small for gestational age was the only APO that did not show significance of association.

	Non-significant	Weak	Suggestive	Highly suggestive	Strong
Preterm Birth (PTB)					
PTB <37 weeks	1	1	1	3	1
Low Birth Weight (LBW)					
LBW <2,500 g	1	1	1	5	1
PTB/LBW				3	
Small for gestational age	1				
Gestational Diabetes Mellitus	1	1	1		1
Preeclampsia	1		1	2	

Figure 3. Evidence grading map of systematic reviews on the association of periodontal disease with adverse pregnancy outocmes (APOs). The information at the top of the map shows the evidence grading scale (from left to right, increasing the evidence level). At the left side of the map, each APO (with detailed information) is presented.

3.3.2. Consistency of Evidence

When analyzing the consistency of the significant estimates (weak to strong) shown in Figure 3, only 8.7% of the estimates (2 out of 23) were likely to change in the future, according to the FSN statistics, indicating a fairly robust consistency (Supplementary Data S3). Of these two, both were classified as weak meta-analyses for PTB (less than 37 weeks) and LBW (less than 2500 g). None of the strong meta-analytic estimates had the potential to change in the future, indicating consistency.

3.4. Periodontal Treatment Effect on APOs

A total of fifteen systematic reviews analyzed the effect of periodontal treatment on APOs, of which 11 conducted meta-analyses (73.3%). A total of 41 meta-analytical estimates were conducted and analyzed below. Overlap was 77.4%, with a CCA of 33.4% (Supplementary Data S6).

3.4.1. Meta-Analytic Strength of Estimates

Of the 41 estimates, periodontal treatment did not have a strong association with APOs (Figure 4). Nevertheless, PTB (less than 37 weeks) showed all the remaining levels of strength, but LBW (less than 2500 g) showed only suggestive and weak evidence. In addition, perinatal mortality was the only APO that showed weak significancant association. The remaining APOs showed no significant association with periodontal treatment.

	Non-significant	Weak	Suggestive	Highly suggestive	Strong
Preterm Birth (PTB)					
PTB <37 weeks	6	3	2	2	
PTB <35 weeks	2				
PTB <32 weeks	2				
Low Birth Weight (LBW)					
LBW <2,500 g	6	1	3		
LBW <1,500	1				
PTB/LBW	1				
Stillbirths	1				
Perinatal mortality	2	1			
Spontaneous death of the fetus	2				
Small for gestational age	1				
Gestational Diabetes Mellitus	2				
Additional analyses					
Gestational age at delivery	1				
Mean Birthweight	2				

Figure 4. Evidence grading map from a meta-analysis studying the association of periodontal treatment with adverse pregnancy outcomes (APOs). The information at the top of the map shows the evidence grading scale (from left to right, increases the evidence level). On the left side of the map, each APO (with detailed information) is presented.

3.4.2. Consistency of Evidence

When analyzing the consistency of the generated estimates shown in Figure 4, 58.3% of the estimates (7 out of 12) were likely to change in the future, according to the FSN statistics, indicating a little robust consistency (Supplementary Data S3). Of these seven, four related to PTB (less than 37 weeks) (one highly suggestive, one suggestive, and two weak), two suggestive meta-analyses for LBW (less than 2500 g), and one weak meta-analysis for perinatal mortality (Supplementary Data S3).

4. Discussion

4.1. Main Findings

The present umbrella review evaluated a total of 43 systematic reviews with a total sample of 67 meta-analytic comparisons to assess the quality of evidence in two main categories: (i) pregnant women with periodontitis have an increased risk of APO; and (ii) periodontal treatment effects on APO. Three associations were supported by strong meta-analytic evidence, endorsing highly significant results with no suggestive bias. These associations were between periodontitis diagnosis and a higher risk of LBW (less than 2500 g) [26] and PTB (less than 37 weeks) [4], as well as GDM [27]. Fourteen associations were supported by highly suggestive evidence, most involving periodontitis and a higher risk of LBW (less than 2500 g) [5,26,28,29],

PTB (less than 37 weeks) [5,28,29], PTB/LBW [28–30], and pre-eclampsia [31,32]. Additionally, periodontal treatment was inversely associated with the risk of PTB (less than 37 weeks) [33,34].

Several factors have been clearly associated with the risk of LBW, PTB, pre-eclampsia, and GDM. Although periodontitis-related factors are an established risk for increasing systemic inflammatory burden, the association of periodontitis with APO risk is less known and potentially biased due to exposure measurement error and reporting bias. To overcome this obstacle, we used statistical tests and sensitivity analyses to search for evidence of bias. A total of 71 meta-analyses were evaluated, but on average, they contained relatively few studies (median = 8). Almost 52% (n = 37) of the included associations between periodontitis diagnosis or treatment and APOs risk reported a statistically significant summary random-effects estimate. Additionally, this proportion of significant associations decreased to 25.4% (n = 18) when a lower p value threshold ($p < 10^{-6}$) was used, pointing to a lack of existing robust associations. One in three associations showed high levels of heterogeneity ($I^2 \geq 50\%$). Moreover, when the FSN research method was used to consider observational studies, the majority of studies (21 out of 23) were unlikely to change the current evidence for associations. Otherwise, when the FSN was calculated in interventional studies, more than 58.3% (7 out of 12) were likely to change the existing research.

The present umbrella supports the notion that there are a limited number of periodontal-related factors and periodontal treatment follow-up data that are robustly associated with APOs risk. Nevertheless, it is critical to continue and increase research efforts in this field because APOs can be life-threatening to both the mother and the fetus/baby.

4.2. Agreement and Disagreement with Previous Umbrella Reviews

To the best of the authors' knowledge, eight umbrella reviews addressed and summarized the available evidence in this association between periodontitis and APOS, and the effect of periodontal disease on pregnancy complications [15–19,35–37]. In all eight published umbrella reviews, the authors only analyzed and interpreted the methodological quality and described the main findings of the included systematic reviews on maternal periodontitis and APOs. This umbrella review goes beyond these very basic aims of a systematic review. We have analyzed the meta-analytic estimates of all systematic reviews with meta-analyses and provide definitive conclusions on whether future research is likely to change the results of existing significant meta-analyses. Briefly stated, we provide solid and enduring evidence maps that will decisively contribute to draw oral and periodontal care strategies for pregnant women with the primary goal of minimizing pregnancy complications. This, to the best of our knowledge, has no equivalent umbrella review conclusion.

Regarding the methodological quality, four of five umbrella reviews used AMSTAR-1 (the first version of this tool, published in 2007), whereas only two umbrella reviews [35,37] used AMSTAR-2 as we did. Furthermore, Condylis et al. [15] did not assess the methodological quality of the evidence of the included studies at all, which can be considered a serious methodological flaw. Lavigne et al. [36] used the PRISMA checklist to assess the quality of systematic reviews, although this checklist was not designed for this purpose.

This umbrella review analyzes the evidence that has been produced in this field. We did not limit our search to a specific area (observational or interventional) or time period. Therefore, we have results from over six APOs associations with periodontitis diagnosis and thirteen effects of periodontal treatment in APOs. In contrast, only one umbrella review [19] examined the association of periodontitis with three APOs (LBW, PTB, and pre-eclampsia) through observational studies, in contrast to ours (six in total: PTB and LBW [both individual or combined outcomes], small for gestational age, gestational diabetes mellitus, and pre-eclampsia). Furthermore, while the previous umbrella reviews examined the effect of periodontal therapy on a few specific APOs (PTB [<37 weeks; <35 weeks], LBW and pre-eclampsia), ours explored this effect on thirteen APOs (PTB [<37 weeks; <35 weeks and <32 weeks], LBW [<2500 g and <1500 g], stillbirth, spontaneous fetal death, small for gestational age, gestational diabetes mellitus, and additional analyses such as gestational age at delivery and mean birth weight).

Overall, 44 systematic reviews from inception to February 2023 were included, while Condylis et al. [15] included 15 RCTs and 5 meta-analyses published until January 2011, Lopez et al. [16] included 6 systematic reviews published between 2003 and March 2012, Vilares-Builes et al. [19] included 19 systematic reviews and did not report the search period, Rangel-Ricon et al. [18] included 18 systematic reviews, and Matei et al. [17] included 9 studies in the periodontal field published between January 2005 and October 2016. Notwithstanding, we included 18 systematic reviews that were not included in previously published umbrella reviews, accounting for nearly 40% of all available meta-evidence.

4.3. Strengths and Limitations

This umbrella review presents strengths and shortcomings worth discussing to help readers interpret these findings. First, it provides a comprehensive overview of the available systematic reviews on the relationship between maternal periodontitis and APOs, following a strict protocol with a transparent and evidence-based methodology. Second, it presents an evidence grid map from nonsignificant to strong associations and distributes information by APO. Third, this umbrella review goes beyond the classical approach by attempting to explore whether the current evidence is likely to change using an FSN methodology. In other words, the application of these metrics demonstrates whether or not further research can influence the existing meta-analytic evidence and therefore provides guidance for future research agendas and public health policy. However, readers must also be aware of the limitations of the FSN methodology. The FSN represents the number of studies required to refute a significant meta-analytic mean, and is purely mathematical estimate, focusing on whether the p-value reaches an arbitrary threshold. It is also highly dependent on the assumed mean intervention effect of the unpublished studies. In this respect, the level of evidence appears to be much more consistent at the observational level (8.7% of estimates are likely to change with future research) than at the interventional level (58.3% of estimates are likely to change with future research).

Nevertheless, the majority of the included systematic reviews are of critically low quality (high risk of bias), and this is the most relevant shortcoming of this review. This conclusion is based on the methodological quality assessment conducted with AMSTAR-2 and will guide future evidence-based research. In addition, this review makes clear that most evidence is based on observational data with a low percentage of longitudinal studies and randomized trials. Additionally, consideration of overlap is critical when conducting systematic reviews [25]. We observed moderate and high levels of overlap for observational and interventional studies, respectively. To address this issue, we presented the overlap as a percentage and the CCA for each outcome and comparison. Hence, the current evidence is based upon more non-inferential evidence than definitive causal assumptions. A further shortcoming is that almost all meta-analyses produced unmeasured estimates for confounding variables, and it is therefore recommended that future studies report effect sizes adjusted for confounding factors.

4.4. Implications for Practice and Research

The results of this umbrella review highlight the importance of periodontal health during pregnancy for the systemic health of both mother and child. The relationship between maternal periodontal status and the risk of APOs, namely PTB, LBW, and GDM, has been demonstrated by a large body of evidence. However, pregnant women do not seek dental care [38] due to unawareness, fear, and/or lack of access. Obstetricians-gynecologists and other obstetric care providers (e.g., nurses, midwives) can play a critical role in changing this paradigm, as they are the health professionals who maintain the closest contact with expectant mothers. For this reason, it is very important that articles on this topic be published in obstetric and gynecologic journals. This information is extremely relevant and allows for a more holistic approach to pregnancy and the integration of oral health programs into prenatal care.

These findings also emphasize that more studies are warranted to further investigate the interplay between maternal periodontitis and APOs, as well as its underlying biological mechanisms. Additionally, the level of evidence found in this umbrella makes clear the need for more trials and increased patient data to face the uncertainty of meta-analytic estimates published so far. Therefore, further exploration of the clinical efficacy of periodontal therapy before and during pregnancy is still a necessary topic of research through intervention studies. The use of the new 2018 Classification for Periodontal and Peri-implant Diseases [39] is highly recommended to improve the standardization of studies and allow future conclusions on this association.

5. Conclusions

Strong and highly suggestive evidence from observational studies supports an association of periodontitis with an increased risk of PTB, LBW, GDM, and pre-eclampsia. Additional similar research is unlikely to change the current evidence for the association between periodontitis status and APOs, with few exceptions, indicating robust consistency. The level of evidence on the effect of periodontal treatment on the prevention of APOs is still uncertain and requires future studies to draw definitive and robust conclusions. These results strongly recommend periodontal primary prevention care as a key health standard in prenatal and perinatal care programs.

Supplementary Materials: The following supporting information can be downloaded at: https://www.mdpi.com/article/10.3390/jcm12113635/s1, Supplementary Data S1. PRISMA Checklist; Supplementary Data S2. List of excluded studies with justification for exclusion.; Supplementary Data S3. Characteristics of the included studies. Supplementary Data S4. AMSTAR 2 results; Supplementary Data S5. Overlap of study results across systematic reviews on the association of periodontal disease with APOs; Supplementary Data S6. Overlap of study results across systematic reviews on the periodontal treatment effect on APOs Refs. [40–68] are cited in the Supplementary Materials.

Author Contributions: Conceptualization, V.M. and J.B.; methodology, V.M. and M.F.; software, V.M. and J.B.; validation, J.J.M. and L.L.; formal analysis, V.M. and J.B.; investigation, V.M. and M.F.; resources, J.J.M.; data curation, V.M., J.B. and M.F.; writing—original draft preparation, V.M. and M.F.; writing—review and editing, J.B., L.L. and J.J.M.; visualization, J.B.; supervision, J.B.; project administration, V.M.; funding acquisition, J.J.M. All authors have read and agreed to the published version of the manuscript.

Funding: This research was funded by Fundação para Ciência e Tecnologia in the Call for R&D Projects un all Scientific Domains 2022, grant number 2022.02119.PTDC.

Institutional Review Board Statement: Not applicable.

Informed Consent Statement: Not applicable.

Conflicts of Interest: The authors declare no conflict of interest.

References

1. Hajishengallis, G.; Lamont, R.J. Polymicrobial Communities in Periodontal Disease: Their Quasi-Organismal Nature and Dialogue with the Host. *Periodontology 2000* **2021**, *86*, 210–230. [CrossRef] [PubMed]
2. Hajishengallis, G.; Chavakis, T. Local and Systemic Mechanisms Linking Periodontal Disease and Inflammatory Comorbidities. *Nat. Rev. Immunol.* **2021**, *21*, 426–440. [CrossRef] [PubMed]
3. Bi, W.G.; Emami, E.; Luo, Z.-C.; Santamaria, C.; Wei, S.Q. Effect of Periodontal Treatment in Pregnancy on Perinatal Outcomes: A Systematic Review and Meta-Analysis. *J. Matern. Fetal Neonatal Med.* **2021**, *34*, 3259–3268. [CrossRef] [PubMed]
4. Manrique-Corredor, E.J.; Orozco-Beltran, D.; Lopez-Pineda, A.; Quesada, J.A.; Gil-Guillen, V.F.; Carratala-Munuera, C. Maternal Periodontitis and Preterm Birth: Systematic Review and Meta-analysis. *Community Dent. Oral Epidemiol.* **2019**, *47*, 243–251. [CrossRef]
5. Moliner-Sánchez, C.A.; Iranzo-Cortés, J.E.; Almerich-Silla, J.M.; Bellot-Arcís, C.; Ortolá-Siscar, J.C.; Montiel-Company, J.M.; Almerich-Torres, T. Effect of per Capita Income on the Relationship between Periodontal Disease during Pregnancy and the Risk

of Preterm Birth and Low Birth Weight Newborn. Systematic Review and Meta-Analysis. *Int. J. Environ. Res. Public Health* **2020**, *17*, 8015. [CrossRef]
6. Teshome, A.; Yitayeh, A. Relationship between Periodontal Disease and Preterm Low Birth Weight: Systematic Review. *Pan Afr. Med. J.* **2016**, *24*, 215. [CrossRef]
7. Bett, J.V.S.; Batistella, E.Â.; Melo, G.; de Munhoz, E.A.; Silva, C.A.B.; da Guerra, E.N.S.; Porporatti, A.L.; De Luca Canto, G. Prevalence of Oral Mucosal Disorders during Pregnancy: A Systematic Review and Meta-analysis. *J. Oral Pathol. Med.* **2019**, *48*, 270–277. [CrossRef]
8. Jang, H.; Patoine, A.; Wu, T.T.; Castillo, D.A.; Xiao, J. Oral Microflora and Pregnancy: A Systematic Review and Meta-Analysis. *Sci. Rep.* **2021**, *11*, 16870. [CrossRef]
9. Borgo, P.V.; Rodrigues, V.A.A.; Feitosa, A.C.R.; Xavier, K.C.B.; Avila-Campos, M.J. Association between Periodontal Condition and Subgingival Microbiota in Women during Pregnancy: A Longitudinal Study. *J. Appl. Oral Sci.* **2014**, *22*, 528–533. [CrossRef]
10. Emmatty, R.; Mathew, J.; Kuruvilla, J. Comparative Evaluation of Subgingival Plaque Microflora in Pregnant and Non-Pregnant Women: A Clinical and Microbiologic Study. *J. Indian Soc. Periodontol.* **2013**, *17*, 47. [CrossRef]
11. Gürsoy, M.; Haraldsson, G.; Hyvönen, M.; Sorsa, T.; Pajukanta, R.; Könönen, E. Does the Frequency of *Prevotella Intermedia* Increase during Pregnancy? *Oral Microbiol. Immunol.* **2009**, *24*, 299–303. [CrossRef] [PubMed]
12. Li, X.; Zheng, J.; Ma, X.; Zhang, B.; Zhang, J.; Wang, W.; Sun, C.; Wang, Y.; Zheng, J.; Chen, H.; et al. The Oral Microbiome of Pregnant Women Facilitates Gestational Diabetes Discrimination. *J. Genet. Genom.* **2021**, *48*, 32–39. [CrossRef] [PubMed]
13. Offenbacher, S.; Katz, V.; Fertik, G.; Collins, J.; Boyd, D.; Maynor, G.; McKaig, R.; Beck, J. Periodontal Infection as a Possible Risk Factor for Preterm Low Birth Weight. *J. Periodontol.* **1996**, *67*, 1103–1113. [CrossRef] [PubMed]
14. Scannapieco, F.A.; Bush, R.B.; Paju, S. Periodontal Disease as a Risk Factor for Adverse Pregnancy Outcomes. A Systematic Review. *Ann. Periodontol.* **2003**, *8*, 70–78. [CrossRef]
15. Condylis, B.; Le Borgne, H.; Demoersman, J.; Campard, G.; Philippe, H.-J.; Soueidan, A. Intérêt du dépistage et du traitement des maladies parodontales chez la femme enceinte: Revue de la littérature. *J. De Gynécologie Obs. Et Biol. De La Reprod.* **2013**, *42*, 511–517. [CrossRef]
16. López, N.J.; Uribe, S.; Martinez, B. Effect of Periodontal Treatment on Preterm Birth Rate: A Systematic Review of Meta-Analyses. *Periodontology 2000* **2015**, *67*, 87–130. [CrossRef]
17. Matei, A.; Saccone, G.; Vogel, J.P.; Armson, A.B. Primary and Secondary Prevention of Preterm Birth: A Review of Systematic Reviews and Ongoing Randomized Controlled Trials. *Eur. J. Obstet. Gynecol. Reprod. Biol.* **2019**, *236*, 224–239. [CrossRef]
18. Rangel-Rincón, L.J.; Vivares-Builes, A.M.; Botero, J.E.; Agudelo-Suárez, A.A. An Umbrella Review Exploring the Effect of Periodontal Treatment in Pregnant Women on the Frequency of Adverse Obstetric Outcomes. *J. Evid. Based Dent. Pract.* **2018**, *18*, 218–239. [CrossRef]
19. Vivares-Builes, A.M.; Rangel-Rincón, L.J.; Botero, J.E.; Agudelo-Suárez, A.A. Gaps in Knowledge About the Association Between Maternal Periodontitis and Adverse Obstetric Outcomes: An Umbrella Review. *J. Evid. Based Dent. Pract.* **2018**, *18*, 1–27. [CrossRef]
20. Page, M.J.; McKenzie, J.E.; Bossuyt, P.M.; Boutron, I.; Hoffmann, T.C.; Mulrow, C.D.; Shamseer, L.; Tetzlaff, J.M.; Akl, E.A.; Brennan, S.E.; et al. The PRISMA 2020 Statement: An Updated Guideline for Reporting Systematic Reviews. *Syst. Rev.* **2021**, *10*, 89. [CrossRef]
21. Shea, B.J.; Reeves, B.C.; Wells, G.; Thuku, M.; Hamel, C.; Moran, J.; Moher, D.; Tugwell, P.; Welch, V.; Kristjansson, E.; et al. AMSTAR 2: A Critical Appraisal Tool for Systematic Reviews That Include Randomised or Non-Randomised Studies of Healthcare Interventions, or Both. *BMJ* **2017**, *358*, j4008. [CrossRef] [PubMed]
22. Papadimitriou, N.; Markozannes, G.; Kanellopoulou, A.; Critselis, E.; Alhardan, S.; Karafousia, V.; Kasimis, J.C.; Katsaraki, C.; Papadopoulou, A.; Zografou, M.; et al. An Umbrella Review of the Evidence Associating Diet and Cancer Risk at 11 Anatomical Sites. *Nat. Commun.* **2021**, *12*, 4579. [CrossRef] [PubMed]
23. Atkins, D.; Eccles, M.; Flottorp, S.; Guyatt, G.H.; Henry, D.; Hill, S.; Liberati, A.; O'Connell, D.; Oxman, A.D.; Phillips, B.; et al. Systems for Grading the Quality of Evidence and the Strength of Recommendations I: Critical Appraisal of Existing Approaches The GRADE Working Group. *BMC Health Serv. Res.* **2004**, *4*, 38. [CrossRef]
24. Rosenberg, M.S. The File-Drawer Problem Revisited: A General Weighted Method for Calculating Fail-Safe Numbers in Meta-Analysis. *Evolution* **2005**, *59*, 464–468. [PubMed]
25. Pieper, D.; Antoine, S.-L.; Mathes, T.; Neugebauer, E.A.M.; Eikermann, M. Systematic Review Finds Overlapping Reviews Were Not Mentioned in Every Other Overview. *J. Clin. Epidemiol.* **2014**, *67*, 368–375. [CrossRef] [PubMed]
26. Porto, E.C.L.; Gomes Filho, I.S.; Batista, J.E.T.; Lyrio, A.O.; Souza, E.S.; Figueiredo, A.C.M.G.; Pereira, M.G.; Cruz, S.S. da Periodontite materna e baixo peso ao nascer: Revisão sistemática e metanálise. *Ciênc. Saúde Coletiva* **2021**, *26*, 5383–5392. [CrossRef]
27. Lima, R.P.E.; Cyrino, R.M.; de Carvalho, B. Association Between Periodontitis and Gestational Diabetes Mellitus: Systematic Review and Meta-Analysis. *J. Periodontol.* **2015**, *16*, 48–57.
28. Corbella, S.; Taschieri, S.; Francetti, L.; De Siena, F.; Del Fabbro, M. Periodontal Disease as a Risk Factor for Adverse Pregnancy Outcomes: A Systematic Review and Meta-Analysis of Case–Control Studies. *Odontology* **2012**, *100*, 232–240. [CrossRef]
29. Corbella, S.; Taschieri, S.; Del Fabbro, M.; Francetti, L.; Weinstein, R.; Ferrazzi, E. Adverse Pregnancy Outcomes and Periodontitis: A Systematic Review and Meta-Analysis Exploring Potential Association. *Quintessence Int.* **2016**, *47*, 193–204. [CrossRef]

30. Chambrone, L.; Guglielmetti, M.R.; Pannuti, C.M.; Chambrone, L.A. Evidence Grade Associating Periodontitis to Preterm Birth and/or Low Birth Weight: I. A Systematic Review of Prospective Cohort Studies: Periodontitis and Adverse Pregnancy Outcomes. *J. Clin. Periodontol.* **2011**, *38*, 795–808. [CrossRef]
31. Conde-Agudelo, A.; Villar, J.; Lindheimer, M. Maternal Infection and Risk of Preeclampsia: Systematic Review and Metaanalysis. *Am. J. Obstet. Gynecol.* **2008**, *198*, 7–22. [CrossRef] [PubMed]
32. Wei, B.-J.; Chen, Y.-J.; Yu, L.; Wu, B. Periodontal Disease and Risk of Preeclampsia: A Meta-Analysis of Observational Studies. *PLoS ONE* **2013**, *8*, e70901. [CrossRef] [PubMed]
33. George, A.; Shamim, S.; Johnson, M.; Ajwani, S.; Bhole, S.; Blinkhorn, A.; Ellis, S.; Andrews, K. Periodontal Treatment during Pregnancy and Birth Outcomes: A Meta-Analysis of Randomised Trials. *Int. J. Evid. Based Healthc.* **2011**, *9*, 122–147. [CrossRef]
34. Uppal, A.; Uppal, S.; Pinto, A.; Dutta, M.; Shrivatsa, S.; Dandolu, V.; Mupparapu, M. The Effectiveness of Periodontal Disease Treatment During Pregnancy in Reducing the Risk of Experiencing Preterm Birth and Low Birth Weight. *J. Am. Dent. Assoc.* **2010**, *141*, 1423–1434. [CrossRef] [PubMed]
35. Khan, N.; Craven, R.; Rafiq, A.; Rafiq, A. Treatment of Periodontal Disease in Pregnancy for the Prevention of Adverse Pregnancy Outcomes: A Systematic Review of Systematic Reviews. *J. Pak. Med. Assoc.* **2023**, *73*, 611–620. [CrossRef]
36. Lavigne, S.E.; Forrest, J.L. An Umbrella Review of Systematic Reviews of the Evidence of a Causal Relationship between Periodontal Disease and Adverse Pregnancy Outcomes: A Position Paper from the Canadian Dental Hygienists Association. *Can. J. Dent. Hyg.* **2020**, *54*, 92–100.
37. Padilla-Cáceres, T.; Arbildo-Vega, H.I.; Caballero-Apaza, L.; Cruzado-Oliva, F.; Mamani-Cori, V.; Cervantes-Alagón, S.; Munayco-Pantoja, E.; Panda, S.; Vásquez-Rodrigo, H.; Castro-Mejía, P.; et al. Association between the Risk of Preterm Birth and Low Birth Weight with Periodontal Disease in Pregnant Women: An Umbrella Review. *Dent. J.* **2023**, *11*, 74. [CrossRef]
38. Onwuka, C.; Onwuka, C.I.; Iloghalu, E.I.; Udealor, P.C.; Ezugwu, E.C.; Menuba, I.E.; Ugwu, E.O.; Ututu, C. Pregnant Women Utilization of Dental Services: Still a Challenge in Low Resource Setting. *BMC Oral Health* **2021**, *21*, 384. [CrossRef]
39. Berglundh, T.; Armitage, G.; Araujo, M.G.; Avila-Ortiz, G.; Blanco, J.; Camargo, P.M.; Chen, S.; Cochran, D.; Derks, J.; Figuero, E.; et al. Peri-Implant Diseases and Conditions: Consensus Report of Workgroup 4 of the 2017 World Workshop on the Classification of Periodontal and Peri-Implant Diseases and Conditions. *J. Clin. Periodontol.* **2018**, *45*, S286–S291. [CrossRef]
40. Merchant, A.T.; Gupta, R.D.; Akonde, M.; Reynolds, M.; Smith-Warner, S.; Liu, J.; Tarannum, F.; Beck, J.; Mattison, D. Association of Chlorhexidine Use and Scaling and Root Planing With Birth Outcomes in Pregnant Individuals With Periodontitis: A Systematic Review and Meta-Analysis. *JAMA Netw. Open* **2022**, *5*, e2247632. [CrossRef]
41. Zhang, Y.; Feng, W.; Li, J.; Cui, L.; Chen, Z.-J. Periodontal Disease and Adverse Neonatal Outcomes: A Systematic Review and Meta-Analysis. *Front. Pediatr.* **2022**, *10*, 799740. [CrossRef] [PubMed]
42. Le, Q.-A.; Eslick, G.D.; Coulton, K.M.; Akhter, R.; Lain, S.; Nassar, N.; Yaacoub, A.; Condous, G.; Leonardi, M.; Eberhard, J.; et al. Differential Impact of Periodontal Treatment Strategies during Pregnancy on Perinatal Outcomes: A Systematic Review and Meta-Analysis. *J. Evid. Based Dent. Pract.* **2022**, *22*, 101666. [CrossRef] [PubMed]
43. Orlandi, M.; Muñoz Aguilera, E.; Marletta, D.; Petrie, A.; Suvan, J.; D'Aiuto, F. Impact of the Treatment of Periodontitis on Systemic Health and Quality of Life: A Systematic Review. *J Clin. Periodontol.* **2022**, *49*, 314–327. [CrossRef]
44. Konopka, T.; Zakrzewska, A. Periodontitis and Risk for Preeclampsia—A Systematic Review. *Ginekol. Pol.* **2020**, *91*, 158–164. [CrossRef] [PubMed]
45. Iheozor-Ejiofor, Z.; Middleton, P.; Esposito, M.; Glenny, A.-M. Treating Periodontal Disease for Preventing Adverse Birth Outcomes in Pregnant Women. *Cochrane Libr. Cochrane Rev.* **2017**, *2017*, CD005297. [CrossRef]
46. da Silva, H.E.C.; Stefani, C.M.; de Santos Melo, N.; de Almeida de Lima, A.; Rösing, C.K.; Porporatti, A.L.; Canto, G.D.L. Effect of Intra-Pregnancy Nonsurgical Periodontal Therapy on Inflammatory Biomarkers and Adverse Pregnancy Outcomes: A Systematic Review with Meta-Analysis. *Syst. Rev.* **2017**, *6*, 197. [CrossRef]
47. Abariga, S.A.; Whitcomb, B.W. Periodontitis and Gestational Diabetes Mellitus: A Systematic Review and Meta-Analysis of Observational Studies. *BMC Pregnancy Childbirth* **2016**, *16*, 344. [CrossRef]
48. Huang, X.; Wang, J.; Liu, J.; Hua, L.; Zhang, D.; Hu, T.; Ge, Z. Maternal Periodontal Disease and Risk of Preeclampsia: A Meta-Analysis. *J. Huazhong Univ. Sci. Technol. [Med. Sci.]* **2014**, *34*, 729–735. [CrossRef]
49. Ide, M.; Papapanou, P.N. Epidemiology of Association between Maternal Periodontal Disease and Adverse Pregnancy Outcomes—Systematic Review. *J. Periodontol.* **2013**, *84*, S181–S194. [CrossRef]
50. Shah, M.; Muley, A.; Muley, P. Effect of Nonsurgical Periodontal Therapy during Gestation Period on Adverse Pregnancy Outcome: A Systematic Review. *J. Matern. Fetal Neonatal Med.* **2013**, *26*, 1691–1695. [CrossRef]
51. Stadelmann, P.; Alessandri, R.; Eick, S.; Salvi, G.E.; Surbek, D.; Sculean, A. The Potential Association between Gingival Crevicular Fluid Inflammatory Mediators and Adverse Pregnancy Outcomes: A Systematic Review. *Clin. Oral Investig.* **2013**, *17*, 1453–1463. [CrossRef] [PubMed]
52. Boutin, A.; Demers, S.; Roberge, S.; Roy-Morency, A.; Chandad, F.; Bujold, E. Treatment of Periodontal Disease and Prevention of Preterm Birth: Systematic Review and Meta-Analysis. *Am. J. Perinatol.* **2012**, *30*, 537–544. [CrossRef] [PubMed]
53. Sgolastra, F.; Petrucci, A.; Severino, M.; Gatto, R.; Monaco, A. Relationship between Periodontitis and Pre-Eclampsia: A Meta-Analysis. *PLoS ONE* **2013**, *8*, e71387. [CrossRef] [PubMed]
54. Rosa, M.I.D.; Pires, P.D.S.; Medeiros, L.R.; Edelweiss, M.I.; Martínez-Mesa, J. Periodontal Disease Treatment and Risk of Preterm Birth: A Systematic Review and Meta-Analysis. *Cad. Saúde Pública* **2012**, *28*, 1823–1833. [CrossRef] [PubMed]

55. Kim, A.J.; Lo, A.J.; Pullin, D.A.; Thornton-Johnson, D.S.; Karimbux, N.Y. Scaling and Root Planing Treatment for Periodontitis to Reduce Preterm Birth and Low Birth Weight: A Systematic Review and Meta-Analysis of Randomized Controlled Trials. *J. Periodontol.* **2012**, *83*, 12. [CrossRef]
56. Tomasz, K.; Anna, P.-S. Periodontitis and Risk of Preterm Birth and Low Birthweight—A Meta-Analysis. *Ginekol Pol.* **2012**, *8*, 446–453.
57. Chambrone, L.; Pannuti, C.M.; Guglielmetti, M.R.; Chambrone, L.A. Evidence Grade Associating Periodontitis with Preterm Birth and/or Low Birth Weight: II. A Systematic Review of Randomized Trials Evaluating the Effects of Periodontal Treatment: Periodontitis and Adverse Pregnancy Outcomes. *J. Clin. Periodontol.* **2011**, *38*, 902–914. [CrossRef]
58. Fogacci, M.F.; Vettore, M.V.; Thomé Leão, A.T. The Effect of Periodontal Therapy on Preterm Low Birth Weight: A Meta-Analysis. *Obstet. Gynecol.* **2011**, *117*, 153–165. [CrossRef]
59. Kunnen, A.; Van Doormaal, J.J.; Abbas, F.; Aarnoudse, J.G.; Van Pampus, M.G.; Faas, M.M. Periodontal Disease and Pre-Eclampsia: A Systematic Review: Periodontal Disease and Pre-Eclampsia. *J. Clin. Periodontol.* **2010**, *37*, 1075–1087. [CrossRef]
60. Pimentel Lopes De Oliveira, G.J.; Amaral Fontanari, L.; Chaves De Souza, J.A.; Ribeiro Costa, M.; Cirelli, J.A. Effect of Periodontal Treatment on the Incidence of Preterm Delivery: A Systematic Review. *Minerva Stomatol.* **2010**, *59*, 543–550.
61. Polyzos, N.P.; Polyzos, I.P.; Mauri, D.; Tzioras, S.; Tsappi, M.; Cortinovis, I.; Casazza, G. Effect of Periodontal Disease Treatment during Pregnancy on Preterm Birth Incidence: A Metaanalysis of Randomized Trials. *Am. J. Obstet. Gynecol.* **2009**, *200*, 225–232. [CrossRef] [PubMed]
62. Rustveld, L.O.; Kelsey, S.F.; Sharma, R. Association Between Maternal Infections and Preeclampsia: A Systematic Review of Epidemiologic Studies. *Matern. Child Health J.* **2008**, *12*, 223–242. [CrossRef] [PubMed]
63. Vergnes, J.-N.; Sixou, M. Preterm Low Birth Weight and Maternal Periodontal Status: A Meta-Analysis. *Am. J. Obstet. Gynecol.* **2007**, *196*, 135.e1–135.e7. [CrossRef] [PubMed]
64. Xiong, X.; Buekens, P.; Vastardis, S.; Yu, S.M. Periodontal Disease and Pregnancy Outcomes: State-of-the-Science. *Obstet. Gynecol. Surv.* **2007**, *62*, 605–615. [CrossRef]
65. Vettore, M.V.; Lamarca, G.D.A.; Leão, A.T.T.; Thomaz, F.B.; Sheiham, A.; Leal, M.D.C. Periodontal Infection and Adverse Pregnancy Outcomes: A Systematic Review of Epidemiological Studies. *Cad. Saúde Pública* **2006**, *22*, 2041–2053. [CrossRef]
66. Xiong, X.; Buekens, P.; Fraser, W.; Beck, J.; Offenbacher, S. Periodontal Disease and Adverse Pregnancy Outcomes: A Systematic Review. *BJOG: Int. J. Obstet. Gynaecol.* **2006**, *113*, 135–143. [CrossRef]
67. Khader, Y.S.; Ta'ani, Q. Periodontal Diseases and the Risk of Preterm Birth and Low Birth Weight: A Meta-Analysis. *J. Periodontol.* **2005**, *76*, 5. [CrossRef]
68. Madianos, P.N.; Bobetsis, G.A.; Kinane, D.F. Is Periodontitis Associated with an Increased Risk of Coronary Heart Disease and Preterm and/or Low Birth Weight Births?: Periodontitis and Systemic Disease. *J. Clin. Periodontol.* **2002**, *29*, 22–36. [CrossRef]

Disclaimer/Publisher's Note: The statements, opinions and data contained in all publications are solely those of the individual author(s) and contributor(s) and not of MDPI and/or the editor(s). MDPI and/or the editor(s) disclaim responsibility for any injury to people or property resulting from any ideas, methods, instructions or products referred to in the content.

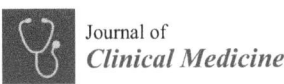

Review

Varicocele: To Treat or Not to Treat?

Antonio Franco [1], Flavia Proietti [2,*], Veronica Palombi [2], Gabriele Savarese [2], Michele Guidotti [3], Costantino Leonardo [2], Fabio Ferro [4], Claudio Manna [5] and Giorgio Franco [2]

[1] Department of Urology, Sant'Andrea Hospital, "Sapienza" University of Rome, 00185 Rome, Italy; antonio.franco@uniroma1.it
[2] Department of Maternal and Child Health and Urological Sciences, Policlinico Umberto I, "Sapienza" University of Rome, 00185 Rome, Italy; veronica.palmbi@uniroma1.it (V.P.); gabriele.savarese@uniroma1.it (G.S.); costantino.leonardo@uniroma1.it (C.L.); giorgio.franco@uniroma1.it (G.F.)
[3] Department of Urology, Nuovo Ospedale dei Castelli, 00040 Rome, Italy; michele.guidotti@gmail.com
[4] Mater Dei Hospital, 00197 Rome, Italy; fabioferro.andrologia@gmail.com
[5] Biofertility IVF and Infertility Center, 00198 Rome, Italy
* Correspondence: flavia.proietti@uniroma1.it

Abstract: Varicocele treatment in infertility still remains controversial. It is clear, in fact, that in many patients, varicocele has no impact on fertility. Recent scientific evidence demonstrated that varicocele treatment is beneficial in improving semen parameters and pregnancy rate when an appropriate selection of patients is made. The purpose of treating varicocele in adults is mainly to improve current fertility status. On the other hand, the goal of treatment in adolescents is to prevent testicular injury and maintain testicular function for future fertility. Hence, the key to the success of varicocele treatment seems to be a correct indication. The aim of this study is to review and summarize current evidence in managing varicocele treatment focusing on the controversies regarding surgical indications in adolescent and adult patients, and in other specific situations such as azoospermia, bilateral or subclinical varicocele, and prior to ART.

Keywords: varicocele repair; varicocelectomy; ART; infertility

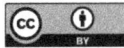

1. Introduction

A varicocele is defined as an abnormal dilatation and/or tortuosity of the pampiniform venous plexus in the scrotum. It is a pathological condition caused by an alteration in the drainage of the testicle due to venous reflux in the internal spermatic vein (ISV). In fact, the left side is mainly affected due to anatomical reasons related to the ISV. In a previous study, using femoral and spermatic venographies, we observed the exclusive involvement of ISV in primary and recurrent varicoceles [1].

The condition occurs in 15% of the healthy general male population, in 35% of men with primary infertility, and in up to 80% of men with secondary infertility [2]. Several different clinical [3] and US sonographic classifications have been proposed for varicocele assessment, but unfortunately, there is no standardization, and a clear consensus has not yet been reached, which obviously also leads to difficulties in comparability [4]. According to the fourth edition of WHO classification [5], there are three grades of varicocele depending on the severity of it, from 1 to 3, with no reference to an absolute measure of the vein diameter or sonographic evidence of reflux with velocity measurement. On the other hand, Sarteschi describes a five-part classification, depending on the presence of dilated veins while supine and/or standing, the anatomical relationships of the dilated veins with the testis, the characteristics of reflux, and testicular size [6]. Cavallini et al. focused on varicocele grade and degree of reflux, showing that surgery to improve OAT and, thus, chances of successful ART should be reserved for Dubin and Amelar grade 2 and grade 3 varicoceles with continuous venous reflux at duplex Doppler assessment [7]. Furthermore, no global consensus has been established on the need for sonographic examination in the diagnosis of varicocele: on the first hand AUA/ASRM guidelines sustain that scrotal ultrasound should not be routinely performed in the initial evaluation of the infertile male; on the other hand, the EAU Guidelines, in accordance with the European Society of Urogenital Radiology Scrotal and Penile Imaging Working Group, consider scrotal Doppler necessary if physical examination is inconclusive or semen analysis remains unsatisfactory after varicocele repair to identify persistent and recurrent varicocele [8–10].

Varicocele may cause spermatogenetic damage resulting in altered seminal parameters, abnormalities in the development and growth of the affected testis, and, rarely, symptoms such as discomfort and pain [11]. Thus observational studies suggest that men with a varicocele tend to have a higher proportion of spermatozoa with fragmented DNA, lower total sperm counts, lower progressive sperm motility, lower sperm vitality, and higher abnormal forms when compared to control groups [12]. The exact pathophysiology and, especially, the cause–effect relationship between the presence of varicocele and abnormalities of the semen analysis has not been clearly established [13]. Conversely, a recent systematic review and meta-analysis provide a high level of evidence in favor of a positive effect of VR to improve conventional semen parameters in infertile men with clinical varicocele [14].

The aim of our study is to review the latest reports on varicocele treatment and provide simple and practical steps for managing a correct indication of treatment, focusing on the controversies on this issue.

2. Surgical Treatment

Several therapeutic options are available for varicocele treatment and may involve an endovascular or surgical approach [13].

In Europe, endovascular techniques are popular due to their minimally invasive nature, despite their higher recurrence rates [15]. They include:

1. Retrograde sclero-embolization, trans-femoral or trans-brachial;
2. Antegrade sclerotherapy (Tauber technique) [16].

Concerning surgical approach, this may be:

- Retroperitoneal;
- Inguinal;
- Sub-inguinal.

The retroperitoneal access involves an incision in the supra inguinal site and the ligation of the ISV immediately above the internal inguinal ring (Ivanissevich technique) or higher up at the level of the anterior iliac spine (Palomo technique).

A recent Palomo technique variant consists of sparing a few lymphatic vessels with the aid of an operating microscope, to avoid post-operative hydrocele which might occur after the standard Palomo procedure [17–20]. The approach is moved from the sub-inguinal to the pre-peritoneal level, just above the internal inguinal ring, as described by Jones for nonpalpable testes [21]. The internal spermatic veins are reached by splitting the muscle plane and thus preserving the integrity of the inguinal channel. The deferential vein can be evaluated but not necessarily ligated, considering that dilation is not synonymous with reflux [17] (Figure 1).

Retroperitoneal repair can also be performed using the laparoscopic technique, particularly in bilateral disease [22]. In our view, laparoscopic repair appears to be more invasive and costly than the other techniques, due to general anesthesia, pneumoperitoneum issues and extremely rare but possible dreadful complications [23]; however, it has the advantage of excellent visibility of the posterior abdominal wall allowing a thorough search of sites known to be responsible for recurrent varicoceles, such as renal, caval and pelvic cross-over veins. Moreover, optical magnification optimizes the surgeon's ability to preserve the testicular artery and lymphatic channels while ligating all veins to minimize the risk of hydrocele formation or varicocele recurrence. Finally, the laparoscopic approach allows a simultaneous correction of bilateral varicocele. Some evidence demonstrates lower recurrence rates

(3–6%), especially when compared to sclero-embolization procedures, which were shown to reach 4–11% of varicocele recurrence [24]; furthermore, sclero-embolization procedures have their specific complications, such as inadvertent femoral artery perforation, radiation exposure, sclerosant agent local irritation or orchitis and coil migration that, despite being very uncommon, should be taken into account [25,26].

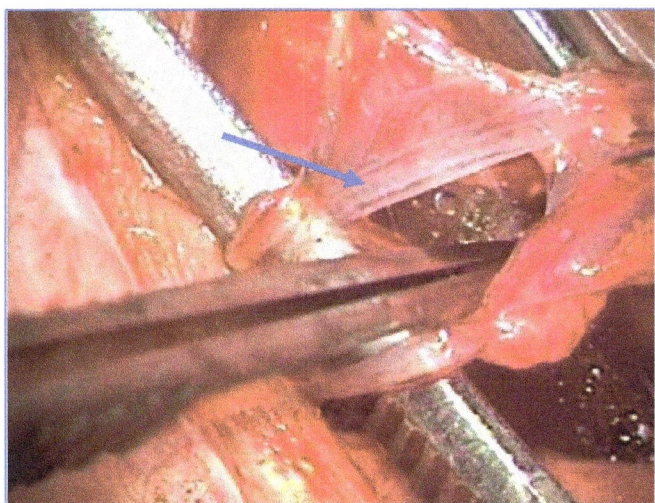

Figure 1. Microsurgical lymphatic sparing Palomo technique (arrow: spared lymphatics).

The sub-inguinal microsurgical technique, instead, is widely used in the United States with very low reported recurrence rates [27,28].

Different subinguinal microsurgical modified approaches have been subsequently proposed [27,29]. According to EAU guidelines and AUA/ASRM [30], the use of an operating microscope makes microsurgical subinguinal varicocelectomy the preferred method of treatment due to its lower incidence of complications and recurrence rates, as well as its potential for greater improvement in semen parameters [30,31]. However, it is technically demanding and needs access to an operating microscope [32].

Regarding the outcomes of the different techniques, there is still debate in the literature: a meta-analysis by Cayan et al. suggested that surgical intervention was better than embolization with regard to spontaneous pregnancy rates (41.97% for microsurgery versus 33.20% for embolization, $p = 0.001$) [23] and recurrence rates (1.05% for microsurgery versus 12.70% for embolization, $p = 0.001$) [23]. A randomized controlled trial (RCT) from Al-Kandari et al. demonstrated that, compared with open inguinal and laparoscopic varicocelectomy, subinguinal microsurgical varicocelectomy offers the best outcome only in terms of complications (hydrocele) and recurrence [33]. In our experience, the modified lymphatic-sparing Palomo technique appears to offer excellent results in terms of outcomes and complication rates: one of the authors (F.F.), in the period January 2009–September 2020, treated 633 children and adolescents using this technique with a recurrence rate of 2.8% and postoperative hydrocele rate of 0.4% (unpublished data). Therefore, no technique has been proven to be certainly superior to the others. Each one of them has its own advantages and disadvantages (Table 1). High-qualities studies comparing different surgical approaches are still missing, and results of the available studies in the literature appear to be inconclusive.

3. Varicocelectomy Indications

The role of varicocele treatment in improving sperm parameters and, most importantly, pregnancy and live birth rate, in other words, in enhancing male fertility, has represented a matter of discussion between authors and specialists.

While initially, some studies and metanalysis denied benefits on fertility in patients treated for varicocele [34,35], recent scientific evidence demonstrated that varicocele treatment improves semen parameters and pregnancy rates, when an appropriate selection of patients is made [22,36,37].

A recent global survey involving 574 experts from 59 countries showed wide disagreement regarding varicocele management and poor adherence to guidelines [37]. Current American Urological Association (AUA) and European Urology Association (EAU) guidelines suggest treating varicocele in well-selected patients when specific conditions are present [9,28].

We will focus on the main indications for varicocelectomy, seeking to answer the relevant question of whether or not varicocelectomy improves the fertility status of the patient. Various clinical scenarios involving varicocele repair (VR) will be discussed below in detail:

- VR in children and adolescents;
- VR in infertile couples, oligoasthenoteratozoospermia and sperm DNA fragmentation;
- VR in azoospermia;
- VR prior to assisted reproductive techniques (ART);
- VR in subclinical varicocele;
- VR in bilateral varicocele.

3.1. Role of Varicocelectomy in Children and Adolescents

A particular situation is represented by the presence of varicocele in children and adolescents. In this delicate period of life, the presence of a varicocele might jeopardize normal testicular growth and impair the spermatogenetic process, and it would be reasonable to believe that the early repair of this vascular anomaly might prevent testicular damage [38]. However, there is still confusion about who should be treated in the pediatric population. Without the aid of a semen analysis, the selection of the children to be treated is only based on the presence of reduced growth of the affected testis (testicular hypotrophy). Instead, in adolescents, current recommendations for VR are based on the clinical findings of impaired testicular growth and/or altered seminal parameters when available [39].

Important studies have focused on this issue; in particular, Cayan et al. evaluated 408 patients (age 12–19) with clinical varicocele undergoing microsurgical varicocelectomy vs. observation only. Their results showed a significant increase in paternity rates, reduced time to conception and no additional treatment necessary to conceive post-operatively in adolescents who received VR compared to ones observed only. In particular, patients with varicocele who underwent microsurgical VR will have better sperm parameters and 3.63 times increased odds of achieving paternity compared to controls not undergoing varicocele surgery and followed conservatively [40].

An interesting meta-analysis by Silay et al. on the treatment of adolescent varicocele states that "moderate evidence exists on the benefits of varicocele treatment in children and adolescents in terms of testicular volume and sperm concentration. Current evidence does not demonstrate the superiority of any of the surgical/interventional techniques regarding treatment success. Long-term outcomes including paternity and fertility still remain unknown" [41]. The editorial of this article, by J. Elder, concludes that RCTs will be necessary to "*prevent a potentially damaging process from going untreated, while at the same time avoiding unnecessary interventions for a highly prevalent condition*" [42].

Current European Association of Urology (EAU) guidelines recommend treating varicocele when one of the following conditions is present: (A) is associated with testicular hypotrophy (size difference >20%), (B) an additional testicular condition affecting fertility is present, (C) is symptomatic and (D) a pathological sperm quality is detected. According to a recent study, varicocelectomy in adolescents may also be associated with increased sperm DNA integrity and mitochondrial activity [43]. Based on current evidence, all these indications are discussed in detail in a recent review by Cannarella et al. who created a flow chart for the management of childhood and adolescent varicocele: conservative management may be suggested in patients with peak retrograde flow (PRF) <30 cm/s, testicular asymmetry <10% and no evidence of sperm and hormonal abnormalities; in patients with 10–20% testicular volume asymmetry or 30 < PRF ≤ 38 cm/s or sperm abnormalities, careful follow-up may ensue. In the case of absent catch-up growth or sperm recovery, varicocele repair should be suggested. Finally, treatment can be proposed at the initial consultation in painful varicocele, testicular volume asymmetry ≥20%, PRF > 38 cm/s, infertility and failure of testicular development [44].

3.2. Role of Varicocelectomy in Infertile Couples, OAT and DNA Fragmentation

Since the Evers and Collins meta-analysis, stating that varicocele treatment had no role in improving couple infertility, a large mass of new studies, including RCTs, global consensus surveys and meta-analyses, have been published, which also demonstrated a significant role of treatment in improving sperm parameters and pregnancy rates [36,37,45,46]. The same Evers and Collins group in 2012 published a new meta-analysis, which concluded that the treatment of varicocele in men from couples with otherwise unexplained subfertility may improve a couple's chance of pregnancy [22]. A meta-analysis from Marmar et al. supporting this hypothesis reported a pregnancy rate of 33% (31 of 96) in surgically treated men compared with 15.5% (27 of 174) in untreated men, corresponding to an OR of 2.87 (95% CI 1.33–6.20). The analysis included two randomized trials and three observational studies comprehending infertile men with an abnormal semen analysis and a palpable varicocele [47]. These data are in line with those obtained in another randomized controlled trial by Abdel-Meguid and colleagues, in which a similar odds ratio for achieving a spontaneous pregnancy after varicocelectomy was reported (OR 3.04; 95% CI 1.33–6.95) [36].

Overall, the available evidence supports a beneficial effect of varicocelectomy on pregnancy outcomes. In fact, the Cochrane reviews denying the beneficial role of VR have been criticized for their inclusion of men with subclinical varicocele and normal semen parameters [22]. Therefore, sufficiently powered RCTs with homogenous patient populations are needed to overcome these partly conflicting results.

The key point, in our view, is the correct indication to treat varicocele, and selecting the right patients to treat will lead to a significant improvement in their fertility.

Both EAU and AUA guidelines suggest the treatment of varicocele in infertile couples [8,9]. However, as far as infertile couples are concerned, EAU guidelines discourage treatment in men who have normal semen analysis and/or subclinical varicocele (grade A recommendation) and suggest treatment in those with clinical varicocele, oligospermia and otherwise unexplained infertility in the couple (grade A recommendation).

Varicocelectomy represents a useful and generally simple procedure for the treatment of men with oligoasthenoteratozoospermia (OAT), and this is often expressed in global practice patterns and in the EAU and AUA/ASRM guidelines. In fact, they recommend surgical treatment if a palpable varicocele and infertility are associated with "abnormal semen parameters, except for azoospermic men". The latest Cochrane review about this issue suggests an improvement in pregnancy rates for men with OAT who underwent VR, but it is uncertain whether live birth rates increase as well [48].

Sperm DNA fragmentation (SDF) has emerged as an important measure of sperm function and a predictor of reproductive outcomes. VR is associated with an improvement in SDF, including both single-strand and double-strand DNA fragmentation, as well as seminal oxidative stress [49–51]. Two recent meta-analyses calculated a mean reduction in SDF after VR of 7.23% and 6.14%, respectively [50,52]. According to a recent study from Yan et al., the possible role of varicocele treatment in improving sperm DNA fragmentation in infertile couples should urge a change in the current guidelines on varicocele treatment [53]. Concerning the guidelines, an important discrepancy between their statements and current evidence must be acknowledged. In fact, AUA/ASRM declare *"there are no well-controlled studies that VR will reduce risk of recurrent pregnancy loss in men with elevated SDF"*. On the other hand, several studies have confirmed the role of varicocelectomy in improving semen quality, increasing the pregnancy rate, and significantly decreasing the miscarriage rate [54,55]. To note, Ghanaie et al. evaluate the effects of varicocelectomy on semen parameters, pregnancy rates, and live birth in couples with first-term recurrent miscarriage in a randomized-control trial and their results showed a significant difference in the varicocele repair arm, in terms of improved outcomes [56]. EAU guidelines report that there is "increasing evidence" that VR may improve SDF and ART outcomes and recommends VR for men with raised SDF and failed ART. Finally, a recent global survey on the management of SDF states that there are no specific recommendations regarding the general approach to managing infertile men with elevated SDF in the guidelines; however, possible first-line treatments consist of lifestyle modification strategies, including maintaining a healthy lifestyle to overcome obesity, the cessation of smoking and alcohol use, as well as treating genital infections and eliminating toxic exposure [57].

Concerning the male age factor, controversy exists as to whether varicocelectomy is as effective in older men, as it is believed that long-standing varicoceles can cause irreversible testicular damage, or that older testes may have limited potential for recovery from varicocele-induced damage [58]. The clinical implication is that if varicocelectomy is less effective in older men, perhaps it should not be offered, with men electing assisted reproduction instead. However, some studies [59,60] showed that age does not necessarily need to be an exclusion factor for varicocele treatment. In fact, evaluating varicocele's outcomes in couples of different ages, Firat and Erdemir [59] found increased semen parameters; although pregnancy rates after varicocelectomy were higher in the younger group compared with the others, this difference was not statistically significant. Therefore, even couples with male partners over 35 years of age might have a reasonable chance of natural pregnancy after VR. Naturally, the female age factor tends to be more important in an infertile couple, and paternal age contributes relatively smaller to the overall age-related decline in the fertility of a couple when compared with maternal age.

In the conclusion of this chapter, very often, the urologist is faced with the dilemma of treating varicocele or sending the couple directly to ART. A flowchart for the treatment of varicocele or ART in infertile couples is presented in Figure 2.

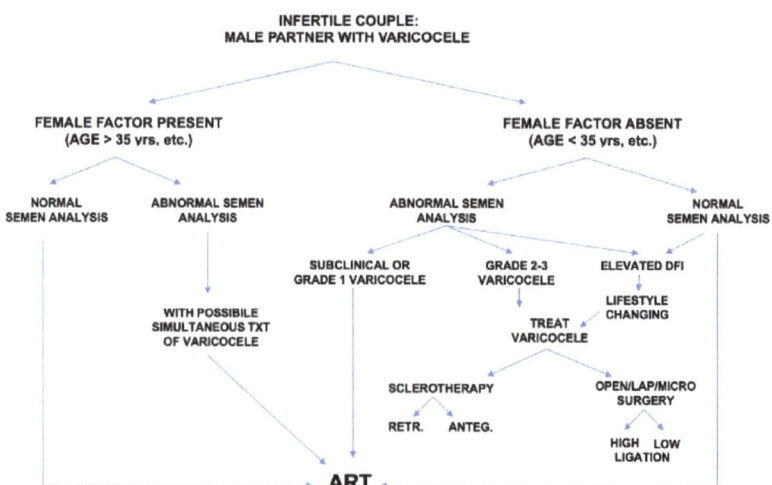

Figure 2. Flow chart analyzing indications to treat varicocele or perform ART.

3.3. Role of Varicocelectomy in Azoospermia

As stated recently in a global consensus on the management of varicocele for male infertility, there is a wide discrepancy in dealing with an azoospermic patient affected by varicocele [37]. Starting from the evidence supported by AUA/ASRM, the guidelines state that "the couple should be informed of the absence of definitive evidence supporting VR prior to ART". The EAU guidelines instead declare that VR in men with NOA may result in the appearance of sperm in the ejaculate (20.8% to 55%) and is associated with improved surgical sperm retrieval rates (OR, 2.65; 95% CI, 1.69–4.14). However, it cautions that the evidence is based on observational studies only and suggests fully discussing the risks and benefits of VR with the patient with NOA and a clinical varicocele. Certainly, clinicians must first evaluate medical history, genetic testing, and hormonal exams to distinguish obstructive azoospermia (OA) from non-obstructive azoospermia (NOA). Then, it is necessary to exclude the possibility that the varicocele is an incidental finding in a patient with azoospermia certainly unrelated to varicocele. If such conditions are excluded, a varicocelectomy may be performed in men with NOA, resulting in beneficial effects on sperm retrieval rates (SRR), as demonstrated in a recent meta-analysis showing an increased SRR in men with NOA who underwent varicocelectomy compared with men with NOA who did not undergo varicocelectomy (OR 2.65; 95% CI 1.69–4.14; $p < 0.001$) [61]. Despite these results, there is still reluctance in offering VR to these patients: a major criticism is that in almost all cases published, the sperm count achieved in the ejaculate is very low, and ICSI is still needed [62]. Sometimes, the appearance of sperm is only transitory [63,64]. Furthermore, none of these studies are controlled, and the appearance of sperm in these men may be due to spontaneous variation and not be due to the VR [9]. A study observed a beneficial effect of VR only in azoospermic patients with a testicular histologic pattern of hypospermatogenesis or late maturation arrest (MA) while those with Sertoli cell-only syndrome (SCOS) showed no change [65]. However, scheduling a testicular biopsy routinely prior to VR in azoospermic patients might be difficult to accept.

In conclusion, we believe that the selection of NOA patients for varicocele repair remains a matter of personal belief and choice. In our view, the advantages of VR in azoospermic patients are very limited and rarely of clinical significance.

3.4. Role of Varicocelectomy Prior to ART

Correcting a varicocele before proceeding with IVF-ICSI is a controversial topic and many ART centers do not even consider the presence of a clinical varicocele.

As previously mentioned, there is fair evidence that the surgical repair of clinical varicocele may improve semen parameters and may decrease seminal oxidative stress and sperm DNA fragmentation, thus increasing the chances of natural conception. However, it is unclear whether performing varicocelectomy in men with clinical varicocele prior to ART may improve treatment outcomes [66].

Support for VR before ART is derived from the fact that surgical VR is certainly a minor and less expensive procedure than ART itself. Furthermore, VR might improve semen quality and facilitate spontaneous pregnancies or enhance the success rate of ART. Positive outcomes are illustrated in a meta-analysis by Esteves et al. who reported increased clinical pregnancies (OR = 1.59, 95% CI: 1.19–2.12, $I^2 = 25\%$) and birth rate (OR = 2.17, 95% CI: 1.55–3.06, $I^2 = 0\%$) in patients who underwent varicocelectomy prior to ART vs. ART without VR [67]. Another meta-analysis by Kirby et al. found that VR improved the ART live birth rate in men with oligospermia (odds ratio [OR], 1.699) [68]. On the other hand, VR might delay the ART procedure by 6 to 12 months for an uncertain benefit; the presence of female factors (age > 35 years, etc.) may induce clinicians to immediately offer ART-avoiding VR. However, our policy in the case of advanced female age and indications of varicocele correction is to offer immediate ART together with VR. In this way, there is no delay in ART, but in the event of an unsuccessful result of it, the couple will benefit from the advantages of VR. It is clear, hence, that the decision to perform VR before ART should be individualized based on other variables such as the female partner's age, history of prior failure, varicocele grade, SDF levels, duration of infertility, etc., and, of course, wide counseling of the infertile couple. As a matter of fact, different studies have investigated several factors implicated in ART success rate after VR [69,70]. EAU guidelines do not indicate whether VR prior to IVF will improve pregnancy rates but suggest VR in men with OAT or when elevated SDF is present [9].

Another aspect that may be considered is the cost-effectiveness of the procedures involved in ART. The cost of the various ART procedures is an important consideration for couples and society, considering that often coverage for these procedures is not provided routinely and there is wide variability of cost-effectiveness when comparing across various ART procedures [71]. For instance, Dubin et al. recently demonstrated through a cost-effectiveness analysis that varicocelectomy increases semen parameters in severely oligospermic patients, thus providing previously ineligible couples an opportunity to elect for intra-uterine insemination (IUI), a less invasive and less expensive alternative to in vitro fertilization (IVF) or intracytoplasmic sperm injection (ICSI) [72].

3.5. Role of Varicocelectomy in Subclinical Varicocele

Another complex topic about the indication of varicocelectomy involves subclinical varicocele. In fact, considerable confusion and diversity of opinion and practice appear to be when it comes to subclinical and grade 1 clinical varicoceles too.

On the one hand, clinicians often do not believe that correcting a grade 1 varicocele is of benefit, and, usually, its repair is not recommended. On the other hand, paradoxically, when there is nothing to offer to a man with idiopathic OAT, for instance, many clinicians would recommend VR if a varicocele was detected through US [37].

Again, even though guidelines are clear in recommending against subclinical varicocele repair, there are nevertheless studies claiming some benefit from varicocelectomy in this type of patient [73,74]. This statement is confirmed by evidence from the literature which analyzed fertility and semen parameters outcomes in subclinical varicocele repair. In a randomized controlled trial by Yamamoto et al., men with subclinical varicocele received either high ligation or no treatment. No difference in terms of pregnancy rates was found (6.7% versus 10%, $p = 0.578$), although those who underwent high ligation demonstrated significant increases in sperm density and total motile sperm ($p < 0.006$ and $p < 0.008$, respectively) [75].

Grasso et al. investigated 68 men with a left-sided subclinical varicocele who randomly underwent either high ligation or no treatment and showed no improvement in semen quality or pregnancy outcomes in either group [76].

Notwithstanding the heterogeneity of these studies, depending on different diagnostic methods, different surgical techniques and different patients' characteristics, these biases highlight the lack of standardization, which makes drawing comparisons difficult. In our opinion, subclinical varicocele seems to be a para-physiological condition and there is no evidence of the efficacy of its treatment on improving semen parameters and pregnancy outcomes; thus, varicocelectomy should only be offered to men presenting with clinically palpable varicoceles, preferably grade 2 or 3.

3.6. Role of Varicocelectomy in Bilateral Varicocele

The bilateral ligation of the spermatic veins has also been debated between urologists and andrologists. Regarding the anatomy, the left gonadal vein drains perpendicularly into the left renal vein, and the "nutcracker" effect on the left renal vein of the compass between the aorta and the superior mesenteric artery results in higher hydrostatic pressure in the left renal vein with increased chances of venous reflux into the left internal spermatic vein when compared to the right one, which drains directly into the inferior vena cava. The study of Pallwein et al. [77] confirms this phenomenon, showing a significantly higher varicocele recurrence rate in patients with left renal vein entrapment compared with patients without. Therefore, venous reflux on the right side seems to be very unlikely. However, particular relevance should be placed on the rare true cases of bilateral clinical varicocele or on the more frequent cases of a left-sided grade 2 or 3 clinical varicocele combined with a subclinical or grade 1 right-sided varicocele [78]. More specifically, an extremely rare case report of isolated right-sided varicocele diagnosed after an extensive work-up was reported in a patient with venous anomalies and a spontaneous portosystemic shunt [79].

Once again, European and American guidelines are not clear on whether or not to treat a subclinical right-side varicocele in the presence of a left-side clinical varicocele.

Recent studies suggested that bilateral varicocelectomy is better than unilateral to improve spontaneous pregnancy rates in patients with left clinical and right subclinical varicocele [80–82]. Among these, a meta-analysis of four RCTs reported no significant difference in sperm concentration and motility between the two groups, but the spontaneous pregnancy rate showed an odds ratio of 1.73, suggesting better results in the bilateral ligation group [82]. Another prospective randomized trial from Sun et al. demonstrated the same results as the previous study, confirming the role of bilateral varicocele treatment [83]. Indeed, there are some limitations upon those trials: only spontaneous pregnancy was evaluated, rather than assisted reproductive pregnancy, and thus it may affect conclusions. Furthermore, as stated by the authors, different surgeons, different surgical techniques and different follow-up times may have led to different rates of spontaneous pregnancy rates.

With this knowledge in mind, a definitive recommendation cannot be made. In our opinion, the rare true clinical bilateral varicocele deserves bilateral treatment, while the more frequent grade 1 or subclinical reflux on the right side accompanying grade 2 or 3 varicocele on the left one should receive repair only on the left side.

Table 1. Varicocele surgical techniques: pros and cons.

Technique	Pros	Cons
Open retroperitoneal high ligation (Palomo) [23,33,48,83]	Complete ligation	General anesthesia, Higher hydrocele risk
Microsurgical lymphatic sparing Palomo [13,17–20]	Complete ligation Lower hydrocele risk	General anesthesia Access to operating microscope
Microsurgical subinguinal or inguinal surgery [23,28,33]	Less invasive (local anesthesia) Lower recurrence rate Lower hydrocele risk	Access to operating microscope Longer surgical time
Laparoscopic surgery [23,32,33]	Bilateral varicocele Higher magnification Lower recurrence rate	High costs More invasive (intraperitoneal) General anesthesia
Sclero-embolization [15,16,23–26,48]	Minimally invasive Short time Outpatient	Limited applicability Higher recurrence rate Radiation exposure

4. Summary

In summary, the strongest recommendations for varicocele repair are represented by couple infertility, OAT, grade 2 or 3 clinical varicocele, partner <37 yrs, patient age <40 yrs and testicular hypotrophy in children and adolescents. Indications are reinforced when OAT is severe and in younger patients. On the other hand, little indication exists to treat varicocele in azoospermic patients. Finally, an additional indication is represented by elevated sperm DNA fragmentation, particularly in partners of women who had undergone an unsuccessful ICSI or repeated miscarriages.

5. Conclusions

A conclusive answer to the Hamletic doubt of the title, to treat or not to treat varicocele, is not yet possible. Varicocele is the most common correctable cause of male infertility. In selected cases, varicocele treatment is beneficial in improving semen parameters and pregnancy rates. On the other hand, the high prevalence of the disease, together with the knowledge that many patients with varicocele are fertile, might lead to overtreatment. Urologists and andrologists, as well as any clinician who plays an important role in dealing with this common disease, must carefully counsel patients after having analyzed their history, physical examination findings and all pertinent clinical parameters before leading them to the operating theatre.

Author Contributions: Conceptualization, A.F. and G.F.; investigation, G.S.; data curation, F.F.; writing—original draft preparation, F.P. and V.P.; writing—review and editing, M.G. and C.L.; supervision, G.F. and C.M. All authors have read and agreed to the published version of the manuscript.

Funding: This research received no external funding.

Institutional Review Board Statement: Not applicable.

Informed Consent Statement: Not applicable.

Data Availability Statement: Not applicable.

Conflicts of Interest: The authors declare no conflict of interest.

References

1. Franco, G.; Iori, F.; De Dominicis, C.; Dal Forno, S.; Mander, A.; Laurenti, C. Challenging the Role of Cremasteric Reflux in the Pathogenesis of Varicocele Using a New Venographic Approach. *J. Urol.* **1999**, *161*, 117–121. [CrossRef] [PubMed]
2. Alsaikhan, B.; Alrabeeah, K.; Delouya, G.; Zini, A. Epidemiology of Varicocele. *Asian J. Androl.* **2016**, *18*, 179. [PubMed]
3. Dubin, L.; Amelar, R.D. Varicocele Size and Results of Varicocelectomy in Selected Subfertile Men with Varicocele. *Fertil. Steril.* **1970**, *21*, 606–609. [CrossRef]
4. Freeman, S.; Bertolotto, M.; Richenberg, J.; Belfield, J.; Dogra, V.; Huang, D.Y.; Lotti, F.; Markiet, K.; Nikolic, O.; Ramanathan, S.; et al. Ultrasound Evaluation of Varicoceles: Guidelines and Recommendations of the European Society of Urogenital Radiology Scrotal and Penile Imaging Working Group (ESUR-SPIWG) for Detection, Classification, and Grading. *Eur. Radiol.* **2020**, *30*, 11–25. [CrossRef]
5. WHO Manual for the Standardized Investigation and Diagnosis of the Infertile Male. Available online: https://www.who.int/publications/i/item/9780521774741 (accessed on 15 May 2023).
6. Sarteschi, L.; Paoli, R.; Bianchini, M.; Menchini Fabris, G. Lo Studio Del Varicocele Con Eco-Color-Doppler. *G Ital. Ultrasonol.* **1993**, *4*, 43–49.
7. Cavallini, G.; Scroppo, F.I.; Colpi, G.M. The Clinical Usefulness of a Novel Grading System for Varicocoeles Using Duplex Doppler Ultrasound Examination Based on Postsurgical Modifications of Seminal Parameters. *Andrology* **2019**, *7*, 62–68. [CrossRef] [PubMed]
8. Schlegel, P.N.; Sigman, M.; Collura, B.; De Jonge, C.J.; Eisenberg, M.L.; Lamb, D.J.; Mulhall, J.P.; Niederberger, C.; Sandlow, J.I.; Sokol, R.Z.; et al. Diagnosis and Treatment of Infertility in Men: AUA/ASRM Guideline Part I. *Fertil. Steril.* **2021**, *115*, 54–61. [CrossRef] [PubMed]
9. Minhas, S.; Bettocchi, C.; Boeri, L.; Capogrosso, P.; Carvalho, J.; Cilesiz, N.C.; Cocci, A.; Corona, G.; Dimitropoulos, K.; Gül, M.; et al. European Association of Urology Guidelines on Male Sexual and Reproductive Health: 2021 Update on Male Infertility. *Eur. Urol.* **2021**, *80*, 603–620. [CrossRef]
10. Su, J.S.; Farber, N.J.; Vij, S.C. Pathophysiology and Treatment Options of Varicocele: An Overview. *Andrologia* **2021**, *53*, e13576. [CrossRef]
11. Dieamant, F.; Petersen, C.G.; Mauri, A.L.; Conmar, V.; Mattila, M.; Vagnini, L.D.; Renzi, A.; Costa, B.P.; Zamara, C.; Oliveira, J.B.A.; et al. Semen Parameters in Men with Varicocele: DNA Fragmentation, Chromatin Packaging, Mitochondrial Membrane Potential, and Apoptosis. *JBRA Assist. Reprod.* **2017**, *21*, 295–301. [CrossRef]
12. Franco, G.; Misuraca, L.; Ciletti, M.; Leonardo, C.; De Nunzio, C.; Palminteri, E.; De Dominicis, C. Surgery of Male Infertility: An Update. *Urologia* **2014**, *81*, 154–164. [CrossRef]
13. Agarwal, A.; Cannarella, R.; Saleh, R.; Boitrelle, F.; Gül, M.; Toprak, T.; Salvio, G.; Arafa, M.; Russo, G.I.; Harraz, A.M.; et al. Impact of Varicocele Repair on Semen Parameters in Infertile Men: A Systematic Review and Meta-Analysis. *World J. Men's Health* **2023**, *41*, 220142. [CrossRef]
14. Crestani, A.; Giannarini, G.; Calandriello, M.; Rossanese, M.; Mancini, M.; Novara, G.; Ficarra, V. Antegrade Scrotal Sclerotherapy of Internal Spermatic Veins for Varicocele Treatment: Technique, Complications, and Results. *Asian J. Androl.* **2016**, *18*, 292–295. [CrossRef]
15. Matsuda, T.; Horii, Y.; Yoshida, O. Should the Testicular Artery Be Preserved at Varicocelectomy? *J. Urol.* **1993**, *149*, 1357–1360. [CrossRef]
16. Ferro, F.; Gentile, V. Il Varicocele in Età Pediatrica Ed Adolescenziale. In *Varicocele e Infertilità Maschile*; Flati, G., Gentile, V., Lenzi, A., Eds.; SEU: Rome, Italy, 2006.
17. Riccabona, M.; Oswald, J.; Koen, M.; Lusuardi, L.; Radmayr, C.; Bartsch, G. Optimizing the Operative Treatment of Boys with Varicocele: Sequential Comparison of 4 Techniques. *J. Urol.* **2003**, *169*, 666–668. [CrossRef] [PubMed]
18. Silveri, M.; Bassani, F.; Adorisio, O. Changing Concepts in Microsurgical Pediatric Varicocelectomy: Is Retroperitoneal Approach Better than Subinguinal One? *Urol. J.* **2015**, *12*, 2032–2035. [PubMed]

19. Zhang, H.; Li, H.; Hou, Y.; Jin, J.; Gu, X.; Zhang, M.; Huo, W.; Li, H. Microscopic Retroperitoneal Varicocelectomy with Artery and Lymphatic Sparing: An Alternative Treatment for Varicocele in Infertile Men. *Urology* **2015**, *86*, 511–515. [CrossRef] [PubMed]
20. Jones, P.F.; Bagley, F.H. An Abdominal Extraperitoneal Approach for the Difficult Orchidopexy. *Br. J. Surg.* **1979**, *66*, 14–18. [CrossRef] [PubMed]
21. Kroese, A.C.; de Lange, N.M.; Collins, J.; Evers, J.L. Surgery or Embolization for Varicoceles in Subfertile Men. *Cochrane Database Syst. Rev.* **2012**, *10*, 67. [CrossRef]
22. Çayan, S.; Shavakhabov, S.; Kadioğlu, A. Treatment of Palpable Varicocele in Infertile Men: A Meta-Analysis to Define the Best Technique. *J. Androl.* **2009**, *30*, 33–40. [CrossRef]
23. Makris, G.C.; Efthymiou, E.; Little, M.; Boardman, P.; Anthony, S.; Uberoi, R.; Tapping, C. Safety and Effectiveness of the Different Types of Embolic Materials for the Treatment of Testicular Varicoceles: A Systematic Review. *Br. J. Radiol.* **2018**, *91*, 20170445. [CrossRef]
24. Halpern, J.; Mittal, S.; Pereira, K.; Bhatia, S.; Ramasamy, R. Percutaneous Embolization of Varicocele: Technique, Indications, Relative Contraindications, and Complications. *Asian J. Androl.* **2016**, *18*, 234–238. [CrossRef]
25. Bebi, C.; Bilato, M.; Minoli, D.G.; De Marco, E.A.; Gnech, M.; Paraboschi, I.; Boeri, L.; Fulgheri, I.; Brambilla, R.; Campoleoni, M.; et al. Radiation Exposure and Surgical Outcomes after Antegrade Sclerotherapy for the Treatment of Varicocele in the Paediatric Population: A Single Centre Experience. *J. Clin. Med.* **2023**, *12*, 755. [CrossRef] [PubMed]
26. Goldstein, M.; Gilbert, B.R.; Dicker, A.P.; Dwosh, J.; Gnecco, C. Microsurgical Inguinal Varicocelectomy with Delivery of the Testis: An Artery and Lymphatic Sparing Technique. *J. Urol.* **1992**, *148*, 1808–1811. [CrossRef]
27. Marmar, J.L.; DeBenedictis, T.J.; Praiss, D. The Management of Varicoceles by Microdissection of the Spermatic Cord at the External Inguinal Ring. *Fertil. Steril.* **1985**, *43*, 583–588. [CrossRef]
28. Colpi, G.M.; Carmignani, L.; Nerva, F.; Piediferro, G.; Castiglioni, F.; Grugnetti, C.; Galasso, G. Surgical Treatment of Varicocele by a Subinguinal Approach Combined with Antegrade Intraoperative Sclerotherapy of Venous Vessels. *BJU Int.* **2006**, *97*, 142–145. [CrossRef]
29. Practice Committee of the American Society for Reproductive Medicine. Report on Varicocele and Infertility. *Fertil. Steril.* **2008**, *90*, S247–S249. [CrossRef] [PubMed]
30. Mehta, A.; Goldstein, M. Microsurgical Varicocelectomy: A Review. *Asian J. Androl.* **2013**, *15*, 56–60. [CrossRef]
31. Wang, H.; Ji, Z.G. Microsurgery Versus Laparoscopic Surgery for Varicocele: A Meta-Analysis and Systematic Review of Randomized Controlled Trials. *J. Investig. Surg.* **2020**, *33*, 40–48. [CrossRef] [PubMed]
32. Al-Kandari, A.M.; Shabaan, H.; Ibrahim, H.M.; Elshebiny, Y.H.; Shokeir, A.A. Comparison of Outcomes of Different Varicocelectomy Techniques: Open Inguinal, Laparoscopic, and Subinguinal Microscopic Varicocelectomy: A Randomized Clinical Trial. *Urology* **2007**, *69*, 417–420. [CrossRef]
33. Evers, J.L.H.; Collins, J.; Clarke, J. Surgery or Embolisation for Varicoceles in Subfertile Men. *Cochrane Database Syst. Rev.* **2009**, *10*, CD000479; Update in: *Cochrane Database Syst. Rev.* **2012**, *10*, CD000479. [CrossRef]
34. Evers, J.L.H.; Collins, J.A. Assessment of Efficacy of Varicocele Repair for Male Subfertility: A Systematic Review. *Lancet* **2003**, *361*, 1849–1852. [CrossRef]
35. Abdel-Meguid, T.A.; Al-Sayyad, A.; Tayib, A.; Farsi, H.M. Does Varicocele Repair Improve Male Infertility? An Evidence-Based Perspective from a Randomized, Controlled Trial. *Eur. Urol.* **2011**, *59*, 455–461. [CrossRef]
36. Shah, R.; Agarwal, A.; Kavoussi, P.; Rambhatla, A.; Saleh, R.; Cannarella, R.; Harraz, A.M.; Boitrelle, F.; Kuroda, S.; Hamoda, T.A.A.A.M.; et al. Consensus and Diversity in the Management of Varicocele for Male Infertility: Results of a Global Practice Survey and Comparison with Guidelines and Recommendations. *World J. Men's Health* **2023**, *41*, 164. [CrossRef] [PubMed]
37. Takihara, H.; Sakatoku, J.; Cockett, A.T.K. The Pathophysiology of Varicocele in Male Infertility. *Fertil. Steril.* **1991**, *55*, 861–868. [CrossRef] [PubMed]
38. Çayan, S.; Woodhouse, C.R.J. The Treatment of Adolescents Presenting with a Varicocele. *BJU Int.* **2007**, *100*, 744–747. [CrossRef] [PubMed]
39. Çayan, S.; Şahin, S.; Akbay, E. Paternity Rates and Time to Conception in Adolescents with Varicocele Undergoing Microsurgical Varicocele Repair vs Observation Only: A Single Institution Experience with 408 Patients. *J. Urol.* **2017**, *198*, 195–201. [CrossRef] [PubMed]
40. Silay, M.S.; Hoen, L.; Quadackaers, J.; Undre, S.; Bogaert, G.; Dogan, H.S.; Kocvara, R.; Nijman, R.J.M.; Radmayr, C.; Tekgul, S.; et al. Treatment of Varicocele in Children and Adolescents: A Systematic Review and Meta-Analysis from the European Association of Urology/European Society for Paediatric Urology Guidelines Panel. *Eur. Urol.* **2019**, *75*, 448–461. [CrossRef] [PubMed]
41. Elder, J. Does the Evidence Support Adolescent Varicocelectomy? *Eur. Urol.* **2019**, *75*, 462–463. [CrossRef]
42. Lacerda, J.I.; Del Giudice, P.T.; Da Silva, B.F.; Nichi, M.; Fariello, R.M.; Fraietta, R.; Restelli, A.E.; Blumer, C.G.; Bertolla, R.P.; Cedenho, A.P. Adolescent Varicocele: Improved Sperm Function after Varicocelectomy. *Fertil. Steril.* **2011**, *95*, 994–999. [CrossRef]
43. Cannarella, R.; Calogero, A.E.; Condorelli, R.A.; Giacone, F.; Aversa, A.; La Vignera, S. Management and Treatment of Varicocele in Children and Adolescents: An Endocrinologic Perspective. *J. Clin. Med.* **2019**, *8*, 1410. [CrossRef] [PubMed]
44. Baazeem, A.; Belzile, E.; Ciampi, A.; Dohle, G.; Jarvi, K.; Salonia, A.; Weidner, W.; Zini, A. Varicocele and Male Factor Infertility Treatment: A New Meta-Analysis and Review of the Role of Varicocele Repair. *Eur. Urol.* **2011**, *60*, 796–808. [CrossRef] [PubMed]

45. Kroese, A.C.J.; Lange, N.M.D.; Collins, J.A.; Evers, J.L.H. Varicocele Surgery, New Evidence. *Hum. Reprod. Update* **2013**, *19*, 317. [CrossRef] [PubMed]
46. Marmar, J.L.; Agarwal, A.; Prabakaran, S.; Agarwal, R.; Short, R.A.; Benoff, S.; Thomas, A.J. Reassessing the Value of Varicocelectomy as a Treatment for Male Subfertility with a New Meta-Analysis. *Fertil. Steril.* **2007**, *88*, 639–648. [CrossRef]
47. Persad, E.; O'Loughlin, C.A.A.; Kaur, S.; Wagner, G.; Matyas, N.; Hassler-Di Fratta, M.R.; Nussbaumer-Streit, B. Surgical or Radiological Treatment for Varicoceles in Subfertile Men. *Cochrane Database Syst. Rev.* **2021**, *4*, CD000479. [CrossRef] [PubMed]
48. Lara-Cerrillo, S.; Gual-Frau, J.; Benet, J.; Abad, C.; Prats, J.; Amengual, M.J.; Ribas-Maynou, J.; García-Peiró, A. Microsurgical Varicocelectomy Effect on Sperm Telomere Length, DNA Fragmentation and Seminal Parameters. *Hum. Fertil.* **2022**, *25*, 135–141. [CrossRef]
49. Lira Neto, F.T.; Roque, M.; Esteves, S.C. Effect of Varicocelectomy on Sperm Deoxyribonucleic Acid Fragmentation Rates in Infertile Men with Clinical Varicocele: A Systematic Review and Meta-Analysis. *Fertil. Steril.* **2021**, *116*, 696–712. [CrossRef]
50. Ribas-Maynou, J.; Yeste, M.; Becerra-Tomás, N.; Aston, K.I.; James, E.R.; Salas-Huetos, A. Clinical Implications of Sperm DNA Damage in IVF and ICSI: Updated Systematic Review and Meta-Analysis. *Biol. Rev. Camb. Philos. Soc.* **2021**, *96*, 1284–1300. [CrossRef]
51. Qiu, D.; Shi, Q.; Pan, L. Efficacy of Varicocelectomy for Sperm DNA Integrity Improvement: A Meta-Analysis. *Andrologia* **2021**, *53*, e13885. [CrossRef]
52. Yan, S.; Shabbir, M.; Yap, T.; Homa, S.; Ramsay, J.; McEleny, K.; Minhas, S. Should the Current Guidelines for the Treatment of Varicoceles in Infertile Men Be Re-Evaluated? *Hum. Fertil.* **2021**, *24*, 78–92. [CrossRef]
53. Jayasena, C.N.; Radia, U.K.; Figueiredo, M.; Revill, L.F.; Dimakopoulou, A.; Osagie, M.; Vessey, W.; Regan, L.; Rai, R.; Dhillo, W.S. Reduced Testicular Steroidogenesis and Increased Semen Oxidative Stress in Male Partners as Novel Markers of Recurrent Miscarriage. *Clin. Chem.* **2019**, *65*, 161–169. [CrossRef]
54. Negri, L.; Levi-Setti, P.E. Pregnancy Rate after Varicocele Repair: How Many Miscarriages? *J. Androl.* **2011**, *32*, 1. [CrossRef]
55. Ghanaie, M.M.; Asgari, S.A.; Dadrass, N.; Allahkhah, A.; Iran-Pour, E.; Safarinejad, M.R. Effects of Varicocele Repair on Spontaneous First Trimester Miscarriage: A Randomized Clinical Trial. *Urol. J.* **2012**, *9*, 505–513.
56. Farkouh, A.; Agarwal, A.; Hamoda, T.A.-A.A.-M.; Kavoussi, P.; Saleh, R.; Zini, A.; Arafa, M.; Harraz, A.M.; Gul, M.; Karthikeyan, V.S.; et al. Controversy and Consensus on the Management of Elevated Sperm DNA Fragmentation in Male Infertility: A Global Survey, Current Guidelines, and Expert Recommendations. *World J. Men's Health* **2023**, *41*, e48. [CrossRef] [PubMed]
57. Lipshultz, L.I.; Corriere, J.N. Progressive Testicular Atrophy in the Varicocele Patient. *J. Urol.* **1977**, *117*, 175–176. [CrossRef]
58. Fırat, F.; Erdemir, F. The Effect of Age on Semen Quality and Spontaneous Pregnancy Rates in Patients Who Treated with Microsurgical Inguinal Varicocelectomy. *Cureus* **2020**, *12*, e7744. [CrossRef] [PubMed]
59. Hsiao, W.; Rosoff, J.S.; Pale, J.R.; Greenwood, E.A.; Goldstein, M. Older Age Is Associated with Similar Improvements in Semen Parameters and Testosterone after Subinguinal Microsurgical Varicocelectomy. *J. Urol.* **2011**, *185*, 620–625. [CrossRef] [PubMed]
60. Esteves, S.C.; Miyaoka, R.; Roque, M.; Agarwal, A. Outcome of Varicocele Repair in Men with Nonobstructive Azoospermia: Systematic Review and Meta-Analysis. *Asian J. Androl.* **2016**, *18*, 246–253. [CrossRef]
61. Berookhim, B.M.; Schlegel, P.N. Azoospermia Due to Spermatogenic Failure. *Urol. Clin. N. Am.* **2014**, *41*, 97–113. [CrossRef]
62. Abdel-Meguid, T.A. Predictors of Sperm Recovery and Azoospermia Relapse in Men with Nonobstructive Azoospermia after Varicocele Repair. *J. Urol.* **2012**, *187*, 222–226. [CrossRef]
63. Lee, J.S.; Park, H.J.; Seo, J.T. What Is the Indication of Varicocelectomy in Men with Nonobstructive Azoospermia? *Urology* **2007**, *69*, 352–355. [CrossRef] [PubMed]
64. Elzanaty, S. Varicocele Repair in Non-Obstructive Azoospermic Men: Diagnostic Value of Testicular Biopsy—A Meta-Analysis. *Scand. J. Urol.* **2014**, *48*, 494–498. [CrossRef]
65. Agarwal, A.; Deepinder, F.; Cocuzza, M.; Agarwal, R.; Short, R.A.; Sabanegh, E.; Marmar, J.L. Efficacy of Varicocelectomy in Improving Semen Parameters: New Meta-Analytical Approach. *Urology* **2007**, *70*, 532–538. [CrossRef]
66. Esteves, S.C.; Roque, M.; Agarwal, A. Outcome of Assisted Reproductive Technology in Men with Treated and Untreated Varicocele: Systematic Review and Meta-Analysis. *Asian J. Androl.* **2016**, *18*, 254–258. [CrossRef] [PubMed]
67. Kirby, E.W.; Wiener, L.E.; Rajanahally, S.; Crowell, K.; Coward, R.M. Undergoing Varicocele Repair before Assisted Reproduction Improves Pregnancy Rate and Live Birth Rate in Azoospermic and Oligospermic Men with a Varicocele: A Systematic Review and Meta-Analysis. *Fertil. Steril.* **2016**, *106*, 1338–1343. [CrossRef] [PubMed]
68. Ghayda, R.A.; El-Doueihi, R.Z.; Lee, J.Y.; Bulbul, M.; Heidar, N.A.; Bulbul, J.; Asmar, S.; Hong, S.H.; Yang, J.W.; Kronbichler, A.; et al. Anthropometric Variables as Predictors of Semen Parameters and Fertility Outcomes after Varicocelectomy. *J. Clin. Med.* **2020**, *9*, 1160. [CrossRef]
69. Sousa, B.P.; Santos-Pereira, J.; Freire, M.J.; Parada, B.; Almeida-Santos, T.; Bernardino, J.; Ramalho-Santos, J. Using Data Mining to Assist in Predicting Reproductive Outcomes Following Varicocele Embolization. *J. Clin. Med.* **2021**, *10*, 3503. [CrossRef]
70. Chiles, K.A.; Schlegel, P.N. Cost-Effectiveness of Varicocele Surgery in the Era of Assisted Reproductive Technology. *Asian J. Androl.* **2016**, *18*, 259–261. [CrossRef]
71. Dubin, J.M.; Greer, A.B.; Kohn, T.P.; Masterson, T.A.; Ji, L.; Ramasamy, R. Men with Severe Oligospermia Appear to Benefit From Varicocele Repair: A Cost-Effectiveness Analysis of Assisted Reproductive Technology. *Urology* **2018**, *111*, 99–103. [CrossRef]
72. Seo, J.T.; Kim, K.T.; Moon, M.H.; Kim, W.T. The Significance of Microsurgical Varicocelectomy in the Treatment of Subclinical Varicocele. *Fertil. Steril.* **2010**, *93*, 1907–1910. [CrossRef]

73. Cantoro, U.; Polito, M.; Muzzonigro, G. Reassessing the Role of Subclinical Varicocele in Infertile Men with Impaired Semen Quality: A Prospective Study. *Urology* **2015**, *85*, 826–830. [CrossRef]
74. Yamamoto, M.; Hibi, H.; Hirata, Y.; Miyake, K.; Ishigaki, T. Effect of Varicocelectomy on Sperm Parameters and Pregnancy Rate in Patients with Subclinical Varicocele: A Randomized Prospective Controlled Study. *J. Urol.* **1996**, *155*, 1636–1638. [CrossRef] [PubMed]
75. Grasso, M.; Lania, C.; Castelli, M.; Galli, L.; Franzoso, F.; Rigatti, P. Low-Grade Left Varicocele in Patients over 30 Years Old:The Effect of Spermatic Vein Ligation on Fertility. *BJU Int.* **2000**, *85*, 305–307. [CrossRef]
76. Pallwein, L.; Pinggera, G.; Schuster, A.H.; Klauser, A.; Weirich, H.G.; Recheis, W.; Herwig, R.; Halpern, E.J.; Bartsch, G.; Zur Nedden, D.; et al. The Influence of Left Renal Vein Entrapment on Outcome after Surgical Varicocele Repair: A Color Doppler Sonographic Demonstration. *J. Ultrasound Med.* **2004**, *23*, 595–601. [CrossRef] [PubMed]
77. Jensen, C.F.S.; Østergren, P.; Dupree, J.M.; Ohl, D.A.; Sønksen, J.; Fode, M. Varicocele and Male Infertility. *Nat. Rev. Urol.* **2017**, *14*, 523–533. [CrossRef]
78. Pinggera, G.M.; Herwig, R.; Pallwein, L.; Frauscher, F.; Judmaier, W.; Mitterberger, M.; Bartsch, G.; Mallouhi, A. Isolated Right-Sided Varicocele as a Salvage Pathway for Portal Hypertension. *Int. J. Clin. Pract.* **2005**, *59*, 740–742. [CrossRef] [PubMed]
79. Elbendary, M.A.; Elbadry, A.M. Right Subclinical Varicocele: How to Manage in Infertile Patients with Clinical Left Varicocele? *Fertil. Steril.* **2009**, *92*, 2050–2053. [CrossRef] [PubMed]
80. Scherr, D.; Goldstein, M. Comparison of Bilateral versus Unilateral Varicocelectomy in Men with Palpable Bilateral Varicoceles. *J. Urol.* **1999**, *162*, 85–88. [CrossRef]
81. Niu, Y.; Wang, D.; Chen, Y.; Pokhrel, G.; Xu, H.; Wang, T.; Wang, S.; Liu, J. Comparison of Clinical Outcome of Bilateral and Unilateral Varicocelectomy in Infertile Males with Left Clinical and Right Subclinical Varicocele: A Meta-Analysis of Randomised Controlled Trials. *Andrologia* **2018**, *50*, e13078. [CrossRef]
82. Sun, X.; Wang, J.; Peng, Y.; Gao, Q.; Song, T.; Yu, W.; Xu, Z.; Chen, Y.; Dai, Y. Bilateral Is Superior to Unilateral Varicocelectomy in Infertile Males with Left Clinical and Right Subclinical Varicocele: A Prospective Randomized Controlled Study. *Int. Urol. Nephrol.* **2018**, *50*, 205–210. [CrossRef]
83. Palomo, A. Radical Cure of Varicocele by a New Technique; Preliminary Report. *J. Urol.* **1949**, *61*, 604–607. [CrossRef] [PubMed]

Disclaimer/Publisher's Note: The statements, opinions and data contained in all publications are solely those of the individual author(s) and contributor(s) and not of MDPI and/or the editor(s). MDPI and/or the editor(s) disclaim responsibility for any injury to people or property resulting from any ideas, methods, instructions or products referred to in the content.

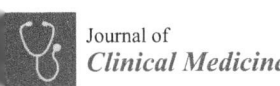

Review

Can Cryopreservation in Assisted Reproductive Technology (ART) Induce Epigenetic Changes to Gametes and Embryos?

Romualdo Sciorio [1,*], Claudio Manna [2], Patricia Fauque [3,4] and Paolo Rinaudo [5]

1. Edinburgh Assisted Conception Programme, Royal Infirmary of Edinburgh, Edinburgh EH16 4SA, UK
2. Biofertility IVF and Infertility Center, 00198 Rome, Italy
3. Université Bourgogne Franche-Comté—Equipe Génétique des Anomalies du Development (GAD) INSERM UMR1231, F-21000 Dijon, France
4. CHU Dijon Bourgogne, Laboratoire de Biologie de la Reproduction—CECOS, F-21000 Dijon, France
5. Department of Obstetrics, Gynecology, and Reproductive Sciences, University of California, San Francisco, CA 92037, USA
* Correspondence: sciorioromualdo@hotmail.com

Abstract: Since the birth of Louise Brown in 1978, more than nine million children have been conceived using assisted reproductive technologies (ARTs). While the great majority of children are healthy, there are concerns about the potential epigenetic consequences of gametes and embryo manipulation. In fact, during the preimplantation period, major waves of epigenetic reprogramming occur. Epigenetic reprogramming is susceptible to environmental changes induced by ovarian stimulation, in-vitro fertilization, and embryo culture, as well as cryopreservation procedures. This review summarizes the evidence relating to oocytes and embryo cryopreservation and potential epigenetic regulation. Overall, it appears that the stress induced by vitrification, including osmotic shock, temperature and pH changes, and toxicity of cryoprotectants, might induce epigenetic and transcriptomic changes in oocytes and embryos. It is currently unclear if these changes will have potential consequences for the health of future offspring.

Keywords: human in-vitro fertilization (IVF); assisted reproductive technology (ART); cryopreservation procedure; vitrification; epigenetics modifications; offspring health

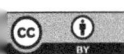

1. Introduction

Over the past forty years, ART has been steadily on the rise, allowing millions of infertile couples to conceive. Currently, it is estimated that over nine million children have been conceived using ART [1,2]. While the number of IVF cycles varies widely worldwide, approximately 5% of births are secondary to the use of ART in some European countries [2]. The main driver of IVF utilization is individuals being affected by infertility (approximately 15% of couples). However, there is a continuous rise in the number of individuals who freeze their eggs or embryos for future use [2–7]. For example, nearly 310,000 frozen embryo transfer (FET) cycles were performed in Europe in 2018 [2].

Current evidence indicates that ART is safe; however, an association between ART and an increased incidence of low birth weight, birth defects, altered growth, and metabolic disorders has been reported [8,9]. These findings might be secondary to epigenetic dysregulation of gametes and embryos [10–12]. Given the continuous rise in the number of cycles that involve oocytes and embryo cryopreservation, it is critical to understand whether cryopreservation is harmful to the future health of children. In this manuscript, we describe the impact that vitrification has on potential epigenetic modifications and consequences for future offspring health.

2. Increased Use of Oocyte and Embryo Vitrification in ART Practice

The advancements in oocyte cryopreservation found a perfect application for fertility preservation for social reasons or in patients affected by cancer. Indeed, societal changes have resulted in the postponement of the age of the first pregnancy [1,2], at the time when diminished ovarian reserve significantly reduces the chance of success. Therefore, multiple patients aim to freeze their eggs for future use. In the UK, elective egg freezing is the fastest growing fertility treatment, with an increase of 10% per year [13]. In Spain, egg freezing cycles increased from 4% of total vitrification procedures to 22% in 10 years [14]. In the USA, fertility preservation cycles increased from 9607 in 2017 to 13,275 in 2018; similar trends have been observed in other countries [15,16].

Egg freezing is also used by young cancer patients, since treatment for malignancies might negatively affect future fertility [17,18]. According to the International Agency for Research on Cancer, in 2020, there were an estimated 19.3 million new cancer cases, with nearly 10 million cancer deaths. Female breast cancer has surpassed lung cancer as the most commonly diagnosed cancer, with more than two million new cases per year [17].

Another important application of oocyte cryopreservation is in egg donor programs [19]. Since the description by Trounson of the first successful pregnancy following oocyte donation in Australia [20], the number of oocyte donation cycles has doubled in the last decade. For example, in the USA, the number of cycles increased from 10,801 in 2000 to 24,300 in 2016 and 49,193 in 2017 [21]. In 2017, 17,099 donors underwent an average of 2.4 oocyte collections [22]. The need for finding a large number of egg donors has resulted in the creation of multiple oocyte banks. In particular, an oocyte bank performs the egg retrieval and cryopreservation of oocytes, which are later transported to the receiving clinic. Then, the imported oocytes, in the IVF laboratory of the recipient center, are warmed, fertilized with the ICSI technique using fresh or frozen sperm, cultured, and transferred to the recipient's uterus or possibly biopsied for PGT procedure and frozen again [23–26].

Several studies have analyzed the efficiency of oocyte vitrification. Importantly, egg donor vitrification provides high survival rates after warming and a similar pregnancy rate compared to cycles performed using fresh donor oocytes (Figure 1) [25–28].

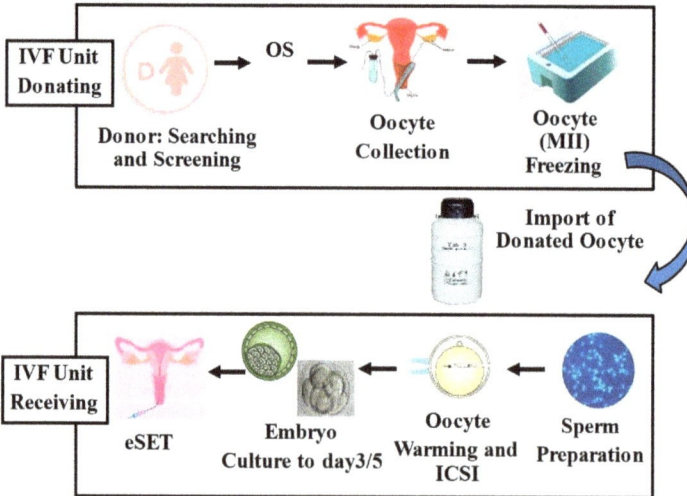

Figure 1. Description of the imported oocyte donation program from a foreign oocyte bank. eSET, elective single embryo transfer; ICSI, intracytoplasmic sperm injection; MII, metaphase II oocyte; OS, ovarian stimulation.

In addition to egg freezing cycles, the ART field has assisted in a significant increase in embryo freeze-all cycles. It has been estimated that 600,000 embryos were stored from 2004 to 2013 in the USA alone, and 309,475 FET were completed in 2018 in Europe (Figure 2) [2]. Reasons for embryo cryopreservation are multiple and include storage of surplus embryos following a fresh transfer [29,30], fertility preservation for cancer patients, and pre-implantation genetic testing (Table 1) [31,32]. Additional reasons include abnormalities of the stimulation cycle, including elevated progesterone at the time of trigger (which has been reported to have a negative impact on pregnancy outcomes [33]) or prevention of ovarian hyperstimulation syndrome, a potentially life-threatening complication [34–36].

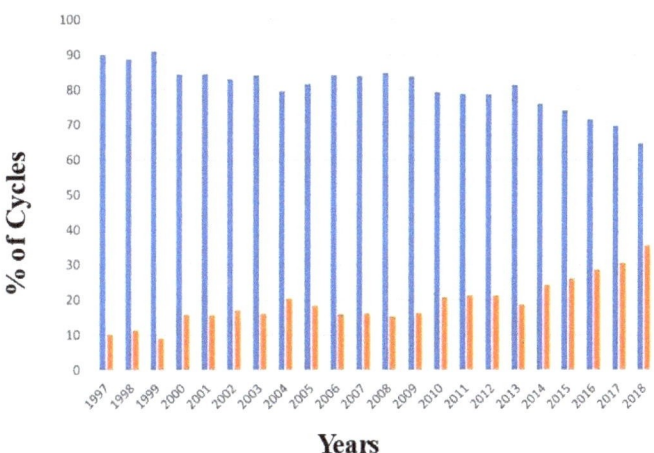

Figure 2. Proportion of fresh and frozen embryo transfers (FETs) performed in Europe (data 1997–2018). Adapted with permission from Wyns and colleagues [2].

Table 1. Main indications for the application of human embryo cryopreservation.

	Embryo Cryopreservation in ART Practice
Preimplantation genetic testing	Genetic assessment is facilitated by the opportunity to utilize the cryopreservation method to store embryos to be transferred in a future cycle, and to overcome the time interval between the blastocyst biopsy and genetic result
Avoiding ovarian hyperstimulation syndrome (OHSS)	When a fresh embryo transfer cannot be performed due to the risk of OHSS, embryos might be cryopreserved and used in a future cycle
Increasing the policy of elective single embryo transfer (eSET)	The cryopreservation of surplus embryos is considered a valid method to reduce the number of embryos transferred during a fresh cycle and to thus minimize the risk of multiple pregnancies and to increase the policy of eSET—as well as to reduce the need for repeated stimulation cycles
Embryo freezing for cancer patients	In women with a stable partner about to go through gonadotoxic/chemotherapy treatment for cancer
Elevated progesterone or other conditions, such as endometriosis	Elevated progesterone in the late follicular phase has a negative impact on pregnancy outcomes; or other conditions and medical pathology that might affect fertility

It is important to note that FET is associated with a higher birth weight compared to fresh embryo transfer and no embryo freezing [37–39]. A meta-analysis of 26 studies reported that singletons born following freezing and thawing had higher birth weights, were large for gestational age, and the pregnancy had an increased risk of hypertensive disorders [40]. An increased birthweight in ART babies conceived following FET has been reported by several authors [41–44]. At present, it is unclear whether the vitrification procedure itself, the use of cryoprotective agents (CPAs), the drugs used for endometrial preparation, or parental infertility are responsible for the higher birthweight in offspring. However, since no difference in birth weight has been observed when embryos are transferred in a natural cycle, it is possible that the drugs applied for endometrial preparation might be responsible for that condition [45].

3. Cryopreservation and Cryoprotectants

Cryopreservation enables the long-term preservation of tissue or cells at ultra-low temperatures (stored in liquid nitrogen at −196 °C) in a state of suspended animation. This process interrupts all biological activities and maintains cell viability and physiological competency for future use. The first report of a live birth following the transfer of a cryopreserved and thawed embryo was recorded in Australia by Trounson and Mohr in 1983 by the "slow freezing" procedure [46]. Later, in the 1990s, a great advancement in the field was achieved with the introduction of the "vitrification" protocol in Japan and Australia [4,5,47]. Vitrification was rapidly adopted since it achieved better outcomes in terms of gamete and embryo survival and higher pregnancy rates, compared to slow freezing [29,30,48]. Vitrification is performed using a high concentration of CPAs. These agents increase viscosity and inhibit ice crystal formation, inducing the solution to enter a "glassy state" [7]. The success of vitrification is correlated with several factors, such as the temperature in the vitrification and warming steps, which depends on the choice of carrier used (open or closed vitrification) and, most importantly, the concentration and type of CPAs used (Table 2). Regarding the temperature, it has been clearly shown that the warming rate is as important as the cooling rate. Seki and Mazur reported that cryo-damage might also be induced by re-crystallization in the warming step. They examined the relationship between cooling versus warming rates in a mouse model and concluded that a warming rate of at least 3000 °C/min is imperative to obtain an acceptable survival rate above 80% [49]. CPAs play a critical role in the success of cryopreservation and are classified into two categories: Permeating and non-permeating agents. The first group includes small molecular weight compounds (less than 400 Da) that can cross cell membranes and, once inside, protect the cell from cryo-induced damage. Permeating agents include ethylene glycol (EG), dimethyl sulfoxide (DMSO; an amphipathic molecule), propylene glycol or 1,2 propanediol (PG), glycerol (GLY), formamide (FMD), methanol (METH), and butanediol (BD; 2,3-butanediol). DMSO and glycerol are the two most used (Table 3). Non-penetrating CPAs are non-diffusible, normally have a higher molecular weight, and therefore cannot cross the cell membrane. Examples are trehalose, sucrose, glucose, mannitol, galactose, and polyvinylpyrrolidone (PVP). These molecules induce an osmotic gradient that removes water from inside to outside the cell (dehydration), reducing the temperature at which ice starts to form and thus preserving membranes and intracellular structures [50,51].

Table 2. Membrane permeability coefficient of some cryoprotectants (Times 10^{-5} cm/s).

Cryoprotectant	Red Blood Cells at 4 °C Study Reference [52]	Sperm Cells at 22 °C Study Reference [53]	Oocytes at 22 °C Study Reference [54]
Methanol	11.35	N/A	N/A
Formamide	8.05	N/A	N/A
Ethylene glycol	3.38	13.2	1.95
Dimethyl sulfoxide	1.30	1.33	2.60
Propylene glycol	1.79	3.83	3.83
Glycerol	0.58	3.50	Low

Table 3. Minimal concentration required to vitrify (C-Vit) for some permeating cryoprotectants at a pressure of 1 atmosphere according to Fahy and colleagues 1984 [55]. PG, propylene glycol; DMSO, dimethyl sulfoxide; EG, ethylene glycol; GLY, glycerol.

Cryoprotectants	Concentration Required to Vitrify (C-Vit) %/Volume
DMSO	49–50
PG	43.5
EG	55
GLY	65

4. Potential Damaging Effects of Cryopreservation

The principal problem that can occur with cryopreservation is the formation of ice crystals. Human embryos and oocytes contain a high content of water, which might be converted into ice, causing irreversible damage and cellular death. This concern was elegantly described by Mazur in 1963 [56]. The sharp reduction of temperature might lead to cold-shock harm and impair the function of several sensible structures located in the oocyte cytoplasm, including membrane permeability, cytoskeleton architecture, and, importantly, the meiotic spindle apparatus [57,58]. The meiotic spindle is a cytoskeletal structure, formed of microtubules and associated proteins [59]. It is considered an indicator of oocyte health; its stability is linked with normal fertilization and is directly responsible for the correct segregation of chromosomes, avoiding errors in chromatin division, accountable for aneuploidies and miscarriage [60]. It is well established that temperature changes can debilitate meiotic spindle stability [61]. At a temperature of 33 °C or lower, the meiotic spindle starts to depolymerize, and only a few minutes of exposure to non-physiologic pH or temperature is sufficient to induce disassembly of the spindle [62]. Several studies on both animals and humans have demonstrated a negative association between temperature, as well as osmolality on normal microtubule disassembly, and spindle alterations [59–63]. Additional impairment following cooling and warming includes premature hardening of the zona pellucida (ZP), which is essential at the time when sperm fertilizes the oocyte. These facts indicate the use of ICSI to fertilize oocytes. However, questions remain concerning the impact of ZP hardening and implantation of the embryo [64]. It is also possible to observe cryo-damage to intracellular organelles, as well as an increased risk of parthenogenetic activation of the oocytes [65]. Oocyte exposure to CPAs might cause ultrastructural modification of the mitochondria and smooth endoplasmic reticulum [66,67]. Animal studies have suggested that oocyte cryopreservation, particularly vitrification, might be associated with increased levels of reactive oxygen species (ROS) and apoptotic events [68–70], which might alter the epigenetic mechanisms associated with oocyte competence and future embryo development and viability [70,71]. In particular, DMSO is a known radical scavenger and, as an antioxidant, helps to protect cells from the damage caused by free radicals. However, at normal or decreased levels of ROS, it may restrict cell metabolism by scavenging the electrons needed for ATP production. Therefore, a decrease in DMSO-induced ATP might cause downstream effects that may disrupt cellular function, fetal development, and implantation potential [72–75]. Finally, over the past few years, several reports have shown the detrimental effects of cryopreservation programs on the epigenetic makeup of the embryo, protein expression, and DNA integrity [76–80], as well as alteration of such genes involved in critical biological processes [79–81], inducing an increase in free radical production and apoptosis [81–85].

5. Epigenetic Changes Occurring during Preimplantation Embryo Development

In 1942, Conrad Waddington, a biologist at Edinburgh University, was the first to emphasize the importance of environmentally directed changes during the early stages of mammalian embryo development and introduced the term "Epigenetics". Epigenetics is a gene-regulatory mechanism that leads to heritable changes in gene function that are not associated with changes in DNA sequence [86]. The importance of epigenetics in the ART field is secondary to the fact that epigenetic changes can be caused by different environmental agents and that important epigenetic changes occur during embryo development. There are two epigenetic reprogramming phases. The first resets DNA methylation marks in primordial germ cells (PGCs) when they migrate to the fetal gonadal ridge. The second wave of DNA methylation changes occurs during the early stage of embryo development, following fertilization; the parental genome is actively demethylated, while the maternal genome is passively demethylated with a wave of re-methylation at the blastocyst stage (Figure 3) [87–89]. In summary, the epigenome of the preimplantation embryo is highly susceptible to external and internal modifications.

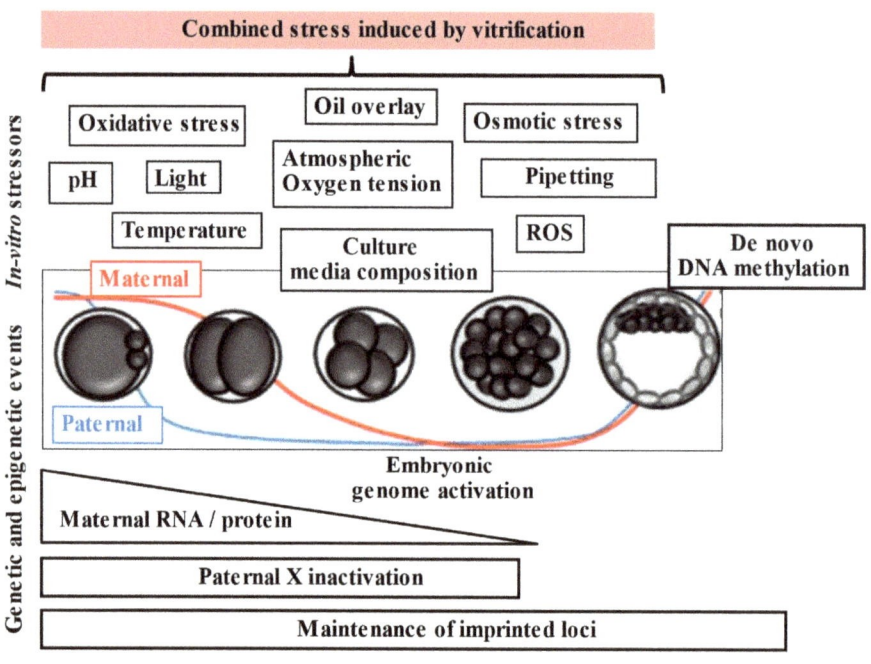

Figure 3. Summary of sensitive genetic and epigenetic events occurring during preimplantation embryo development and when the vitrification procedure is performed. Several stressors exist, and these can act synergistically, causing more negative effects.

DNA methylation is the most investigated epigenetic process and involves the addition of a methyl group at the 5′ carbon position of the cytosine pyrimidine ring in the context of CG dinucleotide (CpG sites). Those epigenetic modifications are maintained by daughter cells throughout cell divisions by DNA methyltransferases (DNMTs). To date, five different types of DNMTs have been identified: Dnmt1, Dnmt2, Dnmt3a, Dnmt3b, and Dnmt3L [90,91]. DNA methylation is generally correlated with gene silencing, but it is also involved in other regulatory mechanisms such as imprinting or X-chromosome inactivation and silencing of centromeric sequences [90–92]. Additional epigenetic regulations comprise post-translational histone modifications, including acetylation, methylation, phosphorylation, and glycosylation ubiquitination [6]. Histone lysine acetylation is particularly important, since it plays a role in cellular differentiation and might be associated with disease processes [93]. This histone modification is regulated by histone acetyltransferases (HATs) and histone deacetylases (HDACs) and is generally associated with transcriptionally active regions of the genome, as it relaxes the chromatin structure, allowing for increased accessibility of the DNA to transcription factors and other regulatory proteins [92–94]. Acetylation leads to open chromatin configuration, enhances transcriptional activity, and encourages transcription factor binding to DNA. On the contrary, deacetylation is correlated with transcriptional inactivation and gene silencing [94]. SUMOylation and de-SUMOylation marks indicate the addition and removal of SUMO (small ubiquitin-related modifier) polypeptides on lysine residues [95], which are essential for the occurrence of oocyte maturation, meiotic resumption, and spindle formation [95–97]. Finally, another newly identified epigenetic modification is lactylation, affected by cellular lactate levels, which directly stimulates gene transcription [98].

An important subgroup of genes affected by epigenetic regulation are imprinted genes [99,100]. Currently, around 150 genes have been identified in mice, and less than 100 in humans [100]. A list of the current mammalian imprinted genes is available online at [https://www.otago.ac.nz/biochemistry/research/facilities/otago652955.html, accessed on 1 January 2023]. These genes are characterized by a monoallelic expression that is dependent on the parental origin of the allele. The parental imprint is linked to differential epigenetic labeling of parental alleles, and importantly is established during gametogenesis and maintained during the early stage of preimplantation embryo development [101–103]. The correct expression of those imprinted genes depicts a critical role in growth and development and are prevalently located in the placenta and brain [104–107]. Examples include loss of imprinted DNA methylation at the Kvdmr icr, found in ART-conceived children with Beckwith–Wiedemann syndrome (BWS) [108] or gain of methylation because of maternal uniparental disomy on chromosome 7 at the Mest icr in approximately 10% of Silver–Russell Syndrome (SRS) cases, as well as Angelman syndrome (AS) and Prader–Willi syndrome [106–113]. While epigenetic changes can affect the individual, new evidence suggests that there could be a transgenerational transmission of epigenetic information [114]. It is therefore possible that the presence of chemical compounds such as cryoprotective agents could alter the reprogramming machinery and cause long-term risk of disease, as postulated by the Developmental Origin of Health and Disease [115–118].

6. Potential Impact of Vitrification on the Epigenome of Oocytes and Embryos

In the past few years, several research groups have investigated the relationship between vitrification and epigenetic disruption in early embryo development [119]. The most studied molecule and the one most widely used is DMSO. DMSO may impact cellular functions, metabolism, enzyme activities, cell growth, and apoptosis, as well as might induce alterations in microRNAs (miRNA) and epigenetic changes [120,121]. Studies have shown that DMSO has temperature-, time-, and concentration-dependent toxic effects [73,74]. Studies focusing on the effect of DMSO and epigenetic changes have reported that DMSO interferes with the activity of the enzyme DNMT3a, even though the specific mechanism is unknown [119–121]. Studies on animal models have shown that following vitrification-warming of mouse oocytes, the expression of the imprinted gene *Kcnq1ot1* decreased significantly [122]. Chen and collaborators reported that following vitrification of mature bovine oocytes, the expression of imprinted genes *Peg10*, *Kcnq1ot1*, and *Xist* in blastocysts obtained by ICSI increased abnormally [123]. The same group in a subsequent publication found that vitrification of mouse MII oocytes affected the expression of the maternally imprinted genes *Peg3*, *Peg10*, and *Igf2r* in oocytes, and maternally imprinted genes *Peg3* and *Peg10* and paternal imprinted gene *Gtl2* in cleavage stage embryos [124]. Another study found that methylation of imprinted genes *H19*, *Peg3*, and *Snrpn* decreased in mouse blastocysts obtained from vitrified mouse oocytes [125]. Comparable results have been reported by other authors, showing a reduction in the overall DNA methylation level in oocytes and early embryos following the vitrification process [126,127]. In summary, animal models suggest that vitrification may affect the normal expression of imprinted genes by changing the DNA methylation level, affecting the regulatory region of those genes (Table 4).

Table 4. Summary of both human and animal studies showing the effects of vitrification on DNA methylation and histone modifications. GV, oocyte at germinal vesicle stage; MII, oocyte at metaphase II stage; IVM, in vitro maturation; 5hmC, 5-hydroxymethylCytosine; 5mC, 5-methylCytosine; DMR, differentially methylated regions.

Study [Ref.]	Materials: Human or Animal	Oocytes or Embryo Analyzed (n)	Technology of Assessment	Studied Sequences or Genes	Main Findings
De Munck et al. [128]	(Human) Mature (MII) donated oocytes	31 embryos (Day 3) from 17 fresh oocytes and 14 after vitrification	Immunofluorescence (5mC, 5hmC)	Global Analysis	No differences in fluorescence intensities between embryos from fresh and vitrified oocytes
Liu et al. [129]	(Human) Vitrified mature oocytes (MII), and MII from GV matured in-vitro	56 in vivo MII, 106 MII from GV matured in-vitro, 122 MII from vitrified GV	Immunofluorescence (5mC)	Global analysis	No significant differences in fluorescence intensities between groups
Al-Khtib et al. [130]	(Human) GV oocytes donated for research and IVM to MII	77 MII after IVM from 184 vitrified GV stage, and 85 MII from 120 fresh GV	Pyrosequencing	Methylation profile of $H19$ and $KCNQ1OT1$, $H19DMR$ and $KvDMR1$	Oocyte vitrification at the GV stage does not affect the methylation profiles of $H19$-DMR and $KvDMR1$
Cantatore et al. [131]	(Mouse) Cleavage stage embryos and blastocysts from vitrified MII oocytes	Two-cell embryos and blastocysts from vitrified oocytes	q-PCR	$Igf2r$ and $Gtl2$	No significant differences observed
Zhao et al. [126]	(Bovine) Oocytes	Vitrified MII oocytes matured in-vitro	Single-cell whole-genome methylation sequencing	Global analysis	$Peg3$ methylation level significantly decreased in the derived blastocysts
Chen et al. [124]	(Mouse) Oocytes	MII oocytes and two-cell embryos	q-PCR and bisulfite sequencing	$Gtl2$, $H19$, $Igf2$, $Peg3$, $Peg10$, $Igf2r$	$Peg3$, $Peg10$, and $Igf2r$ were significantly different in MII oocytes and two-cell embryos after vitrification
Chen et al. [123]	(Bovine) Oocytes	Vitrified MII oocytes matured in vitro	q-PCR	$Peg3$, $Peg10$, $Kcnq1ot1$, $Xist$, $Igf2r$	$Peg10$, $Kcnq1ot1$, and $Xist$ significantly increased after vitrification
Cheng et al. [76]	(Mouse) Blastocysts	Blastocysts from vitrified MII oocytes	Bisulfite sequencing	$H19$, $Peg3$, $Snrpn$	No significant differences in oocytes; decrease in blastocysts after oocyte vitrification
Ma et al. [122]	(Mouse) Oocytes	Mature metaphase II oocytes	WGBS combined with RNA-seq	Global analysis	$Kcnq1ot1$ was significantly downregulated in the vitrified oocytes
Jahangiri et al. [132]	(Mouse) Embryos	Mouse blastocysts from vitrified two-cell embryos	q-PCR	$H3$, $H19$ and $Mest$	The expression level of the chosen imprinted genes increased significantly in experimental groups compared to in vivo blastocysts
Movahed et al. [133]	(Mouse) Embryos	Mouse blastocysts from vitrified two-cell embryos	q-PCR	$Gtl2$ and $Dlk1$	$Gtl2$ was downregulated and $Dlk1$ was upregulated after vitrification

Table 4. Cont.

Study [Ref.]	Materials: Human or Animal	Oocytes or Embryo Analyzed (n)	Technology of Assessment	Studied Sequences or Genes	Main Findings
Barberet et al. [134]	(Human) Placenta	Human placenta	Pyrosequencing and q-PCR	H19, IGF2, KCNQ1OT1 SNURF	The placental DNA methylation levels of H19/IGF2 were lower in the fresh embryo transfer group than in the control (H19/IGF2-seq1) and frozen embryo transfer (H19/IGF2-seq2) groups
Yao et al. [135]	(Human) Placenta	Human placenta obtained from vitrified embryos	q-PCR, Western blotting, and pyrosequencing	SNRPN	The expression level of SNRPN increased after vitrification

Human studies are limited. A study on the effects of DMSO on the DNA methylation profile in human cardiac microtissues found dysregulation of DNA methylation pathways. Methyltransferase DNMT1, a key factor for the maintenance of DNA methylation, as well as DNMT3A, essential for both de novo and maintenance of DNA methylation, were upregulated, while *TET1*, which plays an important role in active de-methylation, was downregulated [121]. Overall, no or limited changes in DNA methylation and imprinted gene expression were found in human oocytes or embryos following vitrification (Table 4). The imprinted genes *H19* and *Kcnq1ot1* showed no differences in DNA methylation in vitrified oocytes. In this study immature oocytes were donated after egg retrieval, and after vitrification warming were in-vitro matured to MII stage [130]. Liu and colleagues estimated the effects of vitrification on nuclear configuration and global DNA methylation in GV-stage oocytes after vitrification warming and in-vitro maturation to MII stage. They found no significant differences in the distribution of mitochondria and global DNA methylation patterns between the groups. However, the authors reported a significantly higher abnormal configuration of the spindle following vitrification [129]. De Munck reported no significant change in the overall DNA methylation level of in-vitro cultured eight-cell embryos derived from vitrified oocytes [128]. Huo and colleagues, using 16 donated human MII oocytes, observed that a total of 1987 genes were differentially expressed following oocyte vitrification warming compared to fresh mature oocytes and found that about 82% of these genes were downregulated, while 18% were upregulated [136]. Those genes involved in several critical biological processes, such as two meiosis-related genes, *Ncapd2* and *Tubgcp5*, were significantly downregulated following oocyte vitrification. In addition, cryopreservation might induce histone changes in oocytes and preimplantation embryos. Suo and colleagues found that the acetylation status of histone H4 at lysine K12 in mouse oocytes was significantly increased in cryopreserved compared to fresh oocytes [137]. Another study evaluated the consequences of mouse embryo vitrification at two cell stages on specific histone marks (H3K9 methylation and H3K9 acetylation) for the genes *Igf2* and *Oct4*. The authors found no significant difference in the expression level of these genes and their histone marks in vitrified and non-vitrified embryos, while only embryo culture induced changes on these loci [138]. Other pathways that were altered following vitrification included several physiological processes, such as oogenesis, cellular response to heat, microtubule-based processes, methylation, ubiquinone biosynthetic processes, sister chromatid migration, DNA repair, oxidative phosphorylation, and ATP metabolic processes [139–142]. The authors also investigated the time of storage of vitrified oocytes in nitrogen and found no alteration in gene expression, suggesting that overall, the potential damage resulting from oocyte vitrification might be associated with the cryopreservation process itself rather than the storage [136]. This finding was confirmed by Stigliani and collaborators, who analyzed the gene expression status between surviving warmed oocytes after three and six years of storage in liquid nitrogen and found no differently expressed genes [143]. The effects of the length of freezing embryos in liquid nitrogen on thawing survival, blastocyst viability, and implantation were recently investigated by Yan and colleagues, who evaluated pregnancy outcomes following different lengths of storage (from less than three years up to 10 years). The authors found a reduced survival rate for blastocysts that were stored for longer than six years. Similarly, clinical pregnancy and live birth rates were significantly decreased in blastocysts stored for more than six years compared with the group frozen for less than three years. No difference was reported in the rates of miscarriage and ectopic pregnancy [144]. In summary, while epigenetic changes in oocytes and embryos following cryopreservation exist, their significance and clinical consequences remain to be fully elucidated [145–148]. Future studies are needed to clarify this important issue [148].

7. Potential Impact of Vitrification on the Epigenome Spermatozoa

Sperm cryopreservation is an essential component of ART that has wide clinical applications while being critical for cancer patients to protect their fertility before receiving chemotherapy or radiotherapy [149–151]. Cryopreservation of human sperm has been practiced for more than 50 years [151]. In the past decade, sperm vitrification has been shown to achieve a higher survival rate and reduced sperm DNA damage compared to slow-freezing protocols [151–154]. Several studies have investigated the impact of sperm cryopreservation on epigenetic markers, including DNA methylation, histone modification, and non-coding RNA molecules [155–162]. De Mello and co-authors investigated the effect of CPA, methanol, ethyl glycol, and glycerol dimethylsulfoxide on DNA methylation of *Colossoma macropomum* sperm and embryo evolution and found that the cryoprotectants investigated induced an overall reduction in DNA methylation levels in spermatozoa, and also caused a significant delay in embryonic development [163]. In contrast, a study by Depince and collaborators reported that DNA methylation of zebrafish spermatozoa significantly increased after cryopreservation with methanol [164]. Salehi and colleagues studied DNA methylation and histone modification, as well as cellular features, including membrane integrity, mitochondria activity and apoptosis, and fertility potential, of rooster semen before and after cryopreservation. The results showed that cryopreservation leads to significantly reduced values of the parameters examined when correlated with fresh samples. Furthermore, there was a significant reduction in H3K9 acetylation and H3K4 methylation compared to the fresh samples [165]. Another study showed that cryoprotectant and freezing–thawing protocols significantly increased global DNA methylation levels in ram spermatozoa [166]. Additionally, a study on humans by Khosravizadeh and co-authors investigated the effects of cryopreservation on DNA methylation in promoter regions of the SNURF–SNRPN and UBE3A imprinted genes, PWS-ICR, and AS-ICR in the chromosome 15q11–q13 region [167]. The authors reported the cryopreservation method to be safe concerning DNA methylation in the chromosome 15q11–q13 region. They found that exposure to cryoprotectants had no significant effect on ROS levels and DNA fragmentation. Neither cryopreservation nor exposure to cryoprotectant significantly affected DNA methylation of the selected gene regions. However, DNA fragmentation had a positive correlation with DNA methylation of AS-ICR [167]. Different mechanisms could lead to epigenetic changes following cryopreservation. First, cryoprotectant agents could be responsible. For example, CPA, a widely used agent for sperm cryopreservation, is cytotoxic and can harm sperm cells, causing osmotic injury and physiological alterations and potentially influencing the epigenetic state of sperm cells indirectly [149,154–157]. Second, raising the level of ROS during the freezing–thawing process [156,159–161] might induce site-specific hypermethylation through either the upregulation of DNA methyltransferases (DNMTs) or the formation of new DNMT-including complexes [158,159]. It is important to emphasize that sperm epigenetic changes could be secondary to additional factors, including sperm manipulation alone or patient characteristics [166–170]. For example, it is well known that oligospermic men have more epigenetic changes than normospermic men [160–162]. However, the number of studies currently available on the topic is still limited. Given the relatively low number of studies conducted using human spermatozoa, additional multicenter studies utilizing the same cryopreservation protocols and DNA methylation analysis are needed to clarify the issue.

8. Conclusions

In the last decade, advancements made in the field of cryobiology have contributed to the increased success of ART. However, concerns about the association between cryopreservation and alteration in epigenetic reprogramming exist. This is relevant, given the association between epigenetic changes and future offspring health. Unfortunately, evidence is lacking, and the number of published reports is limited. Future studies and utilization of novel technologies (such as single-cell sequencing and epigenomics) are needed to fully assess the potential epigenetic aberration that occurs at the time of oocytes or embryo cryopreservation, in order to improve its safety and efficacy in ART.

Author Contributions: R.S. contributed to the conception and designed the manuscript. R.S., C.M., P.F. and P.R. wrote sections of the manuscript and revised it for content. All authors have read and agreed to the published version of the manuscript.

Funding: This research received no external funding.

Institutional Review Board Statement: All procedures performed in studies involving human participants were in accordance with the ethical standards of the institutional and with the 1964 Helsinki Declaration and its later amendments. For this type of study, formal consent was not required.

Informed Consent Statement: Not applicable.

Data Availability Statement: No data is available.

Conflicts of Interest: The authors have no conflict of interest to declare.

References

1. De Geyter, C.; Calhaz-Jorge, C.; Kupka, M.S.; Wyns, C.; Mocanu, E.; Motrenko, T.; Scaravelli, G.; Smeenk, J.; Vidakovic, S.; Goossens, V. ART in Europe, 2015: Results generated from European registries by ESHRE. *Hum. Reprod. Open* **2020**, *2020*, hoz038. [CrossRef]
2. Wyns, C.; De Geyter, C.; Calhaz-Jorge, C.; Kupka, M.S.; Motrenko, T.; Smeenk, J.; Bergh, C.; Tandler-Schneider, A.; Rugescu, I.A.; Goossens, V.; et al. ART in Europe, 2018: Results generated from European registries by ESHRE. *Hum. Reprod. Open* **2022**, *2022*, hoac 022. [CrossRef]
3. Chen, C. Pregnancy after human oocyte cryopreservation. *Lancet* **1986**, *1*, 884–886. [CrossRef] [PubMed]
4. Kuwayama, M.; Vajta, G.; Kato, O.; Leibo, S.P. Highly efficient vitrification method for cryopreservation of human oocytes. *Reprod. Biomed. Online* **2005**, *11*, 300–308. [CrossRef] [PubMed]
5. Rienzi, L.; Gracia, C.; Maggiulli, R.; LaBarbera, A.R.; Kaser, D.J.; Ubaldi, F.M.; Vanderpoel, S.; Racowsky, C. Oocyte, embryo and blastocyst cryopreservation in art: Systematic review and meta-analysis comparing slow-freezing versus vitrification to produce evidence for the development of global guidance. *Hum. Reprod. Update* **2017**, *23*, 139–155. [CrossRef] [PubMed]
6. Potdar, N.; Gelbaya, T.A.; Nardo, L.G. Oocyte vitrification in the 21st century and post-warming fertility outcomes: A systematic review and meta-analysis. *Reprod. Biomed. Online* **2014**, *29*, 159–176. [CrossRef]
7. Hubel, A.; Spindler, R.; Skubitz, A. Storage of Human Biospecimens: Selection of the Optimal Storage Temperature. *Biopreserv. Biobank.* **2014**, *12*, 165–175. [CrossRef] [PubMed]
8. Hart, R.; Norman, R.J. The longer-term health outcomes for children born as a result of IVF treatment: Part I–General health outcomes. *Hum. Reprod. Update* **2013**, *19*, 232–243. [CrossRef]
9. Ventura-Juncá, P.; Irarrázaval, I.; Rolle, A.J.; Gutiérrez, J.I.; Moreno, R.D.; Santos, M.J. In vitro fertilization (IVF) in mammals: Epigenetic and developmental alterations. Scientific and bioethical implications for IVF in humans. *Biol. Res.* **2015**, *18*, 48–68. [CrossRef]
10. Vrooman, L.A.; Bartolomei, M.S. Can assisted reproductive technologies cause adult-onset disease? Evidence from human and mouse. *Reprod. Toxicol.* **2017**, *68*, 72–84. [CrossRef]
11. Hirasawa, R.; Feil, R. Genomic imprinting and human disease. *Essays Biochem.* **2010**, *48*, 187–200. [PubMed]
12. Smith, Z.D.; Chan, M.M.; Humm, K.C.; Karnik, R.; Mekhoubad, S.; Regev, A.; Eggan, K.; Meissner, A. DNA methylation dynamics of the human preimplantation embryo. *Nature* **2014**, *511*, 611–615. [CrossRef] [PubMed]
13. Chronopoulou, E.; Raperport, C.; Sfakianakis, A.; Srivastava, G.; Homburg, R. Elective oocyte cryopreservation for age-related fertility decline. *J. Assist. Reprod. Genet.* **2021**, *38*, 1177–1186. [CrossRef] [PubMed]
14. Cobo, A.; Garcia Velasco, J.; Domingo, J.; Pellicer, A.; Remohí, J. Elective and Onco-fertility preservation: Factors related to IVF outcomes. *Hum. Reprod.* **2018**, *33*, 2222–2231. [CrossRef] [PubMed]

15. Nasab, S.; Ulin, L.; Nkele, C.; Shah, J.; Abdallah, M.E.; Sibai, B.M. Elective egg freezing: What is the vision of women around the globe? *Future Sci. OA* **2020**, *6*, FSO468. [CrossRef] [PubMed]
16. Seyhan, A.; Akin, O.D.; Ertaş, S.; Ata, B.; Yakin, K.; Urman, B. A Survey of Women Who Cryopreserved Oocytes for Non-medical Indications (Social Fertility Preservation). *Reprod. Sci.* **2021**, *28*, 2216–2222. [CrossRef]
17. Sung, H.; Ferlay, J.; Siegel, R.L.; Laversanne, M.; Soerjomataram, I.; Jemal, A.; Bray, F. Global Cancer Statistics 2020: GLOBOCAN Estimates of Incidence and Mortality Worldwide for 36 Cancers in 185 Countries. *CA Cancer J. Clin.* **2021**, *71*, 209–249. [CrossRef]
18. Stearns, V.; Schneider, B.; Henry, N.L.; Hayes, D.F.; Flockhart, D.A. Breast cancer treatment and ovarian failure: Risk factors and emerging genetic determinants. *Nat. Rev. Cancer* **2006**, *6*, 886–893. [CrossRef]
19. Adams, D.; A Clark, R.; Davies, M.; de Lacey, S. A meta-analysis of neonatal health outcomes from oocyte donation. *J. Dev. Orig. Health Dis.* **2015**, *7*, 257–272. [CrossRef]
20. Trounson, A.; Leeton, J.; Besanko, M.; Wood, C.; Conti, A. Pregnancy established in an infertile patient after transfer of a donated embryo fertilised in vitro. *BMJ* **1983**, *286*, 835–838. [CrossRef]
21. Sauer, M.V.; Kavic, S.M. Oocyte and embryo donation 2006: Reviewing two decades of innovation and controversy. *Reprod. Biomed. Online* **2006**, *12*, 153–162. [CrossRef]
22. Kawwass, J.F.; Eyck, P.T.; Sieber, P.; Hipp, H.S.; Van Voorhis, B. More than the oocyte source, egg donors as patients: A national picture of United States egg donors. *J. Assist. Reprod. Genet.* **2021**, *38*, 1171–1175. [CrossRef]
23. Cobo, A.; Garrido, N.; Pellicer, A.; Remohí, J. Six years' experience in ovum donation using vitrified oocytes: Report of cumulative outcomes, impact of storage time, and development of a predictive model for oocyte survival rate. *Fertil. Steril.* **2015**, *104*, 1426–1434. [CrossRef] [PubMed]
24. Cobo, A.; Meseguer, M.; Remoh, J.; Pellicer, A. Use of cryo-banked oocytes in an ovum donation programme: A prospective, randomized, controlled, clinical trial. *Hum. Reprod.* **2010**, *25*, 2239–2246. [CrossRef] [PubMed]
25. Debrock, S.; Peeraer, K.; Gallardo, E.F.; De Neubourg, D.; Spiessens, C.; D'Hooghe, T. Vitrification of cleavage stage day 3 embryos results in higher live birth rates than conventional slow freezing: A RCT. *Hum. Reprod.* **2015**, *30*, 1820–1830. [CrossRef] [PubMed]
26. Rienzi, L.; Cimadomo, D.; Maggiulli, R.; Vaiarelli, A.; Dusi, L.; Buffo, L.; Amendola, M.G.; Colamaria, S.; Giuliani, M.; Bruno, G.; et al. Definition of a clinical strategy to enhance the efficacy, efficiency and safety of egg donation cycles with imported vitrified oocytes. *Hum. Reprod.* **2020**, *35*, 785–795. [CrossRef]
27. Sciorio, R.; Antonini, E.; Engl, B. Live birth and clinical outcome of vitrification-warming donor oocyte programme: An experience of a single IVF unit. *Zygote* **2021**, *29*, 410–416. [CrossRef]
28. Rienzi, L.; Romano, S.; Albricci, L.; Maggiulli, R.; Capalbo, A.; Baroni, E.; Colamaria, S.; Sapienza, F.; Ubaldi, F. Embryo development of fresh 'versus' vitrified metaphase II oocytes after ICSI: A prospective randomized sibling-oocyte study. *Hum. Reprod.* **2009**, *25*, 66–73. [CrossRef]
29. Sciorio, R.; Thong, K.; Pickering, S.J. Single blastocyst transfer (SET) and pregnancy outcome of day 5 and day 6 human blastocysts vitrified using a closed device. *Cryobiology* **2018**, *84*, 40–45. [CrossRef]
30. Sciorio, R.; Thong, K.J.; Pickering, S.J. Increased pregnancy outcome after day 5 versus day 6 transfers of human vitrified-warmed blastocysts. *Zygote* **2019**, *27*, 279–284. [CrossRef]
31. Sciorio, R.; Anderson, R.A. Fertility preservation and preimplantation genetic assessment for women with breast cancer. *Cryobiology* **2019**, *92*, 1–8. [CrossRef] [PubMed]
32. Somigliana, E.; Viganò, P.; Filippi, F.; Papaleo, E.; Benaglia, L.; Candiani, M.; Vercellini, P. Fertility preservation in women with endometriosis: For all, for some, for none? *Hum. Reprod.* **2015**, *30*, 1280–1286. [CrossRef] [PubMed]
33. Santos-Ribeiro, S.; Polyzos, N.; Haentjens, P.; Smitz, J.; Camus, M.; Tournaye, H.; Blockeel, C. Live birth rates after IVF are reduced by both low and high progesterone levels on the day of human chorionic gonadotrophin administration. *Hum. Reprod.* **2014**, *29*, 1698–1705. [CrossRef] [PubMed]
34. Groenewoud, E.R.; Cohlen, B.J.; Macklon, N.S. Programming the endometrium for deferred transfer of cryopreserved embryos: Hormone replacement versus modified natural cycles. *Fertil. Steril.* **2018**, *109*, 768–774. [CrossRef]
35. Sullivan, E.A.; Wang, Y.A.; Hayward, I.; Chambers, G.M.; Illingworth, P.; McBain, J.; Norman, R.J. Single embryo transfer reduces the risk of perinatal mortality, a population study. *Hum. Reprod.* **2012**, *27*, 3609–3615. [CrossRef]
36. Sciorio, R.; Esteves, S.C. Clinical utility of freeze-all approach in ART treatment: A mini-review. *Cryobiology* **2019**, *92*, 9–14. [CrossRef]
37. Belva, F.; Bonduelle, M.; Roelants, M.; Verheyen, G.; Van Landuyt, L. Neonatal health including congenital malformation risk of 1072 children born after vitrified embryo transfer. *Hum. Reprod.* **2016**, *31*, 1610–1620. [CrossRef]
38. Hwang, S.S.; Dukhovny, D.; Gopal, D.; Cabral, H.; Diop, H.; Coddington, C.C.; Stern, J.E. Health outcomes for Massachusetts infants after fresh versus frozen embryo transferr. *Fertil. Steril.* **2019**, *112*, 900–907. [CrossRef]
39. Ainsworth, A.J.; Wyatt, M.A.; Shenoy, C.; Hathcock, M.; Coddington, C.C. Fresh versus frozen embryo transfer has no effect on childhood weight. *Fertil. Steril.* **2019**, *112*, 684–690. [CrossRef]
40. Maheshwari, A.; Pandey, S.; Raja, E.A.; Shetty, A.; Hamilton, M.; Bhattacharya, S. Is frozen embryo transfer better for mothers and babies? Can cumulative meta-analysis provide a definitive answer? *Hum. Reprod. Update* **2017**, *24*, 35–58. [CrossRef]
41. Maheshwari, A.; Raja, E.A.; Bhattacharya, S. Obstetric and perinatal outcomes after either fresh or thawed frozen embryo transfer: An analysis of 112,432 singleton pregnancies recorded in the Human Fertilisation and Embryology Authority anonymized dataset. *Fertil. Steril.* **2016**, *106*, 1703–1708. [CrossRef]

42. Sazonova, A.; Källen, K.; Thurin-Kjellberg, A.; Wennerholm, U.-B.; Bergh, C. Obstetric outcome in singletons after in vitro fertilization with cryopreserved/thawed embryos. *Hum. Reprod.* **2012**, *27*, 1343–1350. [CrossRef]
43. Pelkonen, S.; Koivunen, R.; Gissler, M.; Nuojua-Huttunen, S.; Suikkari, A.-M.; Hydén-Granskog, C.; Martikainen, H.; Tiitinen, A.; Hartikainen, A.-L. Perinatal outcome of children born after frozen and fresh embryo transfer: The Finnish cohort study 1995–2006. *Hum. Reprod.* **2010**, *25*, 914–923. [CrossRef] [PubMed]
44. Pinborg, A.; Henningsen, A.A.; Loft, A.; Malchau, S.S.; Forman, J.; Andersen, A.N. Large baby syndrome in singletons born after frozen embryo transfer (FET): Is it due to maternal factors or the cryotechnique? *Hum. Reprod.* **2014**, *29*, 618–627. [CrossRef]
45. von Versen-Höynck, F.; Narasimhan, P.; Tierney, E.S.S.; Martinez, N.; Conrad, K.P.; Baker, V.L.; Winn, V.D. Absent or Excessive Corpus Luteum Number Is Associated with Altered Maternal Vascular Health in Early Pregnancy. *Hypertension* **2019**, *73*, 680–690. [CrossRef] [PubMed]
46. Trounson, A.; Mohr, L. Human pregnancy following cryopreservation, thawing and transfer of an eight-cell embryo. *Nature* **1983**, *305*, 707–709. [CrossRef] [PubMed]
47. Mukaida, T.; Wada, S.; Takahashi, K.; Pedro, P.; An, T.; Kasai, M. Vitrification of human embryos based on the assessment of suitable conditions for 8-cell mouse embryos. *Hum. Reprod.* **1998**, *13*, 2874–2879. [CrossRef]
48. Li, Z.; Wang, A.Y.; Ledger, W.; Edgar, D.H.; Sullivan, E.A. Clinical outcomes following cryopreservation of blastocysts by vitrification or slow freezing: A population-based cohort study. *Hum. Reprod.* **2014**, *29*, 2794–2801. [CrossRef]
49. Seki, S.; Mazur, P. The dominance of warming rate over cooling rate in the survival of mouse oocytes subjected to a vitrification procedure. *Cryobiology* **2009**, *59*, 75–82. [CrossRef]
50. Karlsson, J.O.; Toner, M. Long-term storage of tissues by cryopreservation: Critical issues. *Biomaterials* **1996**, *17*, 243–256. [CrossRef]
51. Fuller, B.J. Cryoprotectants: The essential antifreezes to protect life in the frozen state. *CryoLetters* **2004**, *25*, 375–388.
52. Naccache, P.; Sha'Afi, R.I. Patterns of Nonelectrolyte Permeability in Human Red Blood Cell Membrane. *J. Gen. Physiol.* **1973**, *62*, 714–736. [CrossRef]
53. Gilmore, J.A.; Liu, J.; Gao, D.Y.; Critser, J.K. Determination of optimal cryoprotectants and procedures for their addition and removal from human spermatozoa. *Hum. Reprod.* **1997**, *12*, 112–118. [CrossRef]
54. Van den Abbeel, E.; Schneider, U.; Liu, J.; Agca, Y.; Critser, J.K.; Van Steirteghem, A. Osmotic responses and tolerance limits to changes in external osmolalities, and oolemma permeability characteristics, of human in vitro matured MII oocytes. *Hum. Reprod.* **2007**, *22*, 1959–1972. [CrossRef]
55. Fahy, G.M.; Macfarlane, D.R.; Angell, C.A.; Meryman, H.T. Vitrification as an approach to cryopreservation. *Cryobiology* **1984**, *21*, 407–426. [CrossRef] [PubMed]
56. Mazur, P. Kinetics of Water Loss from Cells at Subzero Temperatures and the Likelihood of Intracellular Freezing. *J. Gen. Physiol.* **1963**, *47*, 347–369. [CrossRef] [PubMed]
57. Smith, G.D.; Silva, E.S.C.A. Developmental consequences of cryopreservation of mammalian oocytes and embryos. *Reprod. Biomed. Online* **2004**, *9*, 171–178. [CrossRef]
58. Best, B.P. Cryoprotectant toxicity: Facts, issues, and questions. *Rejuvenation Res.* **2015**, *18*, 422–436. [CrossRef]
59. Dal Canto, M.; Guglielmo, M.C.; Mignini Renzini, M.; Fadini, R.; Moutier, C.; Merola, M.; De Ponti, E.; Coticchio, G. Dysmorphic patterns are associated with cytoskeletal alterations in human oocytes. *Hum. Reprod.* **2017**, *32*, 750–757. [CrossRef] [PubMed]
60. Feuer, S.; Rinaudo, P. Preimplantation stress and development. *Birth Defects Res. C Embryo Today* **2012**, *96*, 299–314. [CrossRef]
61. Wang, W.-H.; Meng, L.; Hackett, R.J.; Oldenbourg, R.; Keefe, D.L. Rigorous thermal control during intracytoplasmic sperm injection stabilizes the meiotic spindle and improves fertilization and pregnancy rates. *Fertil. Steril.* **2002**, *77*, 1274–1277. [CrossRef] [PubMed]
62. Montag, M.; van der Ven, H. Symposium: Innovative techniques in human embryo viability assessment. Oocyte assessment and embryo viability prediction: Birefringence imaging. *Reprod. Biomed. Online* **2008**, *17*, 454–460. [CrossRef] [PubMed]
63. Pickering, S.J.; Braude, P.R.; Johnson, M.H.; Cant, A.; Currie, J. Transient cooling to room temperature can cause irreversible disruption of the meiotic spindle in the human oocyte. *Fertil. Steril.* **1990**, *54*, 102–108. [CrossRef] [PubMed]
64. Larman, M.G.; Sheehan, C.B.; Gardner, D.K. Calcium-free vitrification reduces cryoprotectant-induced zona pellucida hardening and increases fertilization rates in mouse oocytes. *Reproduction* **2006**, *131*, 53–61. [CrossRef]
65. Gook, D.A.; Osborn, S.M.; Johnston, W.I. Parthenogenetic activation of human oocytes following cryopreservation using 1,2-propanediol. *Hum. Reprod.* **1995**, *10*, 654–658. [CrossRef]
66. Gualtieri, R.; Iaccarino, M.; Mollo, V.; Prisco, M.; Iaccarino, S.; Talevi, R. Slow cooling of human oocytes: Ultrastructural injuries and apoptotic status. *Fertil. Steril.* **2009**, *91*, 1023–1034. [CrossRef]
67. Jones, A.; VAN Blerkom, J.; Davis, P.; Toledo, A.A. Cryopreservation of metaphase II human oocytes effects mitochondrial membrane potential: Implications for developmental competence. *Hum. Reprod.* **2004**, *19*, 1861–1866. [CrossRef]
68. Kohaya, N.; Fujiwara, K.; Ito, J.; Kashiwazaki, N. Generation of Live Offspring from Vitrified Mouse Oocytes of C57BL/6J Strain. *PLoS ONE* **2013**, *8*, e58063. [CrossRef]
69. Zhao, X.-M.; Hao, H.-S.; Du, W.-H.; Zhao, S.-J.; Wang, H.-Y.; Wang, N.; Wang, D.; Liu, Y.; Qin, T.; Zhu, H.-B. Melatonin inhibits apoptosis and improves the developmental potential of vitrified bovine oocytes. *J. Pineal Res.* **2015**, *60*, 132–141. [CrossRef]
70. Christou-Kent, M.; Dhellemmes, M.; Lambert, E.; Ray, P.F.; Arnoult, C. Diversity of RNA-Binding Proteins Modulating Post-Transcriptional Regulation of Protein Expression in the Maturing Mammalian Oocyte. *Cells* **2020**, *9*, 662. [CrossRef]

71. Sendzikaite, G.; Kelsey, G. The role and mechanisms of DNA methylation in the oocyte. *Essays Biochem.* **2019**, *63*, 691–705. [PubMed]
72. Yu, Z.W.; Quinn, P.J. Dimethyl sulphoxide: A review of its applications in cell biology. *Biosci. Rep.* **1994**, *14*, 259–281. [CrossRef] [PubMed]
73. Hunt, C.J. Cryopreservation of Human Stem Cells for Clinical Application: A Review. *Transfus. Med. Hemother.* **2011**, *38*, 107–123. [CrossRef] [PubMed]
74. Marks, P.A.; Breslow, R. Dimethyl sulfoxide to vorinostat: Development of this histone deacetylase inhibitor as an anticancer drug. *Nat. Biotechnol.* **2007**, *25*, 84–90. [CrossRef] [PubMed]
75. Zorov, D.B.; Juhaszova, M.; Sollott, S.J. Mitochondrial Reactive Oxygen Species (ROS) and ROS-Induced ROS Release. *Physiol. Rev.* **2014**, *94*, 909–950. [CrossRef]
76. Cheng, K.R.; Fu, X.W.; Zhang, R.N.; Jia, G.X.; Hou, Y.P.; Zhu, S.E. Effect of oocyte vitrification on deoxyribonucleic acid methylation of H19, Peg3, and Snrpn differentially methylated regions in mouse blastocysts. *Fertil. Steril.* **2014**, *102*, 1183–1190. [CrossRef]
77. Kader, A.; Agarwal, A.; Abdelrazik, H.; Sharma, R.K.; Ahmady, A.; Falcone, T. Evaluation of post-thaw DNA integrity of mouse blastocysts after ultrarapid and slow freezing. *Fertil. Steril.* **2009**, *91*, 2087–2094. [CrossRef]
78. Kopeika, J.; Thornhill, A.; Khalaf, Y. The effect of cryopreservation on the genome of gametes and embryos: Principles of cryobiology and critical appraisal of the evidence. *Hum. Reprod. Update* **2015**, *21*, 209–227. [CrossRef] [PubMed]
79. Diaferia, G.R.; Dessì, S.S.; DeBlasio, P.; Biunno, I. Is stem cell chromosomes stability affected by cryopreservation conditions? *Cytotechnology* **2008**, *58*, 11–16. [CrossRef]
80. Katkov, I.I.; Kim, M.S.; Bajpai, R.; Altman, Y.S.; Mercola, M.; Loring, J.F.; Terskikh, A.V.; Snyder, E.Y.; Levine, F. Cryopreservation by slow cooling with DMSO diminished production of Oct-4 pluripotency marker in human embryonic stem cells. *Cryobiology* **2006**, *53*, 194–205. [CrossRef]
81. Wagh, V.; Meganathan, K.; Jagtap, S.; Gaspar, J.A.; Winkler, J.; Spitkovsky, D.; Hescheler, J.; Sachinidis, A. Effects of cryopreservation on the transcriptome of human embryonic stem cells after thawing and culturing. *Stem Cell Rev. Rep.* **2011**, *7*, 506–517. [CrossRef] [PubMed]
82. Xu, X.; Cowley, S.; Flaim, C.J.; James, W.; Seymour, L.; Cui, Z. The roles of apoptotic pathways in the low recovery rate after cryopreservation of dissociated human embryonic stem cells. *Biotechnol. Prog.* **2010**, *26*, 827–837. [CrossRef] [PubMed]
83. Li, M.; Feng, C.; Gu, X.; He, Q.; Wei, F. Effect of cryopreservation on proliferation and differentiation of periodontal ligament stem cell sheets. *Stem Cell Res. Ther.* **2017**, *8*, 77. [CrossRef] [PubMed]
84. Estill, M.S.; Bolnick, J.M.; Waterland, R.A.; Bolnick, A.D.; Diamond, M.P.; Krawetz, S.A. Assisted reproductive technology alters deoxyribonucleic acid methylation profiles in bloodspots of newborn infants. *Fertil. Steril.* **2016**, *106*, 629–639.e10. [CrossRef] [PubMed]
85. Cui, M.; Dong, X.; Lyu, S.; Zheng, Y.; Ai, J. The Impact of Embryo Storage Time on Pregnancy and Perinatal Outcomes and the Time Limit of Vitrification: A Retrospective Cohort Study. *Front. Endocrinol.* **2021**, *12*, 724853. [CrossRef]
86. Waddington, C.H. The epigenotype. *Int J. Epidemiol.* **2012**, *41*, 10–13. [CrossRef]
87. Mak, W.; Weaver, J.R.; Bartolomei, M.S. Is ART changing the epigenetic landscape of imprinting? *Anim. Reprod.* **2010**, *7*, 168–176.
88. Marcho, C.; Cui, W.; Mager, J. Epigenetic dynamics during preimplantation development. *Reproduction* **2015**, *150*, R109–R120. [CrossRef]
89. Skinner, M.K. Environmental epigenomics and disease susceptibility. *EMBO Rep.* **2011**, *12*, 620–622. [CrossRef]
90. Rivera, C.M.; Ren, B. Mapping Human Epigenomes. *Cell* **2013**, *155*, 39–55. [CrossRef]
91. Gujar, H.; Weisenberger, D.J.; Liang, G. The Roles of Human DNA Methyltransferases and Their Isoforms in Shaping the Epigenome. *Genes* **2019**, *10*, 172. [CrossRef]
92. Goldberg, A.D.; Allis, C.D.; Bernstein, E. Epigenetics: A Landscape Takes Shape. *Cell* **2007**, *128*, 635–638. [CrossRef] [PubMed]
93. Gallinari, P.; Di Marco, S.; Jones, P.; Pallaoro, M.; Steinkühler, C. HDACs, histone deacetylation and gene transcription: From molecular biology to cancer therapeutics. *Cell Res.* **2007**, *17*, 195–211. [CrossRef] [PubMed]
94. Liu, Y.; Lu, C.; Yang, Y.; Fan, Y.; Yang, R.; Liu, C.-F.; Korolev, N.; Nordenskiöld, L. Influence of Histone Tails and H4 Tail Acetylations on Nucleosome–Nucleosome Interactions. *J. Mol. Biol.* **2011**, *414*, 749–764. [CrossRef]
95. Schatten, H.; Sun, Q.Y. Posttranslationally Modified Tubulins and other Cytoskeletal Proteins: Their Role in Gametogenesis, Oocyte Maturation, Fertilization and Pre-Implantation Embryo Development. In *Posttranslational Protein Modifications in the Reproductive System*; Sutovsky, P., Ed.; Springer: New York, NY, USA, 2014; Volume 59, pp. 57–87.
96. Feitosa, W.B.; Hwang, K.; Morris, P.L. Temporal and SUMO-specific SUMOylation contribute to the dynamics of Polo-like kinase 1 (PLK1) and spindle integrity during mouse oocyte meiosis. *Dev. Biol.* **2017**, *434*, 278–291. [CrossRef] [PubMed]
97. Rodriguez, A.; Briley, S.M.; Patton, B.K.; Tripurani, S.K.; Rajapakshe, K.; Coarfa, C.; Rajkovic, A.; Andrieux, A.; Dejean, A.; Pangas, S.A. Loss of the E2 SUMO-conjugating enzyme Ube2i in oocytes during ovarian folliculogenesis causes infertility in mice. *Development* **2019**, *146*, dev176701. [CrossRef]
98. Zhang, D.; Tang, Z.; Huang, H.; Zhou, G.; Cui, C.; Weng, Y.; Liu, W.; Kim, S.; Lee, S.; Perez-Neut, M.; et al. Metabolic regulation of gene expression by histone lactylation. *Nature* **2019**, *574*, 575–580. [CrossRef]
99. Skaar, D.A.; Li, Y.; Bernal, A.J.; Hoyo, C.; Murphy, S.K.; Jirtle, R.L. The human imprintome: Regulatory mechanisms, methods of ascertainment, and roles in disease susceptibility. *ILAR J.* **2012**, *53*, 341–358. [CrossRef]

100. Glaser, R.L. The imprinted gene and parent-of-origin effect database now includes parental origin of de novo mutations. *Nucleic Acids Res.* **2006**, *34*, D29–D31. [CrossRef]
101. Li, X. Genomic imprinting is a parental effect established in mammalian germ cells. *Curr. Top Dev. Biol.* **2013**, *102*, 35–59. [CrossRef]
102. Das, R.; Lee, Y.K.; Strogantsev, R.; Jin, S.; Lim, Y.C.; Ng, P.Y.; Lin, X.M.; Chng, K.; Yeo, G.S.; Ferguson-Smith, A.C.; et al. DNMT1 and AIM1 Imprinting in human placenta revealed through a genome-wide screen for allele-specific DNA methylation. *BMC Genom.* **2013**, *14*, 685. [CrossRef]
103. Thamban, T.; Agarwaal, V.; Khosla, S. Role of genomic imprinting in mammalian development. *J. Biosci.* **2020**, *45*, 20. [CrossRef] [PubMed]
104. Kalish, J.M.; Jiang, C.; Bartolomei, M.S. Epigenetics and imprinting in human disease. *Int. J. Dev. Biol.* **2014**, *58*, 291–298. [CrossRef]
105. Eggermann, T.; de Nanclares, G.P.; Maher, E.R.; Temple, I.K.; Tümer, Z.; Monk, D.; Mackay, D.J.G.; Grønskov, K.; Riccio, A.; Linglart, A.; et al. Imprinting disorders: A group of congenital disorders with overlapping patterns of molecular changes affecting imprinted loci. *Clin. Epigenet.* **2015**, *7*, 123. [CrossRef] [PubMed]
106. Hiura, H.; Okae, H.; Chiba, H.; Miyauchi, N.; Sato, F.; Sato, A.; Arima, T. Imprinting methylation errors in ART. *Reprod. Med. Biol.* **2014**, *13*, 193–202. [CrossRef] [PubMed]
107. Lazaraviciute, G.; Kauser, M.; Bhattacharya, S.; Haggarty, P.; Bhattacharya, S. A systematic review and meta-analysis of DNA methylation levels and imprinting disorders in children conceived by IVF/ICSI compared with children conceived spontaneously. *Hum. Reprod. Update* **2014**, *20*, 840–852. [CrossRef]
108. Azzi, S.; Habib, A.W.; Netchine, I. Beckwith-Wiedemann and Russell-Silver Syndromes: From New Molecular Insights to the Comprehension of Imprinting Regulation. *Curr. Opin. Endocrinol. Diabetes Obes.* **2014**, *21*, 30–38. [CrossRef]
109. Mabb, A.M.; Judson, M.C.; Zylka, M.J.; Philpot, B.D. Angelman Syndrome: Insights into Genomic Imprinting and Neurodevelopmental Phenotypes. *Trends Neurosci.* **2011**, *234*, 293–303. [CrossRef]
110. Cassidy, S.B.; Schwartz, S.; Miller, J.L.; Driscoll, D.J. Prader-Willi Syndrome. *Genet. Med.* **2012**, *14*, 10–26. [CrossRef]
111. DeBaun, M.R.; Niemitz, E.L.; Feinberg, A.P. Association of In Vitro Fertilization with Beckwith-Wiedemann Syndrome and Epigenetic Alterations of LIT1 and H19. *Am. J. Hum. Genet.* **2003**, *72*, 156–160. [CrossRef] [PubMed]
112. Gicquel, C.; Gaston, V.; Mandelbaum, J.; Siffroi, J.-P.; Flahault, A.; Le Bouc, Y. In Vitro Fertilization May Increase the Risk of Beckwith-Wiedemann Syndrome Related to the Abnormal Imprinting of the KCNQ1OT Gene. *Am. J. Hum. Genet.* **2003**, *72*, 1338–1341. [CrossRef]
113. Halliday, J.; Oke, K.; Breheny, S.; Algar, E.; Amor, D.J. Beckwith-Wiedemann Syndrome and IVF: A Case-Control Study. *Am. J. Hum. Genet.* **2004**, *75*, 526–528. [CrossRef] [PubMed]
114. Russo, V.E.A.; Martiensson, R.A.; Riggs, A.D. *Epigenetic Mechanisms of Gene Regulation*; Monograph 32; Cold Spring Harbor Laboratory Press: Plainview, NY, USA, 1996.
115. Klose, R.J.; Bird, A.P. Genomic DNA methylation: The mark and its mediators. *Trends Biochem. Sci.* **2006**, *31*, 89–97. [CrossRef] [PubMed]
116. Bannister, A.J.; Kouzarides, T. Regulation of chromatin by histone modifications. *Cell Res.* **2011**, *21*, 381–395. [CrossRef]
117. Faulk, C.; Dolinoy, D.C. Timing is everything: The when and how of environmentally induced changes in the epigenome of animals. *Epigenetics* **2011**, *6*, 791–797. [CrossRef]
118. Weaver, J.R.; Susiarjo, M.; Bartolomei, M.S. Imprinting and epigenetic changes in the early embryo. *Mamm. Genome* **2009**, *20*, 532–543. [CrossRef] [PubMed]
119. Iwatani, M.; Ikegami, K.; Kremenska, Y.; Hattori, N.; Tanaka, S.; Yagi, S.; Shiota, K. Dimethyl Sulfoxide Has an Impact on Epigenetic Profile in Mouse Embryoid Body. *Stem Cells* **2006**, *24*, 2549–2556. [CrossRef] [PubMed]
120. Santos, N.C.; Figueira-Coelho, J.; Martins-Silva, J.; Saldanha, C. Multidisciplinary utilization of dimethyl sulfoxide: Pharmacological, cellular, and molecular aspects. *Biochem. Pharmacol.* **2003**, *65*, 1035–1041. [CrossRef]
121. Verheijen, M.; Lienhard, M.; Schrooders, Y.; Clayton, O.; Nudischer, R.; Boerno, S.; Timmermann, B.; Selevsek, N.; Schlapbach, R.; Gmuender, H.; et al. DMSO induces drastic changes in human cellular processes and epigenetic landscape in vitro. *Sci. Rep.* **2019**, *9*, 4641. [CrossRef]
122. Ma, Y.; Long, C.; Liu, G.; Bai, H.; Ma, L.; Bai, T.; Zuo, Y.; Li, S. WGBS combined with RNA-seq analysis revealed that Dnmt1 affects the methylation modification and gene expression changes during mouse oocyte vitrification. *Theriogenology* **2021**, *177*, 11–21. [CrossRef]
123. Chen, H.; Zhang, L.; Deng, T.; Zou, P.; Wang, Y.; Quan, F.; Zhang, Y. Effects of oocyte vitrification on epigenetic status in early bovine embryos. *Theriogenology* **2016**, *86*, 868–878. [CrossRef] [PubMed]
124. Chen, H.; Zhang, L.; Wang, Z.; Chang, H.; Xie, X.; Fu, L.; Zhang, Y.; Quan, F. Resveratrol improved the developmental potential of oocytes after vitrification by modifying the epigenetics. *Mol. Reprod. Dev.* **2019**, *86*, 862–870. [CrossRef] [PubMed]
125. Wang, Z.; Xu, L.; He, F. Embryo vitrification affects the methylation of the H19/Igf2 differentially methylated domain and the expression of H19 and Igf2. *Fertil. Steril.* **2010**, *93*, 2729–2733. [CrossRef] [PubMed]
126. Zhao, Y.-H.; Wang, J.-J.; Zhang, P.-P.; Hao, H.-S.; Pang, Y.-W.; Wang, H.-Y.; Du, W.-H.; Zhao, S.-J.; Ruan, W.-M.; Zou, H.-Y.; et al. Oocyte IVM or vitrification significantly impairs DNA methylation patterns in blastocysts as analysed by single-cell whole-genome methylation sequencing. *Reprod. Fertil. Dev.* **2020**, *32*, 676–689. [CrossRef] [PubMed]

127. Ying, L.; Xiang-Wei, F.; Jun-Jie, L.; Dian-Shuai, Y.; Shi-En, Z. DNA methylation pattern in mouse oocytes and their in vitro fertilized early embryos: Effect of oocyte vitrification. *Zygote* **2014**, *2*, 138–145.
128. De Munck, N.; Petrussa, L.; Verheyen, G.; Staessen, C.; Vandeskelde, Y.; Sterckx, J.; Bocken, G.; Jacobs, K.; Stoop, D.; De Rycke, M. Chromosomal meiotic segregation, embryonic developmental kinetics and DNA (hydroxy) methylation analysis consolidate the safety of human oocyte vitrification. *Basic Sci. Reprod. Med.* **2015**, *21*, 535–544. [CrossRef] [PubMed]
129. Liu, M.-H.; Zhou, W.-H.; Chu, D.-P.; Fu, L.; Sha, W.; Li, Y. Ultrastructural Changes and Methylation of Human Oocytes Vitrified at the Germinal Vesicle Stage and Matured in vitro after Thawing. *Gynecol. Obstet. Investig.* **2017**, *82*, 252–261. [CrossRef]
130. Al-Khtib, M.; Perret, A.; Khoueiry, R.; Ibala-Romdhane, S.; Blachère, T.; Greze, C.; Lornage, J.; Lefèvre, A. Vitrification at the germinal vesicle stage does not affect the methylation profile of H19 and KCNQ1OT1 imprinting centers in human oocytes subsequently matured in vitro. *Fertil. Steril.* **2011**, *95*, 1955–1960. [CrossRef]
131. Cantatore, C.; George, J.S.; Depalo, R.; D'amato, G.; Moravek, M.; Smith, G.D. Mouse oocyte vitrification with and without dimethyl sulfoxide: Influence on cryo-survival, development, and maternal imprinted gene expression. *J. Assist. Reprod. Genet.* **2021**, *38*, 2129–2138. [CrossRef]
132. Jahangiri, M.; Shahhoseini, M.; Movaghar, B. H19 and MEST gene expression and histone modification in blastocysts cultured from vitrified and fresh two-cell mouse embryos. *Reprod. Biomed. Online* **2014**, *29*, 559–566. [CrossRef]
133. Movahed, E.; Shabani, R.; Hosseini, S.; Shahidi, S.; Salehi, M. Interfering effects of in vitro fertilization and vitrification on expression of Gtl2 and Dlk1 in mouse blastocysts. *Int. J. Fertil. Steril.* **2020**, *14*, 110. [PubMed]
134. Barberet, J.; Romain, G.; Binquet, C.; Guilleman, M.; Bruno, C.; Ginod, P.; Chapusot, C.; Choux, C.; Fauque, P. Do frozen embryo transfers modify the epigenetic control of imprinted genes and transposable elements in newborns compared with fresh embryo transfers and natural conceptions? *Fertil. Steril.* **2021**, *116*, 1468–1480. [CrossRef] [PubMed]
135. Yao, J.-F.; Huang, Y.-F.; Huang, R.-F.; Lin, S.-X.; Guo, C.-Q.; Hua, C.-Z.; Wu, P.-Y.; Hu, J.-F.; Li, Y.-Z. Effects of Vitrification on the Imprinted Gene Snrpn in Neonatal Placental Tissue. *Reprod. Dev. Med.* **2020**, *4*, 25–31. [CrossRef]
136. Huo, Y.; Yuan, P.; Qin, Q.; Yan, Z.; Yan, L.; Liu, P.; Li, R.; Yan, J.; Qiao, J. Effects of vitrification and cryostorage duration on single-cell RNA-Seq profiling of vitrified-thawed human metaphase II oocytes. *Front. Med.* **2020**, *15*, 144–154. [CrossRef]
137. Suo, L.; Meng, Q.; Pei, Y.; Fu, X.; Wang, Y.; Bunch, T.D.; Zhu, S. Effect of cryopreservation on acetylation patterns of lysine 12 of histone H4 (acH4K12) in mouse oocytes and zygotes. *J. Assist. Reprod. Genet.* **2010**, *27*, 735–741. [CrossRef] [PubMed]
138. Jahangiri, M.; Shahhoseini, M.; Movaghar, B. The Effect of Vitrification on Expression and Histone Marks of Igf2 and Oct4 in Blastocysts Cultured from Two-Cell Mouse Embryos. *Cell J.* **2018**, *19*, 607–613. [CrossRef]
139. Chatterjee, A.; Saha, D.; Niemann, H.; Gryshkov, O.; Glasmacher, B.; Hofmann, N. Effects of cryopreservation on the epigenetic profile of cells. *Cryobiology* **2016**, *74*, 1–7. [CrossRef]
140. Estudillo, E.; Jiménez, A.; Bustamante-Nieves, P.E.; Palacios-Reyes, C.; Velasco, I.; López-Ornelas, A. Cryopreservation of Gametes and Embryos and Their Molecular Changes. *Int. J. Mol. Sci.* **2021**, *22*, 10864. [CrossRef]
141. Yan, L.-Y.; Yan, J.; Qiao, J.; Zhao, P.-L.; Liu, P. Effects of oocyte vitrification on histone modifications. *Reprod. Fertil. Dev.* **2010**, *22*, 920–925. [CrossRef]
142. Maldonado, M.B.C.; Penteado, J.C.T.; Faccio, B.M.C.; Lopes, F.L.; Arnold, D.R. Changes in tri-methylation profile of lysines 4 and 27 of histone H3 in bovine blastocysts after cryopreservation. *Cryobiology* **2015**, *71*, 481–485. [CrossRef]
143. Stigliani, S.; Moretti, S.; Anserini, P.; Casciano, I.; Venturini, P.L.; Scaruffi, P. Storage time does not modify the gene expression profile of cryopreserved human metaphase II oocytes. *Hum. Reprod.* **2015**, *30*, 2519–2526. [CrossRef] [PubMed]
144. Yan, Y.; Zhang, Q.; Yang, L.; Zhou, W.; Ni, T.; Yan, J. Pregnancy and neonatal outcomes after long-term vitrification of blastocysts among 6900 patients after their last live birth. *Fertil. Steril.* **2022**, *119*, 36–44. [CrossRef]
145. Bouillon, C.; Leandri, R.; Desch, L.; Ernst, A.; Bruno, C.; Cerf, C.; Chiron, A.; Souchay, C.; Burguet, A.; Jimenez, C.; et al. Does Embryo Culture Medium Influence the Health and Development of Children Born after In Vitro Fertilization? *PLoS ONE* **2016**, *11*, e0150857. [CrossRef]
146. Sciorio, R.; Tramontano, L.; Rapalini, E.; Bellaminutti, S.; Bulletti, F.M.; D'Amato, A.; Manna, C.; Palagiano, A.; Bulletti, C.; Esteves, S.C. Risk of genetic and epigenetic alteration in children conceived following ART: Is it time to return to nature whenever possible? *Clin. Genet.* **2022**, *103*, 133–145. [CrossRef] [PubMed]
147. Sciorio, R.; El Hajj, N. Epigenetic Risks of Medically Assisted Reproduction. *J. Clin. Med.* **2022**, *11*, 2151. [CrossRef] [PubMed]
148. Barberet, J.; Barry, F.; Choux, C.; Guilleman, M.; Karoui, S.; Simonot, R.; Bruno, C.; Fauque, P. What impact does oocyte vitrification have on epigenetics and gene expression? *Clin. Epigenet.* **2020**, *12*, 121. [CrossRef] [PubMed]
149. Hezavehei, M.; Sharafi, M.; Kouchesfahani, H.M.; Henkel, R.; Agarwal, A.; Esmaeili, V.; Shahverdi, A. Sperm cryopreservation: A review on current molecular cryobiology and advanced approaches. *Reprod. Biomed. Online* **2018**, *37*, 327–339. [CrossRef] [PubMed]
150. Tran, K.T.D.; Valli-Pulaski, H.; Colvin, A.; E Orwig, K. Male fertility preservation and restoration strategies for patients undergoing gonadotoxic therapies. *Biol. Reprod.* **2022**, *107*, 382–405. [CrossRef]
151. Bunge, R.G.; Sherman, J.K. Fertilizing Capacity of Frozen Human Spermatozoa. *Nature* **1953**, *172*, 767–768. [CrossRef]
152. Riva, N.S.; Ruhlmann, C.; Iaizzo, R.S.; Marcial Lopez, C.A.; Martinez, A.G. Comparative analysis between slow freezing and ultra-rapid freezing for human sperm cryopreservation. *JBRA Assist. Reprod.* **2018**, *22*, 331–337. [CrossRef]

153. Isachenko, V.; Maettner, R.; Petrunkina, A.M.; Sterzik, K.; Mallmann, P.; Rahimi, G.; Sanchez, R.; Risopatron, J.; Damjanoski, I.; Isachenko, E. Vitrification of human ICSI/IVF spermatozoa without cryoprotectants: New capillary technology. *J. Androl.* **2012**, *33*, 462–468. [CrossRef] [PubMed]
154. Aitken, R.; De Iuliis, G. On the possible origins of DNA damage in human spermatozoa. *Mol. Hum. Reprod.* **2009**, *16*, 3–13. [CrossRef]
155. Wu, Q.; Ni, X. ROS-mediated DNA methylation pattern alterations in carcinogenesis. *Curr. Drug Targets* **2015**, *16*, 13–19. [CrossRef] [PubMed]
156. Ziech, D.; Franco, R.; Pappa, A.; Panayiotidis, M.I. Reactive Oxygen Species (ROS)—Induced genetic and epigenetic alterations in human carcinogenesis. *Mutat. Res. Mol. Mech. Mutagen.* **2011**, *711*, 167–173. [CrossRef]
157. Valipour, J.; Nashtaei, M.S.; Khosravizadeh, Z.; Mahdavinezhad, F.; Nekoonam, S.; Esfandyari, S.; Amidi, F. Effect of sulforaphane on apoptosis, reactive oxygen species and lipids peroxidation of human sperm during cryopreservation. *Cryobiology* **2020**, *99*, 122–130. [CrossRef] [PubMed]
158. Kläver, R.; Tüttelmann, F.; Bleiziffer, A.; Haaf, T.; Kliesch, S.; Gromoll, J. DNA methylation in spermatozoa as a prospective marker in andrology. *Andrology* **2013**, *1*, 731–740. [CrossRef]
159. El Hajj, N.; Zechner, U.; Schneider, E.; Tresch, A.; Gromoll, J.; Hahn, T.; Schorsch, M.; Haaf, T. Methylation Status of Imprinted Genes and Repetitive Elements in Sperm DNA from Infertile Males. *Sex. Dev.* **2011**, *5*, 60–69. [CrossRef]
160. Marques, C.J.; Francisco, T.; Sousa, S.; Carvalho, F.; Barros, A.; Sousa, M. Methylation defects of imprinted genes in human testicular spermatozoa. *Fertil. Steril.* **2010**, *94*, 585–594. [CrossRef]
161. Poplinski, A.; Tüttelmann, F.; Kanber, D.; Horsthemke, B.; Gromoll, J. Idiopathic male infertility is strongly associated with aberrant methylation of MEST and IGF2/H19 ICR1. *Int. J. Androl.* **2010**, *33*, 642–649. [CrossRef]
162. Laurentino, S.; Beygo, J.; Nordhoff, V.; Kliesch, S.; Wistuba, J.; Borgmann, J.; Buiting, K.; Horsthemke, B.; Gromoll, J. Epigenetic germline mosaicism in infertile men. *Hum. Mol. Genet.* **2014**, *24*, 1295–1304. [CrossRef]
163. de Mello, F.; Garcia, J.S.; Godoy, L.C.; Depincé, A.; Labbé, C.; Streit, D.P., Jr. The effect of cryoprotectant agents on DNA methylation patterns and progeny development in the spermatozoa of Colossoma macropomum. *Gen. Comp. Endocrinol.* **2017**, *245*, 94–101. [CrossRef]
164. Depincé, A.; Gabory, A.; Dziewulska, K.; Le Bail, P.; Jammes, H.; Labbé, C. DNA methylation stability in fish spermatozoa upon external constraint: Impact of fish hormonal stimulation and sperm cryopreservation. *Mol. Reprod. Dev.* **2019**, *87*, 124–134. [CrossRef] [PubMed]
165. Salehi, M.; Mahdavi, A.H.; Sharafi, M.; Shahverdi, A. Cryopreservation of rooster semen: Evidence for the epigenetic modifications of thawed sperm. *Theriogenology* **2020**, *142*, 15–25. [CrossRef] [PubMed]
166. He, W.; Sun, Y.; Zhang, S.; Feng, X.; Xu, M.; Dai, J.; Ni, X.; Wang, X.; Wu, Q. Profiling the DNA methylation patterns of imprinted genes in abnormal semen samples by next-generation bisulfite sequencing. *J. Assist. Reprod. Genet.* **2020**, *37*, 2211–2221. [CrossRef] [PubMed]
167. Khosravizadeh, Z.; Hassanzadeh, G.; Bazzaz, J.T.; Alizadeh, F.; Totonchi, M.; Salehi, E.; Khodamoradi, K.; Khanehzad, M.; Hosseini, S.R.; Abolhassani, F. The effect of cryopreservation on DNA methylation patterns of the chromosome 15q11–q13 region in human spermatozoa. *Cell Tissue Bank* **2020**, *21*, 433–445. [CrossRef] [PubMed]
168. Bogle, O.A.; Kumar, K.; Attardo-Parrinello, C.; Lewis, S.E.M.; Estanyol, J.M.; Ballescà, J.L.; Oliva, R. Identification of protein changes in human spermatozoa throughout the cryopreservation process. *Andrology* **2016**, *5*, 10–22. [CrossRef]
169. Santi, D.; De Vincentis, S.; Magnani, E.; Spaggiari, G. Impairment of sperm DNA methylation in male infertility: A meta-analytic study. *Andrology* **2017**, *5*, 695–703. [CrossRef]
170. Güngör, İ.H.; Tektemur, A.; Arkali, G.; Cinkara, S.D.; Acisu, T.C.; Koca, R.H.; Önalan, E.E.; Kaya, Ş.Ö.; Kizil, M.; Sönmez, M.; et al. Effect of freeze–thawing process on lipid peroxidation, miRNAs, ion channels, apoptosis and global DNA methylation in ram spermatozoa. *Reprod. Fertil. Dev.* **2021**, *33*, 747–759. [CrossRef]

Disclaimer/Publisher's Note: The statements, opinions and data contained in all publications are solely those of the individual author(s) and contributor(s) and not of MDPI and/or the editor(s). MDPI and/or the editor(s) disclaim responsibility for any injury to people or property resulting from any ideas, methods, instructions or products referred to in the content.

MDPI
St. Alban-Anlage 66
4052 Basel
Switzerland
www.mdpi.com

Journal of Clinical Medicine Editorial Office
E-mail: jcm@mdpi.com
www.mdpi.com/journal/jcm

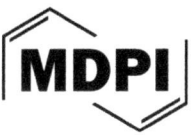

Disclaimer/Publisher's Note: The statements, opinions and data contained in all publications are solely those of the individual author(s) and contributor(s) and not of MDPI and/or the editor(s). MDPI and/or the editor(s) disclaim responsibility for any injury to people or property resulting from any ideas, methods, instructions or products referred to in the content.

www.ingramcontent.com/pod-product-compliance
Lightning Source LLC
LaVergne TN
LVHW070440100526
838202LV00014B/1635